D0536111

Fitness & Wellness

Fourth Edition

Werner W. K. Hoeger
Boise State University

Sharon A. Hoeger
Fitness & Wellness, Inc.

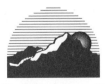

Morton Publishing Company

925 W. Kenyon, Unit 12
Englewood, Colorado 80110
http://www.morton-pub.com

Acknowledgments

Special thanks to Debbie Thompson, Louise Cashmere,
Kaselah Crockett, MeriKarol Welch, Claudia Suastequi,
and Lester Caldwell, who served as models
for the photography in this fourth edition.

Publisher:	Douglas N. Morton
Managing Editor:	Ruth Horton
Designer:	Joanne Saliger
Copyeditor:	Carolyn Acheson
Cover Design:	Bob Schram, Bookends
Typography:	Ash Street Typecrafters, Inc.
Software Developer:	Sharon A. Hoeger

Copyright © 1990, 1993, 1996, 1999 by Morton Publishing Company

All rights reserved. No part of this publication may be reproduced, stored in a retrieval system, or transmitted, in any form or by any means, electronic, mechanical, photocopying, recording, or otherwise, without the prior written permission of the publisher.

Printed in the United States of America

10 9 8 7 6 5 4 3 2 1

ISBN: 0-89582-431-0

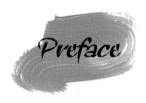
Preface

More than ever before, Americans realize that good health is largely self-controlled and that premature illness and mortality can be prevented through adequate fitness and positive lifestyle behaviors. The current American way of life, unfortunately, does not provide the human body with sufficient physical activity to maintain adequate health. Furthermore, many current lifestyle patterns are such a serious threat to our health that they actually increase the deterioration rate of the human body and often lead to premature morbidity and mortality.

Several major scientific studies have established clearly that people who lead an active and healthy lifestyle live longer and enjoy a better quality of life. As a result, the importance of sound fitness and wellness programs has assumed an entirely new dimension. From an initial fitness fad in the early 1970s, people now accept the value of a sound fitness and wellness program. Most, however, do not reap the benefit because they do not know how to develop their own program. The information in this book has been written to provide you with the necessary guidelines for lifetime exercise and a healthy lifestyle.

Objectives of Fitness and Wellness

Because fitness and wellness needs vary significantly from one person to another, exercise and wellness prescriptions must be personalized to obtain the best results. The information in the following chapters and the worksheets within these chapters set forth guidelines for you to develop a personal lifetime program that will improve your fitness and promote preventive health care and personal wellness.

The worksheets have been prepared on tear-out sheets so you can turn them in to class instructors. As you study this book and complete the respective worksheets, you will learn to:

- Learn behavior modification techniques to help you adhere to a lifetime fitness and wellness program.
- Determine whether medical clearance is needed for you to participate safely in exercise.
- Assess the health-related components of fitness (cardiorespiratory endurance, muscular strength and endurance, muscular flexibility, and body composition).
- Write exercise prescriptions for cardiorespiratory endurance, muscular strength and endurance, and muscular flexibility.
- Conduct nutrient analyses and follow the recommendations for adequate nutrition.
- Write sound diet and weight-control programs.

🐾 Implement a program that will reduce your risk for cardiovascular disease.

🐾 Follow guidelines to reduce your risk of developing cancer.

🐾 Understand stress, lessen your vulnerability to stress, and implement a stress-management program if necessary.

🐾 Implement a smoking cessation program, if applicable.

🐾 Understand the health consequences of chemical dependency and irresponsible sexual behaviors and learn guidelines for preventing sexually transmitted diseases.

🐾 Differentiate myths from facts of exercise and health-related concepts.

What's New in the Fourth Edition

All chapters in the fourth edition of *Fitness and Wellness* have been revised and updated to include new information reported in the literature and at professional health, physical education, and sports medicine meetings. The most significant changes of the fourth edition are the following.

🐾 The book now contains nine chapters instead of eight. A new chapter on stress management (Chapter 8) has been added. This allows for a broader discussion of this important topic.

🐾 Key terms appear in boldface type. Together with their definitions, they appear in boxes within the chapters, as well as a glossary at the end of the book.

🐾 In Chapter 1 we explain the difference between physical activity and exercise, the inverse association between moderate-intensity physical activity and mortality, the importance of the 1996 U.S. Surgeon General's Report on Physical Activity and Health, and present an update on the effects of a healthy lifestyle on quality of life and longevity.

🐾 The Transtheoretical Model, which explains the stages of change as people attempt to modify behavior, has also been included in Chapter 1.

🐾 In Chapter 2 the metabolic fitness concept is introduced and the Body Mass Index (BMI) is included to estimate critical fat values at which the risk for disease increases.

In addition, because of several reports regarding the validity and reliability of the Abdominal Crunch Test and the large number of requests and concerns expressed by course instructors throughout the United States, the Bent-leg Curl-up test has been incorporated again in Chapter 2 as one of the strength test items for the Muscular Endurance Test. The Abdominal Crunch Test remains, as an alternate test item recommended for use by individuals who are at risk for low-back injury.

🐾 The exercise prescription principles in Chapter 3 have been updated to conform with the new 1998 American College of Sports Medicine guidelines. Chapter 3 also covers the benefits of cumulative versus continuous activity, the importance of strength conditioning prior to starting an aerobic exercise program to minimize the risk of exercise-related injuries, and the prescription of flexibility based on the American College of Sports Medicine's guidelines for exercise testing and prescription.

- The topic of Chapter 5, nutrition, has been updated extensively. It contains additional information on fiber and its benefits, the latest information on antioxidant nutrients, and the 1995 Dietary Guidelines for North Americans.

- The controversial association between fitness and obesity is discussed in Chapter 6, Weight Management. A new diet plan is included in this chapter. Incorporating the diet-planning principles of the Dietary Guidelines for Americans and the Food Guide Pyramid, it was designed to meet the current Recommended Dietary Allowances for North Americans. The list of tips for behavior modification and adherence to a lifetime weight management program has been expanded to incorporate techniques used currently to enhance the success rate in weight loss and weight maintenance programs.

- The new chapter on stress management (Chapter 7) contains information on behavior patterns, assessment of stress, sources of stress, anger and hostility, behavior-modification techniques, coping and relaxation techniques, and time management.

- Chapter 8, addressing a healthy lifestyle, has been revised extensively. It contains an update on nutrient guidelines related to the prevention of cardiovascular disease and cancer, the role of homocysteine as a risk factor for heart disease, enhanced sections on the prevention of diabetes and treatment of high blood pressure, the therapeutic effects of polyphenols (for cancer prevention), recommendations by the American Cancer Society for early detection of cancer in asymptomatic people, and a more extensive section on responsible sex and the prevention of sexually transmitted diseases.

- Chapter 9, the final chapter in the book, includes updated information and several new questions and their answers.

- New color photography and graphics give this book a fresh, contemporary look.

Ancillaries

The following ancillaries are provided free of charge to all qualified *Fitness and Wellness* adopters:

- Profile Plus for Windows — The most comprehensive computer software package available with any fitness/wellness textbook. This software, custom-designed for Morton Publishing Company *Fitness and Wellness* textbooks, includes a Fitness and Wellness Profile, a Personalized Cardiorespiratory Exercise Prescription, a Nutrient Analysis, and an Exercise Log. This software package offers a meaningful experience to all participants and greatly decreases the workload of course instructors.

- A video explaining many of the fitness assessment test items used in the book. Instructors can use this video to familiarize themselves with the proper test protocols for each fitness test. This audiovisual aid contains the following test items: 1.5-Mile Run Test, Step Test, Astrand-Ryhming Test, Muscular Strength and Endurance Test, Muscular Endurance Test, Strength-to-Body Weight Ratio Test, Modified Sit-and-Reach Test, Body Rotation Test, Shoulder Rotation Test, Skinfold Thickness Test, and Girth Measurements Test.

🖝 Microtest, edited by Allan S. Cohen Consulting Services, a Fitness and Wellness Computerized Testbank, contains the following options: (a) more than 800 multiple-choice questions; (b) the capability to add or edit test questions; (c) ability to recall previously generated tests — creating new exam versions because multiple-choice answers can be rotated with each new test generated; and (d) the capability to generate tests using a LaserJet printer.

🖝 More than 60 color overhead transparency acetates of the book's most important illustrations and figures to facilitate class instruction and help explain key fitness and wellness concepts.

🖝 An Instructor's Manual to aid with the implementation of your physical fitness and wellness course.

Student Supplement for the World Wide Web

The World Wide Web has emerged as a valuable educational resource. Visiting cyberspace can make for a unique teaching and learning experience. The problem is: How do students identify sites that are academically appropriate and begin to use WWW sites in an educational context?

To make use of the resources of the World Wide Web in a practical way, *Jump-Start with WebLinks: A Guidebook for Fitness/Wellness/Personal Health* is a suggested supplement. Edited by Professor Eileen L. Daniel, Ph.D., this spiral-bound guidebook (approximately 168 pages) contains 36 topics on fitness, wellness, and personal health. For each topic (e.g., cardiovascular endurance, eating disorders), a topic introduction orients users to the topic and concludes with a mix of personal assessment and content-related questions. Following the topic introduction is a directory of WebLinks: the addresses (URLs) of four to six relevant WWW sites and a brief description of each site.

The selected WWW sites are appropriate for students and faculty alike. Each site has been fully verified and approved by a WebAdvisory Board made up of academics from colleges and universities throughout the United States and Canada. A brief *Instructor's Resource Guide* provides general information on how to incorporate *JumpStart with WebLinks* into any classroom setting.

Morton Publishing Company
1-800-348-3777
Web Site http://www.morton-pub.com

Contents

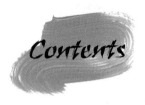

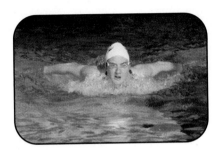

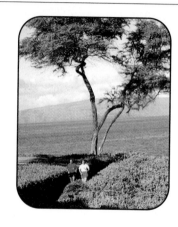

Exercise Prescription   47

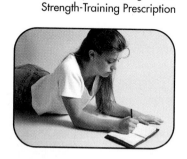

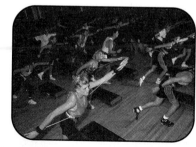

Evaluating Fitness Activities   75

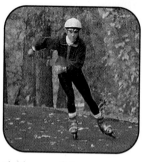

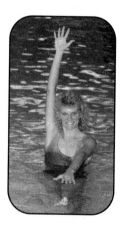

Nutrition for Wellness   **93**

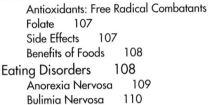

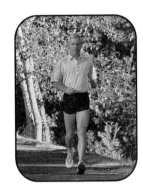

Weight Management   **113**

Stress Management and Assessment   **133**

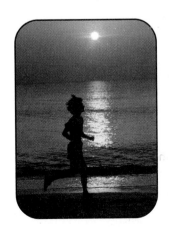

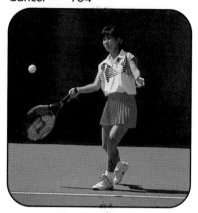

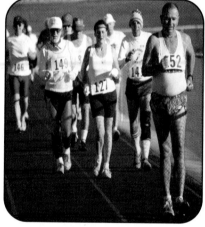

The Importance of Physical Fitness & Wellness

There is no drug in current or prospective use that holds as much promise for sustained health as a lifetime program of physical exercise.[1]

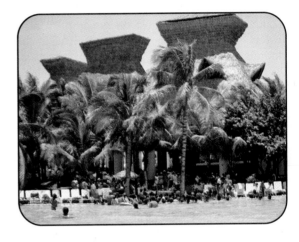

Most people go to school to learn how to make a living. A fitness and wellness course will teach you *how to live* — how to truly live life to its fullest potential. Although some people seem to think that success in life is measured by how much money they make, making a good living will not help you unless you live a wellness lifestyle that will allow you to enjoy what you have. Most people don't know how to reach this objective.

Lifestyle is the most important factor affecting our personal well-being. Even though some people live long because of favorable genetic factors, the quality of life during middle age and the "golden years" is related more often to wise choices initiated during youth and continued throughout life.

During the last three decades the number of people participating in physical fitness programs has increased tremendously. The initial fitness fad in the early 1970s turned into a trend that has become part of the American way of life. The benefits of physical activity have been substantiated by scientific evidence linking increased physical activity and positive lifestyle habits to better health and improved quality of life.

Unfortunately, the current way of life in North America does not provide the human body with sufficient physical exercise to maintain

Objectives

- Understand the importance of physical fitness.
- Understand the wellness concept.
- Define physical fitness and list health-related and skill-related fitness components.
- Learn the benefits of a total fitness and wellness program.
- Learn motivational and behavior modification techniques to enhance compliance with a fitness and wellness program.
- Determine whether medical clearance is required for safe participation in exercise.

adequate health. Furthermore, many lifestyle patterns are such a serious threat to health that they actually speed up deterioration of the human body. In a few short years lack of wellness leads to a loss of vitality and gusto for life, as well as premature morbidity and mortality.

The typical North American is not a good role model when cardiorespiratory fitness is concerned. Almost 60% of U.S. adults engage in little or no leisure-time physical activity. In 1994, only 37% of the adults in the United States exercised strenuously three or more days per week.[2] Even though most people in the United States believe a positive lifestyle has a great impact on health and longevity, most do not implement a fitness and wellness program that will yield the desired results.

Patty Neavill is an example of someone who frequently tried to change her life around but was unable to do so because she did not know how to implement a sound exercise and weight control program. At age 24, Patty, a college sophomore, was discouraged with her weight, level of fitness, self-image, and quality of life in general. She had struggled with weight most of her life. Like thousands of other people, she had made many unsuccessful attempts to lose weight. Patty put her fears aside and decided to enroll in a fitness course. As part of the course requirement, she took a battery of fitness tests at the beginning of the semester. Patty's cardiorespiratory fitness and strength ratings were poor, her flexibility classification was average, she weighed more than 200 pounds, and her percent body fat was 41%.

Following the initial fitness assessment, Patty met with her course instructor, who prescribed an exercise and nutrition program like the one presented in this book. Patty fully committed to carry out the prescription. She walked or jogged five times a week, worked out with weights twice a week, and played volleyball or basketball two to four times each week. Her daily caloric intake was set in the range of 1,500 to 1,700 calories. She took care to meet the minimum required servings from the basic food groups each day, which contributed about 1,200

calories to her diet. The remainder of the calories came primarily from complex carbohydrates. At the end of the 16-week semester, Patty's cardiorespiratory fitness, strength, and flexibility ratings had all improved to the "good" category, she had lost 50 pounds, and her percent body fat had dropped to 22.5!

A thank-you note from Patty to the course instructor at the end of the semester read:

> *Thank you for making me a new person. I truly appreciate the time you spent with me. Without your kindness and motivation, I would have never made it. It's great to be fit and trim. I've never had this feeling before and I wish everyone could feel like this once in their life.*
>
> *Thank you,*
> *Your trim Patty!*

Patty never had been taught the principles governing a sound weight loss program. Not only did she need this knowledge but, like most Americans who never have experienced the process of becoming physically fit, she needed to be in a structured exercise setting to truly feel the joy of fitness.

Of even greater significance, Patty has maintained her aerobic and strength-training programs. A year after ending her calorie-restricted diet, her weight increased by 10 pounds, but her body fat decreased from 22.5% to 21.2%. As discussed in Chapter 6, the weight increase is related mostly to changes in lean tissue, lost during the weight-reduction phase. Despite only a slight drop in weight during the second year following the calorie-restricted diet, the 2-year follow-up revealed a further decrease in body fat, to 19.5%. Patty understands the new quality of life reaped through a sound fitness program.

Physical Activity Versus Exercise

Based on the abundance of scientific research on physical activity and exercise over the last three decades, a clear distinction has been established between physical activity and exercise. **Physical activity** is defined as *bodily movement produced by skeletal muscles that requires energy expenditure and produces progressive health benefits.*[3] Examples of physical activity are walking to and from work and the store, taking stairs (instead of elevators and escalators), gardening, doing household chores, dancing, and washing the car by hand. Physical inactivity, on the other hand, implies a level of activity that is lower than that required to maintain good health.

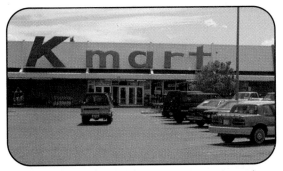

The epitome of physical inactivity is driving around a parking lot for several minutes in search of a parking spot 10 to 20 yards closer to the store's entrance.

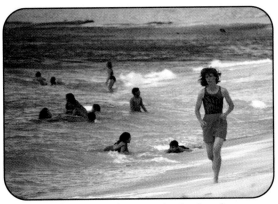

Physical activity and exercise lead to less disease, longer life, and enhanced quality of life.

Exercise is considered *a type of physical activity that requires planned, structured, and repetitive bodily movement done to improve or maintain one or more components of physical fitness.*[4] A regular weekly program of walking, jogging, cycling, aerobics, swimming, strength training, and stretching exercises are all examples of exercise.

Lifestyle, Health, and Quality of Life

Many research findings have shown that physical inactivity and negative lifestyle habits pose a serious threat to health. Movement and physical activity are basic functions for which the human organism was created. Advances in modern technology, however, have all but eliminated the need for physical activity in daily life.

Physical activity no longer is a natural part of our existence. Today we live in an automated society. Most of the activities that used to require strenuous physical exertion can be accomplished by machines with the simple pull of a handle or push of a button. If people need to go to a store that is only a couple of blocks away, most drive their automobiles and then spend a couple of minutes driving around the parking lot to find a spot 10 yards closer to the store's entrance. The groceries do not even have to be carried out any more. A store employee willingly takes them out in a cart and places them in the vehicle. During a visit to a multi-level shopping mall, nearly everyone chooses to ride the escalators instead of taking the stairs. Automobiles, elevators, escalators, telephones, intercoms, remote controls, electric garage door openers — all are modern-day commodities that minimize the amount of movement and effort required of the human body.

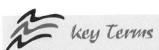

key Terms

Physical activity Bodily movement produced by skeletal muscles that requires energy expenditure and produces progressive health benefits.

Exercise A type of physical activity that requires planned, structured, and repetitive bodily movement done to improve or maintain one or more components of physical fitness.

One of the most significant detrimental effects of modern-day technology has been an increase in **chronic diseases** related to a lack of physical activity. These include hypertension, heart disease, chronic low-back pain, and obesity, among others. They sometimes are referred to as hypokinetic diseases. "Hypo" means low or little, and "kinetic" implies motion. Lack of adequate physical activity is a fact of modern life that most people can avoid no longer, but to enjoy contemporary commodities and still expect to live life to its fullest, a personalized lifetime exercise program must become a part of daily living.

With the developments in technology, three additional factors have changed our lives significantly and have had a negative effect on human health: nutrition, stress, and environment. Fatty foods, sweets, alcohol, tobacco, excessive stress, and environmental hazards such as wastes, noise, and air pollution have detrimental effects on people.

The most prominent causes of death in the United States today are lifestyle-related (see Figure 1.1). More than 64% of all deaths in the United States are caused by cardiovascular disease and cancer.[5] Nearly 80% of these deaths could be prevented by adherence to a healthy lifestyle. The third leading cause of death — chronic and obstructive pulmonary (lung) disease, is related largely to tobacco use. Accidents comprise the fourth leading cause of death. Even though not all accidents are preventable, many are. Fatal accidents often are related to abusing drugs and not wearing seat belts.

As the incidence of chronic diseases increased, the importance of prevention as the best medicine became apparent. Estimates indicate that more than half of disease is lifestyle-related, a fifth is attributed to the environment, and a tenth is influenced by the health care the individual receives. Only 16% is related to genetic factors.[6] Thus, the individual controls 84% of disease and quality of life. Further, according to estimates by the U.S. Surgeon General, 83% of deaths before age 65 are preventable. In essence, most Americans are threatened by the very lives they lead today.

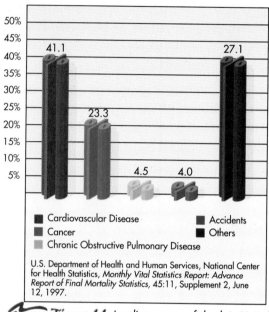

Figure 1.1 Leading causes of death in United States, 1995.

U.S. Department of Health and Human Services, National Center for Health Statistics, *Monthly Vital Statistics Report: Advance Report of Final Mortality Statistics*, 45:11, Supplement 2, June 12, 1997.

Ideally, healthy lifestyle habits should be taught and reinforced in early youth. Unfortunately, many young people are in such poor physical condition that they will add to national health concerns in years to come. Surveys conducted during the past decade have raised public concern regarding the fitness level of American youth. As compared to the 1960s and 1970s, cardiorespiratory endurance and upper body strength have decreased and body fat has increased. These findings suggest that current physical education programs are not promoting lifetime fitness and wellness adequately.

Although the incidence of cardiovascular disease has declined remarkably in the last two decades, concern over youth fitness has led Dr. Kenneth Cooper, Director of the Aerobics Research Institute in Dallas, Texas to state:

> It's discouraging, and I'm afraid that as these kids grow up, we'll see all the gains made against heart disease in the last twenty years wiped out in the next twenty years.[7]

Even 5- and 6-year-old children already have coronary heart disease risk factors such as high blood pressure, excessive body fat, and low fitness.[8] Because of the unhealthy lifestyles of many young adults, physically they may be middle-aged or older! Healthy choices made today influence health a decade or two later. Many physical education programs do not emphasize the necessary skills for our youth to maintain a high level of fitness and health throughout life. The intent of this book is to provide the skills and help to prepare you for a lifetime of physical fitness and wellness. A healthy lifestyle is self-controlled, and people need to be taught how to be responsible for their own health and fitness.

Wellness

After the initial fitness boom swept across the United States in the 1970s, it became clear that improving physical fitness alone was not always enough to lower the risk for disease and ensure better health. For example, individuals who run 3 miles a day, lift weights regularly, participate in stretching exercises, and watch their body weight can be readily classified as having good or excellent fitness. If these same people, however, have high blood pressure, smoke, are under constant stress, consume too much alcohol, and eat too many fatty foods, these are **risk factors** for cardiovascular disease of which they may not be aware.

Good health is no longer viewed as simply the absence of illness. The notion of good health has evolved notably in the last few years and continues to change as scientists learn more about lifestyle factors that bring on illness and affect wellness. Once the idea took hold that fitness by itself would not always decrease the risk for disease and ensure better health, the wellness concept developed in the 1980s.

Wellness is an all-inclusive umbrella covering a variety of health-related factors. Wellness living requires the implementation of positive programs to change behavior and thereby improve health and quality of life, prolong life, and achieve total well-being.

To enjoy a wellness lifestyle, a person needs to practice behaviors that will lead to positive outcomes in six dimensions of wellness: physical, emotional, intellectual, social, environmental, and spiritual (Figure 1.2). These dimensions are interrelated; one frequently affects the others. For example, a person who is emotionally "down" often has no desire to exercise, study, socialize with friends, or attend church.

In looking at the six dimensions of wellness, high-level wellness clearly goes beyond optimum fitness and the absence of disease. Wellness incorporates components such as fitness, proper nutrition, stress management, disease prevention, social support, self-worth, nurturance (sense of being needed), spirituality, personal safety, substance control and not smoking, regular physical examinations, health education, and environmental support.

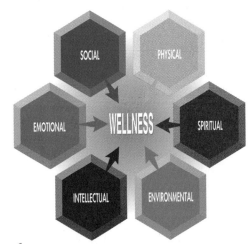

Figure 1.2 The dimensions of wellness.

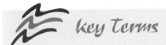

key Terms

Chronic diseases Illnesses that develop and last over a long time.
Risk factors Characteristics that predict the development of a certain disease.
Wellness The constant and deliberate effort to stay healthy and achieve the highest potential for well-being.

For a wellness way of life, individuals must be physically fit and manifest no signs of disease and also must have no risk factors for disease (such as physical inactivity, hypertension, abnormal cholesterol levels, cigarette smoking, excessive stress, faulty nutrition, careless sex). Even though an individual tested in a fitness center may demonstrate adequate or even excellent fitness, indulgence in unhealthy lifestyle behaviors still will increase the risk for chronic diseases and decrease the person's well-being. Additional information on wellness and how to implement a wellness program is discussed in Chapter 8.

Unhealthy behaviors are contributing to the staggering U.S. health-care costs. Risk factors for disease carry a heavy price tag (see Figure 1.3). About 13.6% of the gross national product (GNP), $1.035 trillion, was spent in health-care costs in 1996. Costs averaged $3,759 per person that same year — the highest rate in the world. According to estimates,[9] 1% of Americans account for 30% of these costs. Half of the people use up about 97% of the health-care dollars.

Physical Fitness

Individuals are physically fit when they can meet both the ordinary and the unusual demands of daily life safely and effectively without being overly fatigued and still have energy left for leisure and recreational activities. **Physical fitness** can be classified into health-related and motor-skill-related fitness.

Health-Related Fitness

Health-related fitness has four components (see Figure 1.4)

1. *Cardiorespiratory endurance*: the ability of the heart, lungs, and blood vessels to supply oxygen to the cells to meet the demands of prolonged physical activity (also referred to as aerobic exercise).

2. *Muscular strength and endurance*: the ability of the muscles to generate force.

3. *Muscular flexibility*: the capacity of a joint to move freely through a full range of motion.

4. *Body composition*: the amount of lean body mass and adipose tissue (fat mass) in the human body.

Skill-Related Fitness

Motor **skill-related fitness** is essential in activities such as basketball, racquetball, golf, hiking, soccer, and water skiing. Good skill-related fitness also enhances overall quality of life by helping people cope more effectively in emergency situations (see Chapter 4). The components of skill-related fitness are agility, balance, coordination, power, reaction time, and speed (see Figure 1.5):

1. *Agility*: the ability to change body position and direction quickly and efficiently. Agility

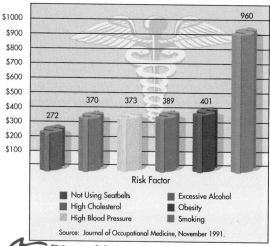

Figure 1.3 Average annual health care costs for leading disease risk factors.

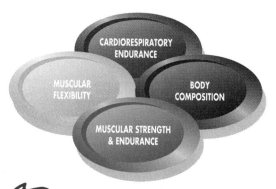

Figure 1.4 Health-related components of physical fitness.

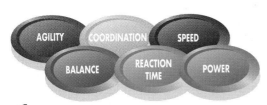

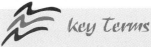 *Figure 1.5* Motor–skill components of physical fitness.

is important in sports such as basketball, soccer, and racquetball, in which the participant must change direction rapidly and at the same time maintain proper body control.

2. *Balance:* the ability to maintain the body in equilibrium. Balance is vital in activities such as gymnastics, diving, ice skating, skiing, and even football and wrestling, in which the athlete attempts to upset the opponent's equilibrium.

3. *Coordination:* integration of the nervous system and the muscular system to produce correct, graceful, and harmonious body movements. This component is important in a wide variety of motor activities such as golf, baseball, karate, soccer, and racquetball, in which hand-eye or foot-eye movements, or both, must be integrated.

4. *Power:* the ability to produce maximum force in the shortest time. The two components of power are *speed* and *force* (strength).

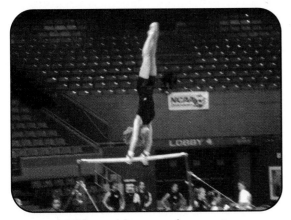

Good skill fitness enhances performance in sports.

An effective combination of these two components allows a person to produce explosive movements such as in jumping, putting the shot, and spiking/throwing/hitting a ball.

5. *Reaction time:* the time required to initiate a response to a given stimulus. Good reaction time is important for starts in track and swimming, to react quickly when playing tennis at the net, and in sports such as ping-pong, boxing, and karate.

6. *Speed:* the ability to propel the body or a part of the body rapidly from one point to another. Examples of activities that require good speed for success include sprints in track, stealing a base in baseball, soccer, and basketball.

In terms of preventive medicine, the main emphasis of fitness programs should be on the health-related components. Although skill-related fitness is crucial for success in sports and athletics, it also contributes to wellness. Improving skill-related fitness not only affords an individual more enjoyment and success in lifetime sports, but regular participation in skill-fitness activities also helps develop health-fitness. Further, total fitness is achieved by taking part in specific programs to improve both health-related and skill-related components.

Benefits of Fitness and Wellness

The benefits to be enjoyed from participating in a regular fitness and wellness program are many.

key Terms

Physical fitness The general capacity to adapt and respond favorably to physical effort.

Health-related fitness A physical state encompassing cardiorespiratory endurance, muscular strength and endurance, muscular flexibility, and body composition.

Skill-related fitness Components of fitness important for successful motor performance in athletic events and in lifetime sports and activities.

In addition to a longer life (see Figures 1.6, 1.7, and 1.8), the greatest benefit of all is that physically fit individuals enjoy a better quality of life. Fit people who lead a positive lifestyle live a better and healthier life. These people live life to its fullest potential and have fewer health problems than inactive individuals who also may indulge in negative lifestyle patterns.

Although compiling an all-inclusive list of the benefits reaped through participation in a fitness and wellness program is difficult, the following list summarizes many of these benefits:

- Improves and strengthens the cardiorespiratory system.
- Maintains better muscle tone, muscular strength, and endurance.
- Improves muscular flexibility.
- Improves your athletic performance.
- Helps maintain recommended body weight.
- Helps preserve lean body tissue.
- Increases resting metabolic rate.
- Improves the body's ability to use fat during physical activity.
- Improves posture and physical appearance.
- Improves functioning of the immune system.
- Lowers the risk for chronic diseases and illness (such as cardiovascular diseases and cancer).
- Decreases the mortality rate from chronic diseases.
- Thins the blood so it doesn't clot as readily (decreasing the risk for coronary heart disease and strokes).
- Helps the body manage cholesterol levels more effectively.
- Prevents or delays the development of high blood pressure and lowers blood pressure in people with hypertension.
- Helps prevent and control diabetes.
- Helps achieve peak bone mass in young adults and maintain bone mass later in life, thereby decreasing the risk for osteoporosis.
- Helps people to sleep better.
- Helps to prevent chronic back pain.
- Relieves tension and helps in coping with life stresses.
- Raises levels of energy and job productivity.
- Extends longevity and slows the aging process.
- Improves self-image and morale and helps fight depression and anxiety.
- Motivates toward positive lifestyle changes (better nutrition, quitting smoking, alcohol and drug-abuse control).
- Speeds recovery time following physical exertion.
- Speeds recovery following injury or disease.
- Regulates and improves overall body functions.
- Improves physical stamina and counteracts chronic fatigue.
- Helps to maintain independent living, especially in older adults.
- Enhances quality of life; makes people feel better and live a healthier and happier life.

In addition to the benefits listed, **epidemiological** research studies linking physical activity habits and mortality rates have shown lower premature mortality rates in physically active people. Work conducted by Dr. Ralph Paffenbarger and colleagues[10] demonstrated that as the amount of weekly physical activity increased, the risk of cardiovascular deaths decreased. In this study, conducted among 16,936 Harvard alumni, the greatest decrease in cardiovascular deaths was observed in alumni who burned more than 2,000 calories per week through physical activity (see Figure 1.6).

Another major study, conducted by Dr. Steve Blair and associates,[11] upheld the findings of the Harvard alumni study. Based on data from 13,344 people who were followed over an average of 8 years, the results confirmed that the level of cardiorespiratory fitness is related to mortality from all causes. These findings showed a graded and consistent inverse relationship between cardiorespiratory fitness and mortality, regardless of age and other risk factors. In

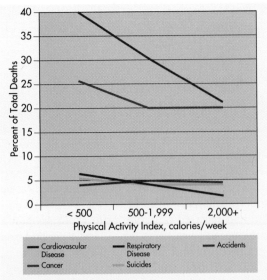

Percent of Total Deaths vs. Physical Activity Index, calories/week (< 500, 500–1,999, 2,000+)

Cardiovascular Disease · Cancer · Respiratory Disease · Suicides · Accidents

NOTE: The graph represents cause-specific death rates per 10,000 man-years of observation among 16,936 Harvard alumni, 1962–1978, by physical activity index; adjusted for differences in age, cigarette smoking, and hypertension.

Source: "A Natural History of Athleticism on Cardiovascular Health," by R. S. Paffenbarger, R. T. Hyde, A. L. Wing,. and C. H. Steinmetz, *Journal of the American Medical Association*, 252 (1989), 491–495. Used by permission.

Figure 1.6 Death rates by physical activity index.

essence, the higher the level of cardiorespiratory fitness, the longer the life (see Figure 1.7).

The death rate from all causes for the least-fit (group 1) men was 3.4 times higher than for the most fit men. For the least-fit women, the death rate was 4.6 times higher than for the most-fit women. The study also reported a greatly reduced rate of premature deaths, even at moderate fitness levels that most adults can achieve easily. People gain further protection when they combine higher fitness levels with reduction in other risk factors such as hypertension, elevated cholesterol, cigarette smoking, and excessive body fat.

Additional research that looked at changes in fitness and mortality found a substantial (44%) reduction in mortality risk when people abandon a sedentary lifestyle and become moderately fit.[12] The lowest death rate was found in people who were fit and remained fit, and the

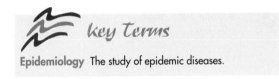

key Terms

Epidemiology The study of epidemic diseases.

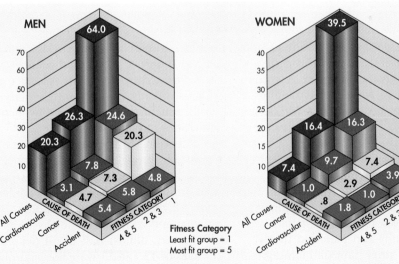

MEN — WOMEN

Fitness Category
Least fit group = 1
Most fit group = 5

Based on data from "Physical Fitness and All-Cause Mortality: A Prospective Study of Healthy Men and Women," by S. N. Blair, H. W. Kohl III, R. S. Paffenbarger, Jr., D. G. Clark, K. H. Cooper, and L. W. Gibbons. *Journal of the American Medical Association*, 262 (1989), 2395–2401.

Figure 1.7 Death rates by physical fitness levels.

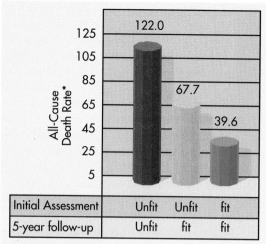

Initial Assessment	Unfit	Unfit	fit
5-year follow-up	Unfit	fit	fit

* Death rate per 10,000 man-years observation. Based on data from "Changes in Physical Fitness and All-Cause Mortality: A Prospective Study of Healthy Men," *Journal of the American Medical Association*, 273 (1995), 1193–1198.

Source: J. E. Enstrom, "Health Practices and Cancer Mortality Among Active California Mormons," *Journal of the National Cancer Institute*, 81 (1989), 1807–1814.

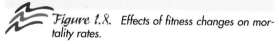

Figure 1.8. Effects of fitness changes on mortality rates.

highest rate was found in men who remained unfit (see Figure 1.8).

Subsequent research published in 1995 in the *Journal of the American Medical Association*[13] substantiated the previous findings and also indicated that primarily vigorous activities are associated with greater longevity. Vigorous activity was defined as activity that requires a MET level equal to or greater than 6 METs (see Chapter 4, Table 4.1). This level represents exercising at an oxygen uptake (VO_2) equal to or greater than 21 ml/kg/min, or the equivalent of 6 times the resting energy requirement.

Examples of vigorous activities used in the previous study include brisk walking, jogging, swimming laps, squash, racquetball, tennis, and shoveling snow. Results also indicated that vigorous exercise is as important as maintaining recommended weight and not smoking.

The results of these studies indicate clearly that fitness improves wellness, quality of life, and longevity. If people are able, vigorous exercise is preferable because it is best associated with longer life.

Surgeon General's Report on Physical Activity and Health

A landmark report on the influence of regular physical activity on health was released in July of 1996 by the U.S. Surgeon General.[14] The significance of this historic document cannot be underestimated. Until 1996, the Surgeon General had released only two prior reports: one on smoking and health, in 1964, and a second one on nutrition and health in 1988. More than 1,000 scientific studies from the fields of epidemiology, exercise physiology, medicine, and the behavioral sciences are summarized in this document on physical activity and health.

The report states that regular moderate physical activity provides substantial benefits in health and well-being for the vast majority of Americans who are not physically active. Among these benefits are a significant reduction in the risk of developing or dying from heart disease, diabetes, colon cancer, and high blood pressure. Regular physical activity also is important for health of muscles, bones, and joints; and it seems to reduce symptoms of depression and anxiety, improve mood, and enhance the ability to perform daily tasks throughout life. If individuals already are moderately active, greater health benefits can be achieved by increasing the amount of physical activity.

According to the Surgeon General, improving health through physical activity is a serious public health problem that we must meet head-on at once. More than 60% of adults had not achieved the recommended amount of physical activity, and 25% were not physically active at all. Further, almost half of all people between the ages of 12 and 21 were not vigorously active on a regular basis. This report became a call to nationwide action. Regular moderate physical activity can prevent premature death, unnecessary illness, and disability. It also can help to control health-care costs and maintain a high quality of life into old age.

In the report, moderate physical activity was defined as physical activity that uses 150 calories of energy per day, or 1,000 calories per week. People should strive to achieve at least 30 minutes of physical activity per day most days of the week. Examples of moderate physical activity are walking, cycling, playing basketball or volleyball, swimming, water aerobics, dancing fast, pushing a stroller, raking leaves, shoveling snow, washing or waxing a car, washing windows or floors, and even gardening.

U.S. Health Objectives for the Year 2000

Every 10 years the U. S. Department of Health and Human Services releases a list of objectives for disease prevention and health promotion. From its onset in 1980, this 10-year plan has helped instill a new sense of purpose and focus for public health and preventive medicine.

The Year 2000 objectives, published in the document *Healthy People 2000*,[15] address three important points:

1. *Personal responsibility.* Individuals need to become ever more health-conscious. Responsible and informed behavior is the key to good health.

2. *Health benefits for all people.* Lower socioeconomic conditions and poor health often are interrelated. Extending the benefits of good health to all people is crucial to the health of the nation.

3. *Health promotion and disease prevention.* A shift from treatment to preventive techniques will cut health-care costs drastically and help Americans achieve a higher quality of life.

Development of the Year 2000 Health Objectives involved more than 10,000 people representing 300 national organizations, including the Institute of Medicine of the National Academy of Sciences, all state health departments, and the federal Office of Disease Prevention and Health Promotion. A summary of key objectives is provided in Figure 1.9. Living the fitness and wellness principles presented here will enhance the quality of your life and also will allow you to be an active participant in achieving the Healthy People 2000 Objectives.

The Path to Fitness and Better Quality of Life

Current scientific data and the fitness movement of the past three decades in the United States have led many people to see the advantages of participating in fitness programs that will improve and maintain health. Because fitness and wellness needs vary significantly from one person to another, all exercise and wellness prescriptions must be personalized for best results. This book provides the necessary guidelines for developing a lifetime program to improve fitness and promote preventive health care and personal wellness. As you study the book and complete the assignments in each chapter, you will learn to:

- Determine whether medical clearance is required for you to participate safely in exercise.
- Assess your overall level of physical fitness, including cardiorespiratory endurance, muscular strength and endurance, muscular flexibility, and body composition.
- Prescribe personal programs for total fitness development.
- Learn behavior modification techniques that will allow you to change unhealthy lifestyle patterns.
- Develop sound diet and weight control programs.
- Implement a healthy lifestyle program that includes prevention of cardiovascular diseases and cancer, stress management, and smoking cessation if applicable.

HEALTHY PEOPLE 2000:
SELECTED HEALTH OBJECTIVES FOR THE YEAR 2000

I. Physical Activity and Fitness

1. Increase the proportion of people who engage regularly, preferably daily, in light to moderate physical activity for at least 30 minutes per day.
2. Increase the proportion of people who engage in vigorous physical activity that promotes the development and maintenance of cardiorespiratory fitness 3 or more days per week for 20 or more minutes per occasion.
3. Increase the proportion of people who regularly perform physical activities that enhance and maintain muscular strength, muscular endurance, and flexibility.
4. Reduce overweight to a prevalence of no more than 20% among people aged 20 and older and no more than 15% among adolescents aged 12 through 19.

II. Nutrition

1. Reduce dietary fat intake to an average of 30% of calories or less and average saturated fat intake to less than 10% of calories among people aged 2 and older.
2. Increase complex carbohydrate and fiber-containing foods in the diets of adults to 5 or more daily servings for vegetables and fruits, and to 6 or more daily servings for grain products.
3. Increase calcium consumption in the diet.
4. Increase to at least 85% the proportion of people aged 18 and older who use food labels to make nutritious selections.

III. Chronic Diseases

1. Increase years of healthy life to at least 65 years.
2. Reduce coronary heart disease deaths.
3. Reduce the mean serum cholesterol level among adults to no more than 200 mg/dL.
4. Increase the proportion of adults with high blood cholesterol who are aware of their condition and are taking action to reduce their blood cholesterol to recommended levels.
5. Increase the proportion of people with high blood pressure whose blood pressure is under control.
6. Increase the proportion of people with high blood pressure who are taking action to help control their blood pressure.
7. Reverse the rise in cancer deaths.
8. Reduce the proportion of people who experience adverse health effects from stress.
9. Decrease the proportion of people who experience stress who do not take steps to reduce or control their stress.

IV. Tobacco

1. Reduce the incidence of cigarette smoking.
2. Reduce the proportion of children who are exposed regularly to tobacco smoke at home.
3. Reduce use of smokeless tobacco.

V. Alcohol and Other Drugs

1. Reduce the proportion of young people who have used alcohol, marijuana, and cocaine.
2. Reduce the proportion of high school seniors and college students engaging in recent occasions of heavy drinking of alcoholic beverages.
3. Reduce alcohol consumption by people aged 14 and older to an annual average of no more than 2 gallons of ethanol per person.
4. Reduce deaths caused by alcohol-related motor vehicle crashes.
5. Reduce drug-related deaths.

VI. AIDS, HIV Infection, and Sexually Transmitted Diseases

1. Confine annual incidence of diagnosed AIDS cases to no more than 98,000 cases.
2. Confine the prevalence of HIV infection to no more than 800 per 100,000 people.
3. Increase the proportion of sexually active, unmarried people who used a condom at last sexual intercourse.
4. Reduce the overall incidence of sexually transmitted diseases.

VII. Family Planning

1. Reduce the number of pregnancies that are unintended.
2. Reduce the proportion of adolescents who have engaged in sexual intercourse.
3. Increase the proportion of sexually active, unmarried people aged 19 and younger who use contraception, especially combined-method contraception that both effectively prevents pregnancy and provides barrier protection against disease.

VIII. Unintentional Injuries

1. Reduce deaths caused by unintentional injuries.
2. Increase use of occupant protection systems, such as safety belts, inflatable safety restraints, and child safety seats among motor vehicle occupants.
3. Increase use of helmets among motorcyclists and bicyclists.

* Adapted from *Healthy People 2000: National Health Promotion and Disease Prevention Objectives*, by U.S. Department of Health and Human Services (Boston: Jones and Bartlett Publishers, 1992). Refer to this publication for further information on these objectives.

Figure 1.9   *Healthy People 2000: Selected health objectives for the year 2000.*

🦅 Discern between myths and facts of exercise and health-related concepts.

Behavior Modification

Scientific evidence of the benefits derived from living a healthy lifestyle continues to mount each day. Although the data are impressive, most people still don't adhere to a healthy lifestyle. To understand why this is so, one has to examine what motivates people and what actions are required to make permanent changes in behavior.

Transtheoretical Model

For most people, changing chronic/unhealthy behaviors to stable/healthy behaviors is often a challenging process. Change usually does not occur all at once, but it is rather a lengthy process that involves several stages. To aid in this process, psychologists James Prochaska, John Norcross, and Carlo DiClemente developed the **Transtheoretical Model** for behavior change.[16] This model includes six stages that are important in understanding the process of willful change. The stages of change describe underlying processes that people go through to change most problem behaviors and adopt healthy behaviors. Most frequently, the model is used to change health-related behaviors such as physical inactivity, smoking, nutrition, weight control, stress, and alcohol abuse.

Stages of Change

The six stages of change in the Transtheoretical Model include precontemplation, contemplation, preparation, action, maintenance, and termination. After years of study, researchers found the applying specific behavioral-change techniques during each stage of the model increases the success rate for change. Understanding each stage of this model will help you determine where you are at in relation to your personal healthy-lifestyle behaviors. It will also help you identify techniques to make successful changes.

Precontemplation

People in this stage are not considering or do not want to change a particular behavior. They typically deny having a problem and have no intent to change in the foreseeable future. These people are usually unaware or underaware of the problem. Other people around them, including family, friends, health care practitioners, and coworkers, however, identify the problem quite clearly. Precontemplators do not care about the problem behavior and may even avoid information and materials that address the issue. They tend to avoid free screenings and workshops that can help identify and change the problem, even if financial compensation is made for attendance. These people frequently have an active resistance to change and seem resigned to accept the unhealthy behavior as their "fate."

Precontemplators are the most difficult people to reach for behavioral change. They often think that change isn't even a possibility. Educating them about the problem behavior is critical to help them start contemplating the process of change. "Knowledge is power" and the challenge is to find ways to help them realize that they will be ultimately responsible for the consequences of their behavior. Frequently, they may initiate change only when under pressure from others.

Contemplation

In this stage people acknowledge that they have a problem and begin to seriously think about overcoming it. Although they are not quite ready yet for change, they are weighing the pros and cons of change. People may remain in this stage for years, but in their minds they are planning to take some action within the next six months. Education and peer support are quite valuable during this stage.

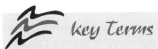

key Terms

Transtheoretical Model A stages of change model that provides framework for studying intentional behavior change.

Preparation

In the preparation stage, people are seriously considering and planning to change a behavior within the next month. They are taking initial steps for change and may even try it for a short while, such as stopping smoking for a day or exercising only a few times during this month. During this stage, people define a general goal for behavioral change (to quit smoking by the last day of the month) and specific objectives are written to accomplish this goal (see Goal Setting discussion later in this chapter). Continued peer and environmental support are recommended during the preparation phase.

Action

This is the stage that requires the greatest commitment of time and energy on the part of the individual. Here people are actively doing things to change or modify the problem behavior or to adopt a new health behavior. The action stage requires that the person follow the specific guidelines set forth for that particular behavior. For example, a person has actually completely stopped smoking, is exercising aerobically three times per week according to exercise prescription guidelines (see Chapter 3), or is maintaining a diet that derives less than 30% of its calories from fat. Relapse is common during this stage and the individual may regress to previous stages. Once people maintain the action stage for six consecutive months, they move into the maintenance stage.

Maintenance

During the maintenance stage the person continues to maintain the behavioral change for a period of up to five years. The maintenance phase requires continued adherence to the specific guidelines that govern the said behavior (complete smoking cessation, exercising aerobically three times per week, or practicing proper stress management techniques). It is at this time that a person works to reinforce the gains made through the various stages of change and strives to prevent lapses and relapse.

Termination

Once a behavior has been maintained for over five years, a person exits from the cycle of change without fear of relapse. Many experts believe that after this period of time, any former addictions, problems, or lack of compliance with healthy behaviors no longer present an obstacle in the quest for wellness. The change has now become a part of one's lifestyle. This phase is the ultimate goal for all people searching for a healthier lifestyle.

You may use the form provided in Figure 1.10 to determine where you stand in respect to behaviors that you want to change or new ones that you wish to adopt. As you use this form, you will realize that you are at different stages for different behaviors. For instance, you may be in the termination stage for aerobic exercise and smoking, in the action stage for strength training, but only in the contemplation stage for a healthy diet. Realizing where you are at with respect to different behaviors will help you design a better action plan for a healthy lifestyle.

Motivation and Locus of Control

Motivation often is used to explain why some people succeed and others do not. Although motivation comes from within, external factors are what trigger the inner desire to accomplish a given task. These external factors, then, control behavior.

When studying motivation, understanding **locus of control** is helpful. People who believe they have control over events in their lives are said to have an *internal locus of control*. People with an *external locus of control* believe that what happens to them is a result of chance, or the environment, and is unrelated to their behavior. These people often have a difficult time getting out of the precontemplation or contemplation stages. People with an internal locus of control generally are healthier and have an easier time initiating and adhering to a wellness program than those who perceive that they have no control and think of themselves as powerless and vulnerable. The latter people also are at greater risk for illness. When illness does strike, restoring a sense of control is vital to regain health.

Few people have either a completely external or a completely internal locus of control. They fall somewhere along a continuum. The more external, the greater is the challenge in changing and adhering to exercise and other healthy lifestyle behaviors. Fortunately, developing a more internal locus of control can be accomplished. Understanding that most events in life are not determined genetically or environmentally helps people to pursue goals and gain control over their lives. Three impediments, however, can keep people from getting into the preparation or action stages: competence, confidence, and motivation.[17]

1. *Problems of competence.* Lacking the skills to get a given task done leads to less competence. If your friends play basketball regularly but you don't know how to play, you might not be inclined to participate. The solution to this problem of competence is to master the skills you need to participate. Most people are not born with all-inclusive natural abilities, including playing sports.

A college professor continuously watched a group of students play an entertaining game of basketball every Friday at noon. Having no basketball skills, he was reluctant to play (contemplation stage). Eventually, however, the desire to join in the fun was strong enough that he enrolled in a beginning course at the college so he

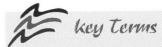

key Terms

Motivation The desire and will to do something.

Locus of control The extent to which a person believes he or she can influence the external environment.

Please indicate which response most accurately describes your current _____ behavior (in the blank space identify the behavior: smoking, physical activity, stress, nutrition, weight control). Next, select the statement below (select only one) that best represents your current behavior pattern. To select the most appropriate statement, fill in the blank for one of the first three statements if your current behavior is a problem behavior. (For example, you may say, "I currently smoke and I do *not* intend to change in the foreseeable future," or "I currently *do not exercise* but I am contemplating changing in the next 6 months.") If you have already started to make changes, fill in the blank in one of the last three statements. (In this case, you may say: "I currently *eat a low-fat diet* but I have only done so within the last 6 months," or "I currently *practice adequate stress management techniques* and I have done so for over 6 months.") As you can see, you may use this form to identify your stage of change for any type of health-related behavior.

☐ 1. I currently _____ and I do not intend to change in the foreseeable future.

☐ 2. I currently _____ but I am contemplating changing in the next 6 months.

☐ 3. I currently _____ regularly but I intend to change in the next month.

☐ 4. I currently _____ but I have done so only within the last 6 months.

☐ 5. I currently _____ and I have done so for more than 6 months.

☐ 6. I currently _____ and I have done so for more than 5 years.

Stages of Change

1 = Precontemplation   4 = Action
2 = Contemplation   5 = Maintenance
3 = Preparation   6 = Termination

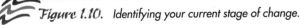

Figure 1.10. Identifying your current stage of change.

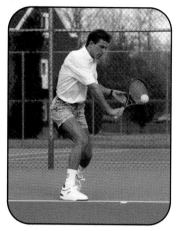

Many people refrain from physical activity because they lack the necessary skills to enjoy and reap the benefits of regular participation.

would learn to play the game (preparation stage). To his surprise, most of the students were impressed that he was willing to do this. Now, with greater competence, he is able to join in on Friday's "pick-up" games (action phase).

Another alternative is to select an activity in which you are skilled. It may not be basketball, but it well could be aerobics. Don't be afraid, however, to try new activities. Similarly, if your body weight is a problem, you could learn to cook low-fat meals. Try different recipes until you find foods that you like.

Patty's story at the beginning of this chapter exemplifies a lack of competence. Patty was motivated and knew she could do it, but she lacked the skills to reach her goal. All along Patty was fluctuating between the contemplation and action stages. Once she mastered the skills, she was able to achieve and maintain her goal.

2. *Problems of confidence.* Problems with confidence arise when the skills are there but you don't believe you can get it done. Fear and feelings of inadequacy often interfere with the ability to perform the task.

You shouldn't talk yourself out of something until you have given it a fair try. If the skills are there, the sky is the limit. Initially, try to visualize yourself doing the task and getting it done. Repeat this several times, then actually give it a try. You will surprise yourself.

Sometimes lack of confidence develops when the task appears to be insurmountable. In

these situations dividing a goal into smaller, realistic objectives helps to accomplish the task. You may know how to swim, but to swim a continuous mile may take several weeks to accomplish. Set up your training program so that each day you swim a little farther until you are able to swim the entire mile. If on a given day you don't meet your objective, try it again, reevaluate, cut back a little, and, most important, don't give up.

3. *Problems of motivation.* In problems of motivation, both the competence and the confidence are there, but the individuals are unwilling to change because the reasons for change are not important to them. For example, people begin contemplating a smoking cessation program when the reasons for quitting outweigh the reasons for smoking.

When considering quality of life, lack of knowledge and lack of goals are the primary causes of unwillingness to change (precontemplators). Knowledge often determines goals, and goals determine motivation. How badly you want something dictates how hard you'll work at it. Many people are unaware of the magnitude of the benefits of a wellness program. When it comes to a healthy lifestyle, however, there may not be a second chance. A stroke, a heart attack, or cancer can have irreparable or fatal consequences. Greater understanding of what leads to disease may be all that is needed to initiate change.

Also, feeling physically fit is difficult to explain unless you have experienced it yourself. What Patty expressed to her instructor — feelings of fitness, self-esteem, confidence, health, and quality of life — cannot be conveyed to someone who is constrained by sedentary living. In a way, wellness is like reaching the top of a mountain. The quietness, the clean air, the lush vegetation, the flowing water in the river, the wildlife, and the majestic valley below are difficult to explain to someone who has spent a lifetime within city limits.

Behavior Modification Principles

Over the course of many years, we all develop habits that at some point we would like to change. The adage "old habits die hard," comes to mind. Acquiring positive behaviors that will lead to better health and well-being requires continual effort. When wellness is concerned, the sooner we implement a healthy lifestyle program, the greater are the health benefits and quality of life that lie ahead. The following **behavior modification** principles can be adopted to help change behavior.

Self-Analysis

The first step in modifying behavior is a decisive desire to do so. If you have no interest in changing a behavior, you won't do it (precontemplator). A person who has no intention of quitting smoking will not quit, regardless of what anyone may say or how strong the evidence is against it. In your self-analysis you may want to prepare a list of reasons for continuing or discontinuing the behavior. When the reasons for changing outweigh the reasons for not changing, you are ready for the next step (contemplation stage).

Behavior Analysis

Next you have to determine the frequency, circumstances, and consequences of the behavior to be altered or implemented. If the desired outcome is to consume less fat, you first must find out what foods in your diet are high in fat, when you eat them, and when you don't eat them (preparation stage). Knowing when you don't eat them points to circumstances under which you exert control of your diet and will help as you set goals.

Goal Setting

Goals motivate change in behavior. The stronger the goal, or desire, the more motivated you'll be either to change unwanted behaviors or to implement new healthy behaviors. The discussion on goal setting (page 18) will help you write goals and prepare an action plan to achieve those goals. This will aid with behavior modification.

Social Support

Surrounding yourself with people who will work toward a common goal with you or will encourage you along the way will be helpful. Attempting to quit smoking, for instance, is easier when the person is around others who are trying as well. The person also may get help from friends who already have quit. Peer support is a strong incentive for behavioral change. During this process, people who will not be supportive should be avoided. Friends who have no desire to quit smoking may tempt one to smoke and encourage relapse of unwanted behaviors. People who have achieved the same goal already may not be supportive either. For instance, someone may say, "I can do six consecutive miles." The response should be, "I'm proud that I can jog three consecutive miles."

Monitoring

During the action and maintenance stages, continuous behavior monitoring increases awareness of the desired outcome. Sometimes this principle in itself is sufficient to cause change. For example, keeping track of daily food intake reveals sources of fat in the diet. This can help you cut down gradually or completely eliminate high-fat foods prior to consuming them. If the goal is to increase daily intake of fruit and vegetables, keeping track of the number of servings consumed each day raises awareness and may help increase their intake.

Positive Outlook

Having a positive outlook means taking a positive approach from the beginning and believing in yourself. Following the guidelines in this chapter will help you pace yourself so you can work toward change. Also, you may become motivated by looking at the outcomes — how much healthier you will be, how much better you will look, or being able to jog a certain distance.

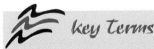

key Terms

Behavior modification The process of changing actions permanently.

Reinforcement

People tend to repeat behaviors that are rewarded and disregard those that are not rewarded or are punished. If you have successfully cut down your fat intake during the week, reward yourself by going to a show or buying a new pair of shoes. Do not reinforce yourself with destructive behaviors such as eating a high-fat dinner. If you fail to change a desired behavior (or to implement a new one), you may want to put off buying those new shoes you had planned for that week. When a positive behavior becomes habitual, give yourself an even better reward. Treat yourself to a weekend away from home or go on a short trip.

Goal Setting

To initiate change, goals are essential. Goals motivate behavioral change and provide a plan of action. Goals are most effective when they are:

1. *Well planned.* Only a well conceived action plan will help you attain your goal. The items below, as well as others discussed in different chapters, will help you design your plan of action. You also should write specific objectives to help you reach each goal. Examples of specific objectives are provided in Chapter 3 under "Setting Fitness Goals."

2. *Personalized.* Goals that you set for yourself are more motivational than goals that someone else sets for you.

3. *Written.* An unwritten goal is simply a wish. A written goal, in essence, becomes a contract with yourself. Show this goal to a friend or an instructor, and have him or her witness with his or her signature the contract you made with yourself.

4. *Realistic.* Goals should be within reach. If you have not exercised regularly, it would be unrealistic to start a daily exercise program consisting of 45 minutes of step aerobics at a vigorous intensity level. Unattainable goals lead to discouragement and loss of interest. To set smaller, attainable goals is better.

At times problems arise even with realistic goals. Try to anticipate potential difficulties as much as possible, and plan for ways to deal with them. If your goal is to jog for 30 minutes on 6 consecutive days, what are the alternatives if the weather turns bad? Possible solutions are to jog in the rain, find an indoor track, jog at a different time of day when the weather improves, or participate in a different aerobic activity such as stationary cycling, swimming, or step aerobics.

5. *Measurable.* Write your goals so they are clear, and state specifically the objective to accomplish. "I will lose weight" is not clear enough and is not measurable. A better example is: "I will decrease my body fat to 17%."

6. *Time-specific.* A goal always should have a specific date set for completion. This date should be realistic but not too distant in the future.

7. *Monitored.* Monitoring your progress as you move toward a goal reinforces behavior. Keeping an exercise log or doing a body composition assessment periodically determines where you are at at any given time.

8. *Evaluated.* Periodic reevaluations are vital for success. You may find that a given goal is unreachable. If so, reassess the goal. On the other hand, if a goal is too easy, you may lose interest and stop working toward it. Once you achieve a goal, set a new one to improve upon or maintain what you have achieved. Goals keep you motivated.

In addition to the previous guidelines, you will find additional information on behavioral change throughout this book. For example, the Exercise Readiness Questionnaire, tips to start and adhere to an exercise program, and how to set your fitness goals are provided in Chapter 3; tips to enhance your aerobic workout are given in Chapter 4; tips to adhere to a lifetime weight management program are found in Chapter 6; stress management techniques are provided in Chapter 7; and a six-step smoking cessation plan is given in Chapter 8.

A Word of Caution Before You Start Exercise

Even though exercise testing and participation is relatively safe for most apparently healthy individuals under age 45, a small but real risk exists for exercise-induced abnormalities in people with a history of cardiovascular problems and those who are at higher risk for disease.[18] These people should be screened before initiating or increasing the intensity of an exercise program.

Before you start an exercise program or participate in any exercise testing, you should fill out the health history questionnaire provided in Figure 1.11. A "yes" answer to any of these questions may signal the need for a physician's approval before you participate. If you don't have any "yes" responses, you can proceed to Chapter 2 to assess your current level of fitness.

http://www.fitlife.com/

FITLIFE *An electronic resource of fitness, health promotion, wellness and lifestyle*

Notes

1. W. M. Bortz II, "Disuse and Aging," *Journal of the American Medical Association,* 248(1982), 1203–1208.

2. Editors of Prevention Magazine, *The Prevention Index 1995: A Report Card on the Nation's Health* (Emmaus, PA: Prevention Magazine, 1995).

3. National Institutes of Health, Consensus Development Conference Statement: Physical Activity and Cardiovascular Health (Washington, DC, NIH, December 18–20, 1995).

4. National Institutes of Health.

5. U.S. Department of Health and Human Services, National Center for Health Statistics, *Monthly Vital Statistics Report: Advance Report of Final Mortality Statistics,* 45:11, Supplement 2, June 12, 1997.

6. T. A. Murphy and D. Murphy, *The Wellness for Life Workbook* (San Diego: Fitness Publications, 1987).

7. P. E. Allsen, J. M. Harrison, and B. Vance, *Fitness for Life* (Madison, WI: Brown & Benchmark, 1993), p. 3.

8. B. Gutin et al., "Blood Pressure, Fitness, and Fitness in 5- and 6-Year-Old Children," *Journal of the American Medical Association,* 264(1990), 1123–1127.

9. "Wellness Facts," University of California at Berkeley *Wellness Letter* (Palm Coast, FL: The Editors, April, 1995).

10. R. S. Paffenbarger, Jr., R. T. Hyde, A. L. Wing, and C. H. Steinmetz, "A Natural History of Athleticism and Cardiovascular Health," *Journal of the American Medical Association,* 252(1984), 491–495.

11. S. N. Blair, H. W. Kohl III, R. S. Paffenbarger, Jr., D. G. Clark, K. H. Cooper, and L. W. Gibbons, "Physical Fitness and All-Cause Mortality: A Prospective Study of Healthy Men and Women," *Journal of the American Medical Association,* 262(1989), 2395–2401.

12. S. N. Blair, H. W. Kohl III, C. E. Barlow, R. S. Paffenbarger, Jr., L. W. Gibbons, and C. A. Macera, "Changes in Physical Fitness and All-Cause Mortality: A Prospective Study of Healthy and Unhealthy Men," *Journal of the American Medical Association,* 273(1995), 1193–1198.

13. I. Lee, C. Hsieh, and R. S. Paffenbarger, Jr., "Exercise Intensity and Longevity in Men: The Harvard Alumni Health Study," *Journal of the American Medical Association,* 273(1995), 1179–1184.

14. U.S. Department of Health and Human Services, "Physical Activity and Health: A Report of the Surgeon General" (Atlanta: U.S. Department of Health and Human Services, Centers for Disease Control and Prevention, National Center for Chronic Disease Prevention and Health Promotion, 1996).

15. U.S. Department of Health and Human Services, Public Health Service, *Healthy People 2000: National Health Promotion and Disease Prevention Objectives* (Boston: Jones and Bartlett Publishers, 1992).

16. J. O. Prochaska, J. C. Norcross, and C. C. DiClemente, *Changing for Good* (New York: William Morrow and Company, 1994).

17. G. S. Howard, D. W. Nance, and P. Myers, *Adaptive Counseling and Therapy* (San Francisco: Jossey-Bass, 1987).

18. American College of Sports Medicine, *Guidelines for Exercise Testing and Prescription* (Baltimore: Williams & Wilkins, 1995).

Health History Questionnaire

Even though exercise participation is relatively safe for most apparently healthy individuals, the reaction of the cardiovascular system to increased levels of physical activity cannot always be totally predicted. Consequently, there is a small but real risk of certain changes occurring during exercise participation. These changes include abnormal blood pressure, irregular heart rhythm, fainting, and in rare instances a heart attack or cardiac arrest. Therefore, you must provide honest answers to this questionnaire. Exercise may not be recommended under some of the conditions listed below; others may simply indicate special consideration. If any of the conditions apply, you should consult your physician before participating in an exercise program. You also should promptly report to your instructor any exercise-related abnormalities experienced during the course of the semester.

Have you ever had or do you now have any of the following conditions?

☐ Yes ☐ No   1. Cardiovascular disease (any type of heart or blood vessel disease, including strokes)

☐ Yes ☐ No   2. Elevated blood lipids (cholesterol and triglycerides)

☐ Yes ☐ No   3. Chest pain at rest or during exertion

☐ Yes ☐ No   4. Shortness of breath or other respiratory problems

☐ Yes ☐ No   5. Uneven, irregular, or skipped heartbeats (including a racing or fluttering heart)

☐ Yes ☐ No   6. Elevated blood pressure

☐ Yes ☐ No   7. Often feel faint or have spells of severe dizziness

☐ Yes ☐ No   8. Diabetes

☐ Yes ☐ No   9. Any joint, bone, or muscle problems (e.g., arthritis, low-back pain, rheumatism)

☐ Yes ☐ No 10. An eating disorder (anorexia, bulimia)

☐ Yes ☐ No 11. Any other concern regarding your ability to participate safely in an exercise program? If so, explain:

Indicate if any of the following two conditions apply:

☐ Yes ☐ No 12. Do you smoke cigarettes?

☐ Yes ☐ No 13. Men — Are you age 40 or older?

☐ Yes ☐ No 14. Women — Are you age 50 or older?

Student's Signature: _____   Date: _____

Figure 1.11 Health history questionnaire.

Assessment of Physical Fitness

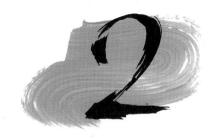

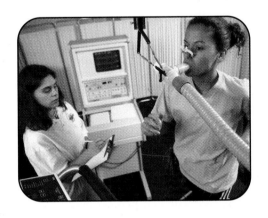

The health-related components of physical fitness — cardiorespiratory endurance, muscular strength and endurance, muscular flexibility, and body composition — are the topics of this chapter, along with basic techniques used frequently in their assessment. Through these assessment techniques you will be able to determine your level of physical fitness regularly as you engage in an exercise program. You are encouraged to conduct fitness assessments at least twice: once as a pre-test, which will serve as a starting point, and later as a post-test, to assess improvements in fitness following 10 to 14 weeks of participation in exercise.

A personal fitness profile is provided in Appendix A, Figure A.1,* for you to record the results of each fitness test in this chapter (pre-test). Figure A.2 can be used at the end of the term to record the results of your post-test.

In Chapter 3 you will learn to write personal fitness goals for this course (see Figure 3.9). These goals should be based on the actual results of your initial fitness assessments. As you proceed with your exercise program, you should allow a minimum of 8 weeks before doing your post-fitness assessments.

As discussed in Chapter 1, exercise testing or exercise participation is not advised for people with certain medical or physical conditions. Therefore, before starting an exercise program or participating in any exercise testing, you should fill out the Health History Questionnaire given in Figure 1.11. A "yes" answer to any of the questions suggests that you consult with a

Objectives

- Identify the health-related components of physical fitness.
- Be able to assess cardiorespiratory fitness.
- Understand the difference between muscular strength and muscular endurance.
- Learn to assess strength fitness.
- Be able to assess muscular flexibility.
- Understand the components of body composition.
- Be able to assess body composition.
- Learn to determine recommended body weight.
- Learn to assess disease risk based on Body Mass Index (BMI) and waist-to-hip ratio.

---

* You may obtain a computerized fitness profile by using the software for this book available to your instructor from Morton Publishing Company, 925 W. Kenyon, Unit 12, Englewood, CO 80110.

physician before initiating, continuing, or increasing your level of physical activity.

Fitness Assessment Battery

No single test can provide a complete measure of physical fitness. Because health-related fitness has four components, a battery of tests is necessary to determine an individual's overall level of fitness. In the next few pages are several tests used to assess the health-related fitness components. When interpreting fitness test results, two standards can be applied: health fitness and physical fitness.

As illustrated in Figure 2.1, although fitness (VO_{2max} — see discussion on cardiorespiratory endurance below) improvements with a moderate aerobic activity program are not as notable, significant health benefits are reaped with such a program. These improvements are quite striking, and only slightly greater benefits are obtained through a more intense exercise program. Health benefits include a reduction in blood lipids, lower blood pressure, decreased risk for diabetes, weight loss, stress release, and lower risk for disease and premature mortality.

More specifically, improvements in the **metabolic profile** (better insulin sensitivity and glucose tolerance and improved cholesterol levels) can be notable in spite of little or no improvement in aerobic capacity or weight loss. These improvements in the metabolic profile

through an active lifestyle and moderate physical activity are referred to as **metabolic fitness.**

The health fitness or criterion-referenced standards used in this book are based on epidemiological data linking minimum fitness values to disease prevention and health. Attaining the **health fitness standards** requires only moderate amounts of physical activity. For example, a 2-mile walk in less than 30 minutes, five to six times per week, seems to be sufficient to achieve the health-fitness standard for cardiorespiratory endurance.

The **physical fitness standard** is set higher than the health fitness standard and requires a more vigorous exercise program. Physically fit people of all ages have the freedom to enjoy most of life's daily and recreational activities to their fullest potential. Current health fitness standards may not be enough to achieve these objectives.

Sound physical fitness gives the individual a level of independence throughout life that many people no longer enjoy. Most older people should be able to carry out activities similar to those they conducted in their youth, though not with the same intensity. Although a person does not have to be an elite athlete, activities such as changing a tire, chopping wood, climbing several flights of stairs, playing a vigorous game of basketball, mountain biking, playing soccer with grandchildren, walking several miles around a lake, and hiking through a national park require

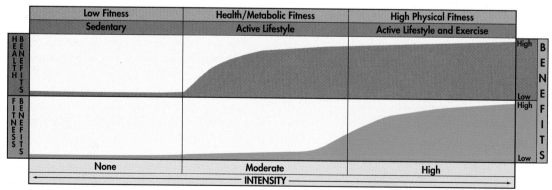

© Fitness & Wellness, Inc.

Figure 2.1. Health and fitness benefits based on lifestyle and physical activity program.

more than the "average fitness" level of the American people.

If the main objective of the fitness program is to lower the risk for disease, attaining the health fitness standards may be enough to ensure better health. In contrast, if the individual wants to participate in moderate to vigorous fitness activities, achieving a high physical fitness standard is recommended. For the purposes of this book, both health fitness and physical fitness standards are given for each fitness test. You will have to decide your personal objectives for the fitness program.

Cardiorespiratory Endurance

As a person breathes, part of the oxygen in the air is taken up in the lungs and transported in the blood to the heart. The heart then pumps the oxygenated blood through the circulatory system to all organs and tissues of the body. At the cellular level, oxygen is used to convert food substrates, primarily carbohydrates and fats, into the energy necessary to conduct body functions, maintain a constant internal equilibrium, and perform physical tasks.

Some examples of activities that promote **cardiorespiratory endurance**, or aerobic fitness, are walking, jogging, cycling, rowing, swimming, cross-country skiing, aerobic dance, soccer, basketball, and racquetball. Guidelines to develop a lifetime cardiorespiratory endurance exercise program are given in Chapter 3, and an introduction and description of benefits of leading aerobic activities are given in Chapter 4.

A sound cardiorespiratory endurance program contributes greatly to good health. The typical American is not exactly a good role model when physical fitness is concerned. A poorly conditioned heart that has to pump more often just to keep a person alive is subject to more wear-and-tear than a well conditioned heart is. In situations that place strenuous demands on the heart, such as doing yard work, lifting heavy objects or weights, or running to catch a bus, the unconditioned heart may not be able to sustain the strain.

Everyone who initiates a cardiorespiratory exercise program can expect a number of benefits from training. Among these are lower resting heart rate, blood pressure, blood lipids (cholesterol and triglycerides), recovery time following exercise, and risk for hypokinetic diseases (those associated with physical inactivity and sedentary living). Simultaneously, cardiac muscle strength and oxygen-carrying capacity increase.

Cardiorespiratory endurance is determined by the **maximal oxygen uptake** or VO_{2max}, *the maximum amount of oxygen the human body is able to utilize per minute of physical activity.* The VO_{2max} usually is expressed in ml/kg/min. Because all tissues and organs of the body utilize oxygen to function, more oxygen consumption means a more efficient cardiorespiratory system.

During physical exertion more energy is needed to perform the activity. As a result, the heart, lungs, and blood vessels have to deliver more oxygen to the cells to supply the required energy. During prolonged exercise an individual with a high level of cardiorespiratory endurance is able to deliver the required amount of oxygen to the tissues with relative ease. The cardiorespiratory system of a person with a low level of endurance has to work much harder, as the heart

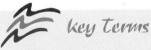

key Terms

Metabolic profile Result of the assessment of diabetes and cardiovascular disease risk through plasma insulin, glucose, lipid, and lipoprotein levels.

Metabolic fitness Denotes improvements in the metabolic profile through a moderate-intensity exercise program in spite of little or no improvements in health-related fitness.

Health fitness standards The lowest fitness requirements for maintaining good health, decreasing the risk for chronic diseases, and lowering the incidence of muscular-skeletal injuries.

Physical fitness standard Required criteria to achieve a high level of physical fitness, ability to do moderate to vigorous physical activity without undue fatigue.

Cardiorespiratory endurance Ability of the lungs, heart, and blood vessels to deliver adequate amounts of oxygen to the cells to meet the demands of prolonged physical activity.

Maximal oxygen uptake (VO_{2max}) Maximum amount of oxygen the human body is able to utilize per minute of physical activity.

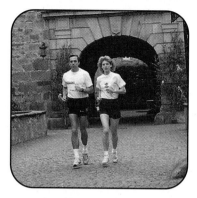

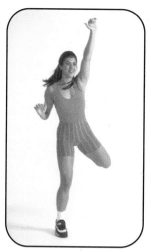

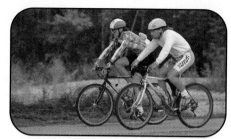

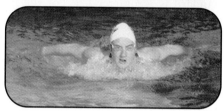

Aerobic activities promote cardiorespiratory development and help decrease the risk for chronic diseases.

has to pump more often to supply the same amount of oxygen to the tissues and consequently fatigues faster. Hence, a higher capacity to deliver and utilize oxygen (oxygen uptake) indicates a more efficient cardiorespiratory system.

Even though most cardiorespiratory endurance tests probably are safe to administer to apparently healthy individuals (those with no major coronary risk factors or symptoms), the American College of Sports Medicine recommends that a physician be present for all maximal exercise tests on apparently healthy men over age 40 and women over age 50.[1] A maximal test is any test that requires the participant's all-out or nearly all-out effort, such as the 1.5-mile run test or a maximal exercise treadmill test

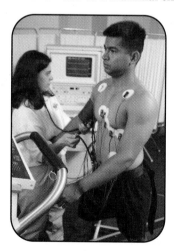

Exercise tolerance test with 12-lead electrocardiographic monitoring (stress ECG).

(stress electrocardiogram). For submaximal exercise tests (such as a walking test) a physician should be present when testing higher risk/symptomatic individuals or people with medical conditions, regardless of the participant's age.

1.5-Mile Run Test

The test used most often to determine cardiorespiratory endurance is the 1.5-Mile Run Test. The fitness category is determined according to the time a person takes to run or walk a 1.5-mile course. The only equipment necessary to conduct this test is a stopwatch and a track or premeasured 1.5-mile course.

Although the 1.5-Mile Run Test is quite simple to administer, a note of caution is in order: As the objective is to cover the distance in the shortest time, it is considered a maximal exercise test. The 1.5-Mile Run Test should be limited to conditioned individuals who have been cleared for exercise. It is not recommended for unconditioned beginners, symptomatic individuals, those with known cardiovascular disease or heart disease risk factors, and men over age 40 and women over age 50. Unconditioned beginners are encouraged to have at least 6 weeks of aerobic training before they take the test.

Prior to taking the 1.5-Mile Run Test, you should do a few warm-up exercises — some stretching exercises, some walking, and slow jogging. Next, time yourself during the 1.5-Mile Run to see how fast you cover the distance. If any unusual symptoms arise during the test, do not continue. Stop immediately and see your physician, or retake the test after another 6 weeks of aerobic training. At the end of the test, cool down by walking or jogging slowly for another 3 to 5 minutes. Referring to your performance time, look up your estimated VO_{2max} in Table 2.1 and the corresponding fitness category in Table 2.2.

For example, a 20-year-old female runs the 1.5-mile course in 12 minutes and 40 seconds. Table 2.1 shows a VO_{2max} of 39.8 ml/kg/min for a time of 12:40. According to Table 2.2, this VO_{2max} places her in the good cardiorespiratory fitness category.

1.0-Mile Walk Test*

The walking test calls for a 440-yard track (four laps to a mile) or a premeasured 1.0-mile course. Body weight in pounds must be determined prior to the walk. A stopwatch is required to measure total walking time and exercise heart rate.

You can proceed to walk the 1-mile course at a brisk pace so the exercise heart rate at the end of the test is above 120 beats per minute. At the end of the 1.0-Mile Walk, check your walking time and immediately count your pulse for 10 seconds. You can take your pulse on the

* "Estimation of VO_{2max} from a One-Mile Track Walk, Gender, Age, and Body Weight," by G. Kline et al., *Medicine and Science in Sports and Exercise*, 19(3):253–259, 1987. © American College of Sports Medicine.

Table 2.1 Estimated Maximal Oxygen Uptake in ml/kg/min for 1.5-Mile Run Test

Time	VO_{2max}	Time	VO_{2max}	Time	VO_{2max}	Time	VO_{2max}
6:10	80.0	9:30	54.7	12:50	39.2	16:10	30.5
6:20	79.0	9:40	53.5	13:00	38.6	16:20	30.2
6:30	77.9	9:50	52.3	13:10	38.1	16:30	29.8
6:40	76.7	10:00	51.1	13:20	37.8	16:40	29.5
6:50	75.5	10:10	50.4	13:30	37.2	16:50	29.1
7:00	74.0	10:20	49.5	13:40	36.8	17:00	28.9
7:10	72.6	10:30	48.6	13:50	36.3	17:10	28.5
7:20	71.3	10:40	48.0	14:00	35.9	17:20	28.3
7:30	69.9	10:50	47.4	14:10	35.5	17:30	28.0
7:40	68.3	11:00	46.6	14:20	35.1	17:40	27.7
7:50	66.8	11:10	45.8	14:30	34.7	17:50	27.4
8:00	65.2	11:20	45.1	14:40	34.3	18:00	27.1
8:10	63.9	11:30	44.4	14:50	34.0	18:10	26.8
8:20	62.5	11:40	43.7	15:00	33.6	18:20	26.6
8:30	61.2	11:50	43.2	15:10	33.1	18:30	26.3
8:40	60.2	12:00	42.3	15:20	32.7	18:40	26.0
8:50	59.1	12:10	41.7	15:30	32.2	18:50	25.7
9:00	58.1	12:20	41.0	15:40	31.8	19:00	25.4
9:10	56.9	12:30	40.4	15:50	31.4		
9:20	55.9	12:40	39.8	16:00	30.9		

Adapted from "A Means of Assessing Maximal Oxygen Intake," by K. H. Cooper, *Journal of the American Medical Association*, 203 (1968), 201–204; *Health and Fitness Through Physical Activity*, by M. L. Pollock (New York: John Wiley and Sons, 1978); and *Training for Sport Activity*, by J. H. Wilmore (Boston: Allyn and Bacon, 1982).

Table 2.2 *Cardiorespiratory Fitness Classification According to Maximal Oxygen Update in ml/kg/min*

Gender	Age	Fitness Classification				
		Poor	**Fair**	**Average**	**Good**	**Excellent**
Men	≤29	≤24.9	25–33.9	34–43.9	44–52.9	≥53
	30–39	≤22.9	23–30.9	31–41.9	42–49.9	≥50
	40–49	≤19.9	20–26.9	27–38.9	39–44.9	≥45
	50–59	≤17.9	18–24.9	25–37.9	38–42.9	≥43
	60–69	≤15.9	16–22.9	23–35.9	36–40.9	≥41
Women	≤29	≤23.9	24–30.9	31–38.9	39–48.9	≥49
	30–39	≤19.9	20–27.9	28–36.9	37–44.9	≥45
	40–49	≤16.9	17–24.9	25–34.9	35–41.9	≥42
	50–59	≤14.9	15–21.9	22–33.9	34–39.9	≥40
	60–69	≤12.9	13–20.9	21–32.9	33–36.9	≥37

☐ High physical fitness standard   Health fitness or criterion referenced standard

wrist by placing two fingers over the radial artery (inside of the wrist on the side of the thumb) or over the carotid artery in the neck just below the jaw next to the voice box.

Next multiply the 10-second pulse count by 6 to obtain the exercise heart rate in beats per minute. Now convert the walking time from minutes and seconds to minute units. Each minute has 60 seconds, so the seconds are divided by 60 to obtain the fraction of a minute. For instance, a walking time of 12 minutes and 15 seconds equals 12 + (15 ÷ 60), or 12.25 minutes.

To obtain the estimated VO_{2max} in ml/kg/min for the 1.0-Mile Walk Test, plug in your values in the following equation:

$$VO_{2max} = 132.853 - (.0769 \times W) - (.3877 \times A) + (6.315 \times G) - (3.2649 \times T) - (.1565 \times HR)$$

where:

- W = weight in pounds
- A = age in years
- G = gender; use 0 for women and 1 for men
- T = total time for the 1-mile walk in minutes
- HR = exercise heart rate in beats per minute at the end of the 1-mile walk

For example, a 19-year-old female who weighs 140 pounds completed the 1-mile walk in 14 minutes and 39 seconds and with an exercise heart rate of 148 beats per minute. The estimated VO_{2max} is:

- W = 140 lbs
- A = 19
- G = 0 (female gender)
- T = 14:39 = 14 + (39 ÷ 60) = 14.65 min.
- HR = 148 bpm

$$VO_{2max} = 132.853 - (.0769 \times 140) - (.3877 \times 19) + (6.315 \times 0) - (3.2649 \times 14.65) - (.1565 \times 148)$$

$$VO_{2max} = 43.7 \text{ ml/kg/min}$$

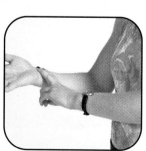

The pulse can be taken at the radial artery, at the wrist.

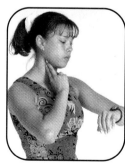

The pulse can be taken at the carotid artery, at the neck.

As with the 1.5-Mile Run Test, the fitness categories based on VO_{2max} are found in Table 2.2. Record your cardiorespiratory fitness test results on your fitness profile in Appendix A, Figure A.1.

Muscular Strength and Endurance

Many people are under the impression that muscular strength and endurance are necessary only for athletes and those who hold jobs that require heavy muscular work. Strength and endurance, however, are important components of total physical fitness and have been shown to be essential to everyone.

Adequate levels of strength enhance a person's health and well-being throughout life. Strength is crucial for top performance in daily activities such as sitting, walking, running, lifting and carrying objects, doing housework, and even enjoying recreational activities. Strength is also valuable in improving personal appearance and self-image, developing sports skills, and meeting certain emergencies in life in which strength is necessary to cope effectively.

Muscular strength also seems to be the most important health-related component of physical fitness in the older-adult population. Whereas proper cardiorespiratory endurance helps maintain a healthy heart, good strength levels do more toward independent living than any other fitness component.

More than anything else, older adults want to enjoy good health and function independently. Many, however, are confined to nursing homes because they lack sufficient strength to move about. They cannot walk very far or need to be helped in and out of beds, chairs, and tubs.

A strength-training program can have a tremendous impact on quality of life. Research has shown leg strength improvements as high as 200% in previously inactive adults over age 90.[2] As strength improves, so does the ability to move about, the capacity for independent living, and life enjoyment during the "golden years."

More specifically, good strength enhances quality of life in the following ways:

- It improves balance and restores mobility.
- It makes lifting and reaching easier.
- It decreases the risk for injuries and falls.
- It stresses the bones, preserves bone density, and decreases the risk for osteoporosis.

Perhaps one of the most significant benefits of maintaining good strength is its relationship to human **metabolism**. A major result of a strength-training program is **muscle hypertrophy**.

Muscle tissue uses energy even at rest, whereas fatty tissue uses very little energy and may be considered metabolically inert from the standpoint of caloric use. As muscle size increases, so does resting metabolic rate, or the amount of energy (expressed in milliliters of oxygen per minute or total calories per day) an individual requires during nonactive conditions to sustain proper body function. Even small increases in muscle mass may affect **resting metabolism**.

Each additional pound of muscle tissue increases resting metabolism by an estimated 35 calories per day.[3] All other factors being equal, if two individuals who weigh 150 pounds each but have different amounts of muscle mass — let's say 5 pounds — the one with the greater muscle mass will have a higher resting metabolic rate, allowing this person to eat more calories to maintain the muscle tissue.

Although muscular strength and endurance are interrelated, the two have a basic difference. **Muscular strength** is the *ability to exert*

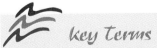

key Terms

Metabolism All energy and material transformations that take place within living cells.

Muscle hypertrophy An increase in muscle mass or size.

Resting metabolism The amount of energy a person requires while at rest to sustain proper body function.

Muscular strength Ability to exert maximum force against resistance.

maximum force against resistance. **Muscular endurance** (also called localized muscular endurance) is the *ability of the muscle to exert submaximal force repeatedly over a period of time.* Muscular endurance depends to a large extent on muscular strength and to a lesser extent on cardiorespiratory endurance. Weak muscles cannot repeat an action several times or sustain it for long. Keeping these concepts in mind, strength tests and training programs have been designed to measure and develop absolute muscular strength, muscular endurance, or a combination of the two.

Determining Strength

Muscular strength usually is determined using the **one repetition maximum** technique. This assessment gives a good measure of absolute strength, but it does require a considerable amount of time to administer. Muscular endurance commonly is established by the number of repetitions an individual can perform against a submaximal resistance or by the length of time a person can sustain a given contraction.

Muscular Endurance Test

We live in a world in which muscular strength and endurance both are required, and muscular endurance depends to a large extent on muscular strength. Accordingly, a muscular endurance test has been selected to determine the level of strength. Three exercises that help assess endurance of the upper body, lower body, and abdominal muscle groups have been selected for your muscular endurance test. To perform the test, you will need a stopwatch, a metronome, a bench or gymnasium bleacher 16¼ inches high, and a partner.

The exercises conducted for this test are the bench jump, modified dip (men) or modified push-up (women), and bent-leg curl-up. Individuals who are susceptible to low-back injury may do the abdominal crunch instead of the bent-leg curl-up test (see discussion below). All exercises should be conducted with the aid of a partner. The correct procedures for performing these exercises follow.

Bench Jump

Using a bench or gymnasium bleacher 16¼" high, attempt to jump up and down on the bench as many times as you can in 1 minute. If you cannot jump the full minute, step up and down. A repetition is counted each time both feet return to the floor.

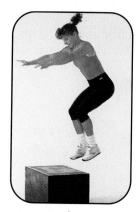

Bench jump.

Modified Dip

This upper-body exercise is done by men only. Using a bench or gymnasium bleacher, place your hands on the bench with the fingers pointing forward. Have a partner hold your feet in front of you. Bend your hips at approximately 90° (you also may use three sturdy chairs; put your hands on two chairs placed by the sides of your body and your feet on the third chair in front of you).

Next, lower your body by flexing the elbows until you reach a 90° angle at this joint, and then return to the starting position. The repetition does not count if you fail to reach 90°. Perform the repetitions to a two-step cadence (down-up), regulated with a metronome set at 56 beats per minute. Perform as many continuous repetitions as possible. If you fail to follow the metronome cadence, you no longer can count the repetitions.

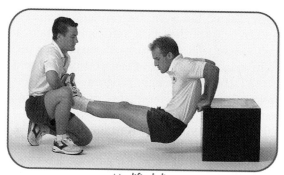

Modified dip.

Modified Push-Up

Women perform the modified push-up exercise instead of the modified dip. Lie down on the floor (face down), bend the knees (feet up in the air), and place the hands on the floor by the shoulders with the fingers pointing forward. The lower body will be supported at the knees (rather than the feet) throughout the test. The chest must touch the floor on each repetition.

Perform the repetitions to a two-step cadence (up-down) regulated with a metronome set at 56 beats per minute. Do as many continuous repetitions as possible. If you fail to follow the metronome cadence, you cannot count any more repetitions.

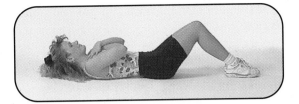

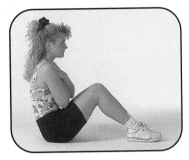

Bent-leg curl-up.

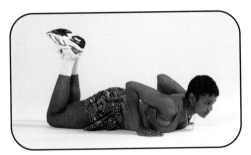

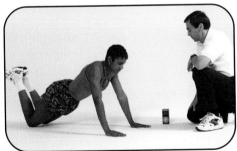

Modified push-up.

Bent-leg Curl-Up

Lie down on the floor (face up), and bend both legs at the knees at approximately 100°. The feet should be on the floor, and you must hold them in place yourself throughout the test. Cross your arms in front of the chest, each hand on the opposite shoulder.

Now raise your head off the floor, placing the chin against the chest. This is the starting and finishing position for each curl-up. *The*

back of the head may not come in contact with the floor; the hands cannot be removed from the shoulders; nor may the feet or hips be raised off the floor at any time during the test. The test is terminated if any of these four conditions occur. When you curl up, the upper body must come to an upright position before going back down. The repetitions are performed to a two-step cadence (up-down) regulated with the metronome set at 40 beats per minute.

For this exercise, you should allow a brief practice period of 5 to 10 seconds to familiarize yourself with the cadence (the *up* movement is initiated with the first beat, then you must wait for the next beat to initiate the *down* movement; one repetition is accomplished every two beats of the metronome). Count as many repetitions as you are able to perform following the proper cadence. The test also is terminated if you fail to maintain the appropriate cadence or if you accomplish 100° repetitions. Have your partner check the angle at the knees throughout the test

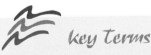

key terms

Muscular endurance The ability of a muscle to exert sub-maximal force repeatedly over a period of time.

One repetition maximum (1 RM) The maximal amount of resistance a person is able to lift in a single effort.

to make sure that you maintain the 100° angle as closely as possible.

Abdominal Crunch

This test is recommended only for individuals who are unable to perform the bent-leg curl-up test because of susceptibility to low-back injury. Exercise form must be monitored carefully during the test.

Several authors and researchers[4,5,6,7] have indicated that proper form during this test is extremely difficult to control. The participants often slide their bodies, bend their elbows, or shrug their shoulders during the test. These actions make the test easier and misrepresent performance. Biomechanical factors also limit the ability to perform this test.[8] Further, lack of spinal flexibility does not allow some individuals to move the full 3½" range of motion.[9,10] Others are unable to keep their heels on the floor during the test. The validity of this test as an effective measure of abdominal strength or abdominal endurance has been questioned in recent research.[11,12] With these caveats in mind, the procedure is as follows.

Tape a 3½" × 30" strip of cardboard onto the floor. Lie down on the floor in a supine position (face up) with the knees bent at approximately 100° and the legs slightly apart. The feet should be on the floor, and you must hold them

in place yourself throughout the test. Straighten your arms, and place them on the floor alongside the trunk with the palms down and the fingers fully extended. The fingertips of both hands should barely touch the closest edge of the cardboard. Bring your head off the floor until the chin is 1" to 2" away from your chest. Keep your head in this position during the entire test. (Do not move the head by flexing or extending the neck.) You now are ready to begin the test.

Perform the repetitions to a two-step cadence (up-down) regulated with a metronome set at 60 beats per minute. As you curl up, slide the fingers over the cardboard until the fingertips reach the far end (3½") of the board, then return to the starting position.

Allow a brief practice period of 5 to 10 seconds to familiarize yourself with the cadence. Initiate the *up* movement with the first beat and the *down* movement with the next beat. Accomplish one repetition every two beats of the metronome. Count as many repetitions as you are able to perform following the proper cadence. You may not count a repetition if the fingertips fail to reach the distant end of the cardboard.

Terminate the test if: (a) you fail to maintain the appropriate cadence, (b) bend the elbows, (c) shrug the shoulders, (d) slide the body, (e) the heels come off the floor, (f) the chin is not kept

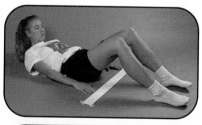

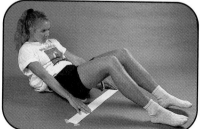

Abdominal crunch.

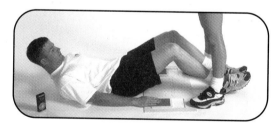

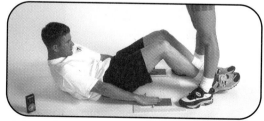

Abdominal crunch test using Crunch-Ster Curl-Up Tester.

close to the chest, (g) you accomplish 100 repetitions, or (h) you no longer can perform the test. Have your partner check the angle at the knees throughout the test to make sure the 100°-angle is maintained as closely as possible. For this test you may also use a Crunch-Ster Curl-Up Tester, available from Novel Products.*

Interpretation of Strength Test

According to the number of repetitions performed on each test item, look up the percentile rank for each exercise in the far left column of Table 2.3. Based on your percentile ranks, you can determine your muscular endurance fitness category for each exercise using the guidelines provided in Table 2.4. Next, look up the number of points assigned for each fitness category in Table 2.4. Now total the points and determine your overall strength endurance fitness category according to the ratings provided in Table 2.5.

---

*Novel Products, Inc., Figure Finder Collection, P.O. Box 408, Rockton, IL 61072-0408; 1-800-323-5143.

Table 2.4 Fitness Categories Based on Percentile Ranks

Percentile Rank	Fitness Category	Points
≥90	Excellent	5
70–80	Good	4
50–60	Average	3
30–40	Fair	2
≤20	Poor	1

Table 2.5 Muscular Strength/Endurance Fitness Categories by Total Points

Total Points	Strength Endurance Category
≥13	Excellent
10–12	Good
7–9	Average
4–6	Fair
≤3	Poor

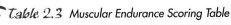

Table 2.3 Muscular Endurance Scoring Table

	MEN							WOMEN						
Percentile Rank	Lat Pull-Down	Leg Extension	Bench Press	Bent-Leg Curl-Up	Abdominal Crunch	Leg Curl	Arm Curl	Lat Pull-Down	Leg Extension	Bench Press	Bent-Leg Curl-Up	Abdominal Crunch	Leg Curl	Arm Curl
99	30	25	26	100	100	24	25	30	25	27	100	100	20	25
95	25	20	21	81	100	20	21	25	20	21	100	100	17	21
90	19	19	19	65	100	19	19	21	18	20	97	69	12	20
80	16	15	16	51	66	15	15	16	13	16	77	49	10	16
70	13	14	13	44	45	13	12	13	11	13	57	37	9	14
60	11	13	11	31	38	11	10	11	10	11	45	34	7	12
50	10	12	10	28	33	10	9	10	9	10	37	31	6	10
40	9	10	7	25	29	8	8	9	8	5	28	27	5	8
30	7	9	5	22	26	6	7	7	7	3	22	24	4	7
20	6	7	3	17	22	4	5	6	5	1	17	21	3	6
10	4	5	1	10	18	3	3	3	3	0	9	15	1	3
5	3	3	0	3	16	1	2	2	1	0	4	0	0	2

■ High physical fitness standard   ☐ Health fitness standard

Muscular Flexibility

Muscular flexibility is highly specific and varies from one joint to the other (hip, trunk, shoulder), as well as from one individual to the next. Muscular flexibility relates primarily to genetic factors and the index of physical activity. Beyond that, factors such as joint structure, ligaments, tendons, muscles, skin, tissue injury, adipose (fat) tissue, body temperature, age, and gender influence the range of motion about a joint.

On the average, women are more flexible than men and seem to retain this advantage throughout life. Aging decreases the extensibility of soft tissue, decreasing flexibility in both genders. The most significant contributors to loss of flexibility, however, are sedentary living and lack of physical activity.

Developing and maintaining some level of flexibility are important factors in all health enhancement programs, and even more so as we age. Sportsmedicine specialists say that many muscular/skeletal problems and injuries, especially in adults, are related to a lack of flexibility.

Most experts agree that participating in a regular flexibility program has the following benefits.

- It helps to maintain good joint mobility.
- It increases resistance to muscle injury and soreness.
- It prevents low-back and other spinal column problems.
- It improves and maintains good postural alignment.
- It enhances proper and graceful body movement.
- It improves personal appearance and self-image.
- It facilitates the development of motor skills throughout life.

Flexibility exercises also have been used successfully in treating patients with dysmenorrhea (painful menstruation) and general neuromuscular tension. Stretching exercises, in conjunction with calisthenics, are helpful in warm-up routines to prepare for more vigorous aerobic or strength-training exercises, as well as subsequent cool-down routines to help the body return to the normal resting state.

Assessment of Flexibility

Two flexibility tests are used to determine one's flexibility profile. These are the Modified Sit-and-Reach Test and the Total Body Rotation Test.

Modified Sit-and-Reach Test

To perform this test, you will need the Acuflex I* sit-and-reach flexibility tester, or you may simply place a yardstick on top of a box approximately 12" high. The procedure to administer this test is as follows:

1. Be sure to warm up properly before the first trial.

2. Remove your shoes for the test. Sit on the floor with your hips, back, and head against a wall, legs fully extended, and the bottom of the feet against the Acuflex I or the sit-and-reach box.

3. Place your hands one on top of the other, and reach forward as far as possible without letting the hips, back, or head come off the wall. Another person then should slide the

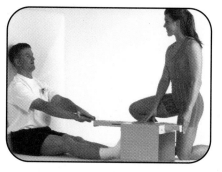

Starting position for Modified Sit-and-Reach Test.

*The Acuflex I and II flexibility testers for the Modified Sit-and-Reach and the Total Body Rotation tests can be obtained from Novel Products, Inc., Figure Finder Collection, P.O. Box 408, Rockton, IL 61072-0408; 1-800-323-5143.

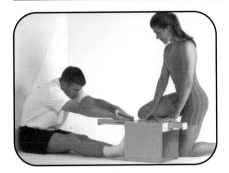

Modified Sit-and-Reach Test.

least 2 seconds. Be sure to keep the back of your knees against the floor throughout the test. Record the final number of inches reached to the nearest half inch.

You are allowed two trials, and an average of the two scores is used as the final test score. The percentile ranks and fitness categories for this test are given in Tables 2.6 and 2.4, respectively.

Total Body Rotation Test

An Acuflex II total body rotation flexibility tester or a measuring scale with a sliding panel is needed to administer this test. The Acuflex II or scale is placed on the wall at shoulder

reach indicator on the Acuflex I (or yardstick) along the top of the box until the end of the indicator touches the tips of your fingers. The indicator then must be held firmly in place throughout the rest of the test.

4. The head and back now can come off the wall, and you may reach forward gradually three times, the third time stretching forward as far as possible on the indicator (or yardstick), holding the final position for at

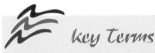

key Terms

Muscular flexibility Ability of a joint to move freely through its full range of motion.

Table 2.6 *Modified Sit-and-Reach Scoring Table*

	MEN						WOMEN				
Percentile Rank	Age Category				Fitness Category	Percentile Rank	Age Category				Fitness Category
	<18	19–35	36–49	>50			<18	19–35	36–49	>50	
99	20.8	20.1	18.9	16.2		99	22.6	21.0	19.8	17.2	
95	19.6	18.9	18.2	15.8	Excellent	95	19.5	19.3	19.2	15.7	Excellent
90	18.2	17.2	16.1	15.0		90	18.7	17.9	17.4	15.0	
80	17.8	17.0	14.6	13.3	Good	80	17.8	16.7	16.2	14.2	Good
70	16.0	15.8	13.9	12.3		70	16.5	16.2	15.2	13.6	
60	15.2	15.0	13.4	11.5	Average	60	16.0	15.8	14.5	12.3	Average
50	14.5	14.4	12.6	10.2		50	15.2	14.8	13.5	11.1	
40	14.0	13.5	11.6	9.7	Fair	40	14.5	14.5	12.8	10.1	Fair
30	13.4	13.0	10.8	9.3		30	13.7	13.7	12.2	9.2	
20	11.8	11.6	9.9	8.8		20	12.6	12.6	11.0	8.3	
10	9.5	9.2	8.3	7.8	Poor	10	11.4	10.1	9.7	7.5	Poor
05	8.4	7.9	7.0	7.2		05	9.4	8.1	8.5	3.7	
01	7.2	7.0	5.1	4.0		01	6.5	2.6	2.0	1.5	

High physical fitness standard

Health fitness or criterion referenced standard

From *Lifetime Physical Fitness & Wellness: A Personalized Program*, by W. W. K. Hoeger (Englewood, CO: Morton Publishing Company, 1998).

height and should be adjustable to accommodate individual differences in height.

If an Acuflex II is not available, you can build your own scale. Glue or tape a measuring tape above the sliding panel and another below it, centered at the 15" mark. Each tape should be at least 30" long. Draw a line on the floor, centered with the 15" mark. Use the following procedure:

1. Warm up properly before beginning this test.

2. To start, stand sideways, an arm's length away from the wall, with the feet straight ahead, slightly separated, and the toes right up to the corresponding line drawn on the floor. Hold out the arm opposite the wall horizontally from the body, making a fist. The Acuflex II, measuring scale, or tapes should be shoulder height at this time.

3. Now rotate the body, the extended arm going backward (always maintaining a horizontal plane) and making contact with the panel, gradually sliding it forward as far as possible. If no panel is available, slide the fist alongside the tapes as far as possible. Hold the final position at least 2 seconds.

Position the hand with the little finger-side forward during the entire sliding movement. The proper hand position is crucial. Some people attempt to open the hand or push with extended fingers or slide the panel with the knuckles — none of which is acceptable. During the test the knees can be bent slightly, but the feet cannot be moved; they always must point straight forward. The body must be kept as straight (vertical) as possible.

4. Conduct the test on either the right or the left side of the body. Two trials are allowed on the selected side. The farthest point reached, measured to the nearest half inch and held for at least 2 seconds, is recorded. The average of the two trials is the final test score. Referring to Tables 2.7 and 2.4, you can determine the respective percentile rank and flexibility fitness classification for this test.

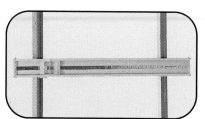

Acuflex II measuring device for Total Body Rotation test.

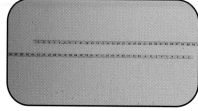

Use of measuring tapes for Total Body Rotation test.

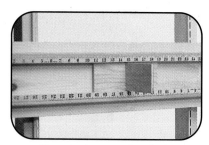

Homemade measuring device for Total Body Rotation test.

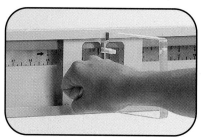

Proper hand position for Total Body Rotation Test.

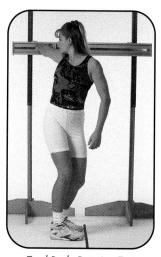

Total Body Rotation Test.

Interpretation of Flexibility Tests

The fitness classification for each flexibility test is obtained based on your percentile rank for each test, using the guidelines provided in Table 2.4. You also should look up the number of points assigned for each fitness category in this table. Your overall flexibility fitness classification is obtained by totaling these points and using the ratings provided in Table 2.8.

Table 2.7 Total Body Rotation: Scoring Table

	Percentile Rank	Left Rotation				Right Rotation				Fitness Category
		Age Category				Age Category				
		<18	19–35	36–49	>50	<18	19–35	36–49	>50	
Men	99	29.1	28.0	26.6	21.0	28.2	27.8	25.2	22.2	
	95	26.6	24.8	24.5	20.0	25.5	25.6	23.8	20.7	Excellent
	90	25.0	23.6	23.0	17.7	24.3	24.1	22.5	19.3	
	80	22.0	22.0	21.2	15.5	22.7	22.3	21.0	16.3	Good
	70	20.9	20.3	20.4	14.7	21.3	20.7	18.7	15.7	
	60	19.9	19.3	18.7	13.9	19.8	19.0	17.3	14.7	Average
	50	18.6	18.0	16.7	12.7	19.0	17.2	16.3	12.3	
	40	17.0	16.8	15.3	11.7	17.3	16.3	14.7	11.5	Fair
	30	14.9	15.0	14.8	10.3	15.1	15.0	13.3	10.7	
	20	13.8	13.3	13.7	9.5	12.9	13.3	11.2	8.7	
	10	10.8	10.5	10.8	4.3	10.8	11.3	8.0	2.7	Poor
	05	8.5	8.9	8.8	0.3	8.1	8.3	5.5	0.3	
	01	3.4	1.7	5.1	0.0	6.6	2.9	2.0	0.0	
Women	99	29.3	28.6	27.1	23.0	29.6	29.4	27.1	21.7	
	95	26.8	24.8	25.3	21.4	27.6	25.3	25.9	19.7	Excellent
	90	25.5	23.0	23.4	20.5	25.8	23.0	21.3	19.0	
	80	23.8	21.5	20.2	19.1	23.7	20.8	19.6	17.9	Good
	70	21.8	20.5	18.6	17.3	22.0	19.3	17.3	16.8	
	60	20.5	19.3	17.7	16.0	20.8	18.0	16.5	15.6	Average
	50	19.5	18.0	16.4	14.8	19.5	17.3	14.6	14.0	
	40	18.5	17.2	14.8	13.7	18.3	16.0	13.1	12.8	Fair
	30	17.1	15.7	13.6	10.0	16.3	15.2	11.7	8.5	
	20	16.0	15.2	11.6	6.3	14.5	14.0	9.8	3.9	
	10	12.8	13.6	8.5	3.0	12.4	11.1	6.1	2.2	Poor
	05	11.1	7.3	6.8	0.7	10.2	8.8	4.0	1.1	
	01	8.9	5.3	4.3	0.0	8.9	3.2	2.8	0.0	

High physical fitness standard
Health fitness or criterion referenced standard

From *Lifetime Physical Fitness & Wellness: A Personalized Program*, by W. W. K. Hoeger (Englewood, CO: Morton Publishing Company, 1998).

Table 2.8 Muscular Flexibility Fitness Categories by Total Points

Total Points	Flexibility Category
≥9	Excellent
7–8	Good
5–6	Average
3–4	Fair
≤3	Poor

Body Composition

Currently, starting at age 25, the average man and woman in the United States gains 1 pound of weight per year. Thus, by age 65, the average American will have gained 40 pounds of weight. Because of the typical reduction in physical activity in our society, however, each year the average person also loses a half pound of lean tissue. Therefore, this span of 40 years has resulted in an actual fat gain of 60 pounds accompanied by a 20-pound loss of lean body mass[13] (see Figure 2.2). These changes cannot be detected unless body composition is assessed periodically.

Body composition refers to *the fat and nonfat components of the human body.* The fat component of the body usually is called fat mass or **percent body fat.** *The nonfat component of the body* is termed **lean body mass.**

Total fat in the human body is classified into two types: essential fat and storage fat. **Essential fat** *is the body fat needed for normal physiological functions.* Essential fat constitutes about 3% of the total weight in men and 12% in women. The percentage is higher in women because it includes gender-specific fat, such as that found in the breast tissue, the uterus, and other gender-related fat deposits. Without it, human health deteriorates. **Storage fat,** *the body fat stored in adipose tissue,* is found mostly beneath the skin (subcutaneous fat) and around major organs in the body.

Obesity is a health hazard of epidemic proportions in most developed countries around the world. Obesity by itself has been associated with

several serious health problems and accounts for 15% to 20% of the annual U.S. mortality rate. It is one of the 5 major risks for coronary heart disease. It is also a risk factor for other diseases of the cardiovascular system, including hypertension, congestive heart failure, elevated blood lipids, atherosclerosis, strokes, thromboembolitic disease, varicose veins, and intermittent claudication.

Underweight people, too, have health problems and a higher mortality rate. Although the social pressure to be thin has waned slightly in recent years, pressure to attain model-like thinness is still with us and contributes to the gradual increase in eating disorders (anorexia nervosa and bulimia nervosa, discussed in Chapter 5). Extreme weight loss can spawn medical conditions such as heart damage, gastrointestinal problems, shrinkage of internal organs, immune system abnormalities, disorders of the reproductive system, loss of muscle tissue, damage to the nervous system, and even death.

For many years people relied on height/weight charts to determine **recommended body weight,** but we now know that these tables are highly inaccurate for many people. The standard height/weight tables, first published in 1912,

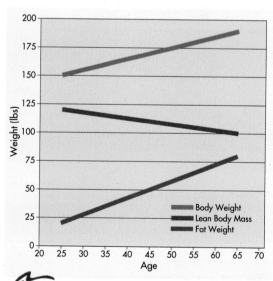

Figure 2.2. *Typical body composition changes for adults in United States.*

were based on average weights (including shoes and clothing) for men and women who obtained life insurance policies between 1888 and 1905. The recommended weight on height/weight tables is obtained according to gender, height, and frame size. As no scientific guidelines are given to determine frame size, most people choose their frame size based on the column where the weight comes closest to their own.

The proper way to determine recommended weight is to find out what percent of total body weight is fat and what amount is lean tissue (body composition). Once the fat percentage is known, recommended weight can be calculated from recommended body fat.

Obesity is related to an excess of body fat. If body weight is the only criterion, an individual easily can be considered overweight according to height/weight charts, yet not be genuinely obese. Football players, body builders, weight lifters, and other athletes with large muscle size are typical examples. Some athletes who appear to be 20 or 30 pounds overweight really have little body fat.

At the other end of the spectrum, some people who weigh very little and are viewed by many as "skinny" or underweight actually can be classified as obese because of their high body fat content. People who weigh as little as 100 pounds but are more than 30% fat (about a third of their total body weight) are not uncommon. These people are often sedentary or dieting constantly. Physical inactivity and constant negative caloric balance both lead to a loss in lean body mass (see Chapter 6). Body weight alone clearly does not always tell the true story.

Assessment of Body Composition

Skinfold Thickness

Assessment of body composition is done most frequently using skinfold thickness. This technique is based on the principle that approximately half of the body's fatty tissue is directly beneath the skin. Valid and reliable estimates of this tissue give a good indication of percent body fat.

The skinfold thickness test is performed with the aid of pressure calipers. To reflect the total percentage of fat, several sites must be measured: triceps, suprailium, and thigh skinfolds for women; and chest, abdomen, and thigh for men. All measurements should be taken on the right side of the body with the person standing. The correct anatomical landmarks for skinfolds are as follows and as shown in Figure 2.3.

Chest: a diagonal fold halfway between the shoulder crease and the nipple

Abdomen: a vertical fold about 1" to the right of the umbilicus

Triceps: a vertical fold on the back of the upper arm, halfway between the shoulder and the arm

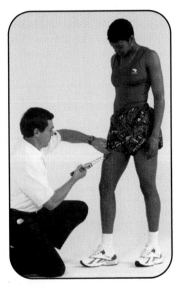

Skinfold thickness technique for assessment of body composition.

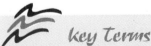

key Terms

Body composition The fat and nonfat components of the human body.

Percent body fat (fat mass) Fat component of the body.

Lean body mass Nonfat component of the body.

Essential fat Body fat needed for normal physiological functions.

Storage fat Body fat stored in adipose tissue.

Recommended body weight The weight at which there appears to be no harm to human health.

Thigh: a vertical fold on the front of the thigh, midway between the knee and the hip

Suprailium: a diagonal fold above the crest of the ilium (on the side of the hip)

Each site is measured by grasping a double thickness of skin firmly with the thumb and forefinger, pulling the fold slightly away from the muscle tissue. Hold the calipers perpendicular to the fold, and take the measurements ½" below the finger hold. Measure each site three times, and read the values to the nearest .1 to .5 mm. Record the average of the two closest readings as the final value. Take the readings without delay to avoid excessive compression of the skinfold. Releasing and refolding the skinfold is required between readings. Be sure to wear shorts, a loose fitting t-shirt (no leotards), and do not use lotion on your skin the day when skinfolds are to be taken.

After determining the average value for each site, percent fat can be obtained by adding together all three skinfold measurements and looking up the respective values in Table 2.9 for women, Table 2.10 for men under age 40, and Table 2.11 for men over 40. Then compute your recommended body weight using the range given in Table 2.10 and the computation form in Figure 2.4.

The recommended percent body fat values given in Table 2.12 include essential fat and storage fat, discussed previously. For example, the recommended body fat range for women under age 30 is 17% to 25%. This indicates that only 5% to 13% of the total recommended fat is storage fat, and the other 12% is essential fat. The recommended range has been selected based on research indicating that some storage fat is required for optimal health and greater longevity.

The recommended body fat range selected in this book incorporates the recommendations

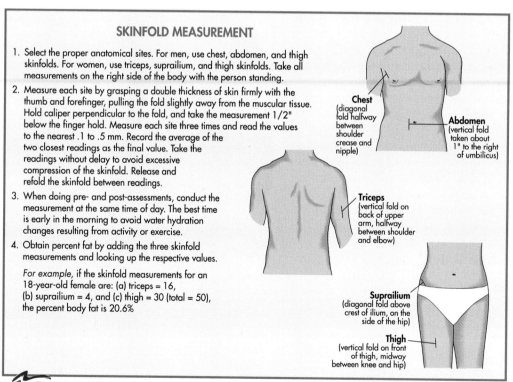

SKINFOLD MEASUREMENT

1. Select the proper anatomical sites. For men, use chest, abdomen, and thigh skinfolds. For women, use triceps, suprailium, and thigh skinfolds. Take all measurements on the right side of the body with the person standing.

2. Measure each site by grasping a double thickness of skin firmly with the thumb and forefinger, pulling the fold slightly away from the muscular tissue. Hold caliper perpendicular to the fold, and take the measurement 1/2" below the finger hold. Measure each site three times and read the values to the nearest .1 to .5 mm. Record the average of the two closest readings as the final value. Take the readings without delay to avoid excessive compression of the skinfold. Release and refold the skinfold between readings.

3. When doing pre- and post-assessments, conduct the measurement at the same time of day. The best time is early in the morning to avoid water hydration changes resulting from activity or exercise.

4. Obtain percent fat by adding the three skinfold measurements and looking up the respective values.

For example, if the skinfold measurements for an 18-year-old female are: (a) triceps = 16, (b) suprailium = 4, and (c) thigh = 30 (total = 50), the percent body fat is 20.6%

Chest
(diagonal fold halfway between shoulder crease and nipple)

Abdomen
(vertical fold taken about 1" to the right of umbilicus)

Triceps
(vertical fold on back of upper arm, halfway between shoulder and elbow)

Suprailium
(diagonal fold above crest of ilium, on the side of the hip)

Thigh
(vertical fold on front of thigh, midway between knee and hip)

Figure 2.3. Anatomical landmarks for skinfolds.

Table 2.9 Percent Fat Estimates for Women Calculated from Triceps, Suprailium, and Thigh Skinfold Thickness

Sum of 3 Skinfolds	Under 22	23 to 27	28 to 32	33 to 37	38 to 42	43 to 47	48 to 52	53 to 57	Over 58
23– 25	9.7	9.9	10.2	10.4	10.7	10.9	11.2	11.4	11.7
26– 28	11.0	11.2	11.5	11.7	12.0	12.3	12.5	12.7	13.0
29– 31	12.3	12.5	12.8	13.0	13.3	13.5	13.8	14.0	14.3
32– 34	13.6	13.8	14.0	14.3	14.5	14.8	15.0	15.3	15.5
35– 37	14.8	15.0	15.3	15.5	15.8	16.0	16.3	16.5	16.8
38– 40	16.0	16.3	16.5	16.7	17.0	17.2	17.5	17.7	18.0
41– 43	17.2	17.4	17.7	17.9	18.2	18.4	18.7	18.9	19.2
44– 46	18.3	18.6	18.8	19.1	19.3	19.6	19.8	20.1	20.3
47– 49	19.5	19.7	20.0	20.2	20.5	20.7	21.0	21.2	21.5
50– 52	20.6	20.8	21.1	21.3	21.6	21.8	22.1	22.3	22.6
53– 55	21.7	21.9	22.1	22.4	22.6	22.9	23.1	23.4	23.6
56– 58	22.7	23.0	23.2	23.4	23.7	23.9	24.2	24.4	24.7
59– 61	23.7	24.0	24.2	24.5	24.7	25.0	25.2	25.5	25.7
62– 64	24.7	25.0	25.2	25.5	25.7	26.0	26.2	26.4	26.7
65– 67	25.7	25.9	26.2	26.4	26.7	26.9	27.2	27.4	27.7
68– 70	26.6	26.9	27.1	27.4	27.6	27.9	28.1	28.4	28.6
71– 73	27.5	27.8	28.0	28.3	28.5	28.8	29.0	29.3	29.5
74– 76	28.4	28.7	28.9	29.2	29.4	29.7	29.9	30.2	30.4
77– 79	29.3	29.5	29.8	30.0	30.3	30.5	30.8	31.0	31.3
80– 82	30.1	30.4	30.6	30.9	31.1	31.4	31.6	31.9	32.1
83– 85	30.9	31.2	31.4	31.7	31.9	32.2	32.4	32.7	32.9
86– 88	31.7	32.0	32.2	32.5	32.7	32.9	33.2	33.4	33.7
89– 91	32.5	32.7	33.0	33.2	33.5	33.7	33.9	34.2	34.4
92– 94	33.2	33.4	33.7	33.9	34.2	34.4	34.7	34.9	35.2
95– 97	33.9	34.1	34.4	34.6	34.9	35.1	35.4	35.6	35.9
98–100	34.6	34.8	35.1	35.3	35.5	35.8	36.0	36.3	36.5
101–103	35.2	35.4	35.7	35.9	36.2	36.4	36.7	36.9	37.2
104–106	35.8	36.1	36.3	36.6	36.8	37.1	37.3	37.5	37.8
107–109	36.4	36.7	36.9	37.1	37.4	37.6	37.9	38.1	38.4
110–112	37.0	37.2	37.5	37.7	38.0	38.2	38.5	38.7	38.9
113–115	37.5	37.8	38.0	38.2	38.5	38.7	39.0	39.2	39.5
116–118	38.0	38.3	38.5	38.8	39.0	39.3	39.5	39.7	40.0
119–121	38.5	38.7	39.0	39.2	39.5	39.7	40.0	40.2	40.5
122–124	39.0	39.2	39.4	39.7	39.9	40.2	40.4	40.7	40.9
125–127	39.4	39.6	39.9	40.1	40.4	40.6	40.9	41.1	41.4
128–130	39.8	40.0	40.3	40.5	40.8	41.0	41.3	41.5	41.8

Body density is calculated based on the generalized equation for predicting body density of women developed by A. S. Jackson, M. L. Pollock, and A. Ward, reported in *Medicine and Science in Sports and Exercise*, 12 (1980), 175–182. Percent body fat is determined from the calculated body density using the Siri formula.

Table 2.10 Percent Fat Estimates for Men Under Age 40 Calculated from Chest, Abdomen, and Thigh Skinfold Thickness

Sum of 3 Skinfolds	Age							
	Under 19	20 to 22	23 to 25	26 to 28	29 to 31	32 to 34	35 to 37	38 to 40
8– 10	.9	1.3	1.6	2.0	2.3	2.7	3.0	3.3
11– 13	1.9	2.3	2.6	3.0	3.3	3.7	4.0	4.3
14– 16	2.9	3.3	3.6	3.9	4.3	4.6	5.0	5.3
17– 19	3.9	4.2	4.6	4.9	5.3	5.6	6.0	6.3
20– 22	4.8	5.2	5.5	5.9	6.2	6.6	6.9	7.3
23– 25	5.8	6.2	6.5	6.8	7.2	7.5	7.9	8.2
26– 28	6.8	7.1	7.5	7.8	8.1	8.5	8.8	9.2
29– 31	7.7	8.0	8.4	8.7	9.1	9.4	9.8	10.1
32– 34	8.6	9.0	9.3	9.7	10.0	10.4	10.7	11.1
35– 37	9.5	9.9	10.2	10.6	10.9	11.3	11.6	12.0
38– 40	10.5	10.8	11.2	11.5	11.8	12.2	12.5	12.9
41– 43	11.4	11.7	12.1	12.4	12.7	13.1	13.4	13.8
44– 46	12.2	12.6	12.9	13.3	13.6	14.0	14.3	14.7
47– 49	13.1	13.5	13.8	14.2	14.5	14.9	15.2	15.5
50– 52	14.0	14.3	14.7	15.0	15.4	15.7	16.1	16.4
53– 55	14.8	15.2	15.5	15.9	16.2	16.6	16.9	17.3
56– 58	15.7	16.0	16.4	16.7	17.1	17.4	17.8	18.1
59– 61	16.5	16.9	17.2	17.6	17.9	18.3	18.6	19.0
62– 64	17.4	17.7	18.1	18.4	18.8	19.1	19.4	19.8
65– 67	18.2	18.5	18.9	19.2	19.6	19.9	20.3	20.6
68– 70	19.0	19.3	19.7	20.0	20.4	20.7	21.1	21.4
71– 73	19.8	20.1	20.5	20.8	21.2	21.5	21.9	22.2
74– 76	20.6	20.9	21.3	21.6	22.0	22.2	22.7	23.0
77– 79	21.4	21.7	22.1	22.4	22.8	23.1	23.4	23.8
80– 82	22.1	22.5	22.8	23.2	23.5	23.9	24.2	24.6
83– 85	22.9	23.2	23.6	23.9	24.3	24.6	25.0	25.3
86– 88	23.6	24.0	24.3	24.7	25.0	25.4	25.7	26.1
89– 91	24.4	24.7	25.1	25.4	25.8	26.1	26.5	26.8
92– 94	25.1	25.5	25.8	26.2	26.5	26.9	27.2	27.5
95– 97	25.8	26.2	26.5	26.9	27.2	27.6	27.9	28.3
98–100	26.6	26.9	27.3	27.6	27.9	28.3	28.6	29.0
101–103	27.3	27.6	28.0	28.3	28.6	29.0	29.3	29.7
104–106	27.9	28.3	28.6	29.0	29.3	29.7	30.0	30.4
107–109	28.6	29.0	29.3	29.7	30.0	30.4	30.7	31.1
110–112	29.3	29.6	30.0	30.3	30.7	31.0	31.4	31.7
113–115	30.0	30.3	30.7	31.0	31.3	31.7	32.0	32.4
116–118	30.6	31.0	31.3	31.6	32.0	32.3	32.7	33.0
119–121	31.3	31.6	32.0	32.3	32.6	33.0	33.3	33.7
122–124	31.9	32.2	32.6	32.9	33.3	33.6	34.0	34.3
125–127	32.5	32.9	33.2	33.5	33.9	34.2	34.6	34.9
128–130	33.1	33.5	33.8	34.2	34.5	34.9	35.2	35.5

Body density is calculated based on the generalized equation for predicting body density of men developed by A. S. Jackson and M. L. Pollock, *British Journal of Nutrition*, 40 (1978), 497–504. Percent body fat is determined from the calculated body density using the Siri formula.

Table 2.11 Percent Fat Estimates for Men Over Age 40 Calculated from Chest, Abdomen, and Thigh Skinfold Thickness

Sum of 3 Skinfolds	Age							
	41 to 43	44 to 46	47 to 49	50 to 52	53 to 55	56 to 58	59 to 61	Over 62
8– 10	3.7	4.0	4.4	4.7	5.1	5.4	5.8	6.1
11– 13	4.7	5.0	5.4	5.7	6.1	6.4	6.8	7.1
14– 16	5.7	6.0	6.4	6.7	7.1	7.4	7.8	8.1
17– 19	6.7	7.0	7.4	7.7	8.1	8.4	8.7	9.1
20– 22	7.6	8.0	8.3	8.7	9.0	9.4	9.7	10.1
23– 25	8.6	8.9	9.3	9.6	10.0	10.3	10.7	11.0
26– 28	9.5	9.9	10.2	10.6	10.9	11.3	11.6	12.0
29– 31	10.5	10.8	11.2	11.5	11.9	12.2	12.6	12.9
32– 34	11.4	11.8	12.1	12.4	12.8	13.1	13.5	13.8
35– 37	12.3	12.7	13.0	13.4	13.7	14.1	14.4	14.8
38– 40	13.2	13.6	13.9	14.3	14.6	15.0	15.3	15.7
41– 43	14.1	14.5	14.8	15.2	15.5	15.9	16.2	16.6
44– 46	15.0	15.4	15.7	16.1	16.4	16.8	17.1	17.5
47– 49	15.9	16.2	16.6	16.9	17.3	17.6	18.0	18.3
50– 52	16.8	17.1	17.5	17.8	18.2	18.5	18.8	19.2
53– 55	17.6	18.0	18.3	18.7	19.0	19.4	19.7	20.1
56– 58	18.5	18.8	19.2	19.5	19.9	20.2	20.6	20.9
59– 61	19.3	19.7	20.0	20.4	20.7	21.0	21.4	21.7
62– 64	20.1	20.5	20.8	21.2	21.5	21.9	22.2	22.6
65– 67	21.0	21.3	21.7	22.0	22.4	22.7	23.0	23.4
68– 70	21.8	22.1	22.5	22.8	23.2	23.5	23.9	24.2
71– 73	22.6	22.9	23.3	23.6	24.0	24.3	24.7	25.0
74– 76	23.4	23.7	24.1	24.4	24.8	25.1	25.4	25.8
77– 79	24.1	24.5	24.8	25.2	25.5	25.9	26.2	26.6
80– 82	24.9	25.3	25.6	26.0	26.3	26.6	27.0	27.3
83– 85	25.7	26.0	26.4	26.7	27.1	27.4	27.8	28.1
86– 88	26.4	26.8	27.1	27.5	27.8	28.2	28.5	28.9
89– 91	27.2	27.5	27.9	28.2	28.6	28.9	29.2	29.6
92– 94	27.9	28.2	28.6	28.9	29.3	29.6	30.0	30.3
95– 97	28.6	29.0	29.3	29.7	30.0	30.4	30.7	31.1
98–100	29.3	29.7	30.0	30.4	30.7	31.1	31.4	31.8
101–103	30.0	30.4	30.7	31.1	31.4	31.8	32.1	32.5
104–106	30.7	31.1	31.4	31.8	32.1	32.5	32.8	33.2
107–109	31.4	31.8	32.1	32.4	32.8	33.1	33.5	33.8
110–112	32.1	32.4	32.8	33.1	33.5	33.8	34.2	34.5
113–115	32.7	33.1	33.4	33.8	34.1	34.5	34.8	35.2
116–118	33.4	33.7	34.1	34.4	34.8	35.1	35.5	35.8
119–121	34.0	34.4	34.7	35.1	35.4	35.8	36.1	36.5
122–124	34.7	35.0	35.4	35.7	36.1	36.4	36.7	37.1
125–127	35.3	35.6	36.0	36.3	36.7	37.0	37.4	37.7
128–130	35.9	36.2	36.6	36.9	37.3	37.6	38.0	38.5

Body density is calculated based on the generalized equation for predicting body density of men developed by A. S. Jackson and M. L. Pollock, *British Journal of Nutrition*, 40 (1978), 497–504. Percent body fat is determined from the calculated body density using the Siri formula.

of most health and fitness experts throughout the United States. If you desire to have just one target weight, you may select your body weight according to your personal preference, as long as it falls within the recommended range. The lower end of the range constitutes the physical fitness standard; the high end represents the health fitness standard.

Body Mass Index

Another technique scientists use to determine thinness and excessive fatness is the **Body Mass Index (BMI)**, *a table incorporating height and weight to estimate critical fat values at which the risk for disease increases.* BMI is calculated by dividing the weight in kilograms by the square of the height in meters or multiplying your weight in pounds by 705 and dividing this figure by the square of the height in inches. For

Table 2.12 *Recommended Body Composition According to Percent Body Fat*

Age	Males	Females
≤29	12–20%	17–25%
30–49	13–21%	18–26%
≥50	14–22%	19–27%

    High physical fitness standard
    Health fitness or criterion referenced standard

example, the BMI for an individual who weighs 172 pounds (78 kg) and is 67 inches (1.7 mts) tall would be 27 [78 ÷ (1.7)^2] or [172 × 705 ÷ (67)^2]. You can compute and record your own BMI using the form provided in Figure 2.5. You also can obtain your BMI for selected weights and heights by looking it up in Table 2.13.

Recommended Body Weight Determination

A. Current Body Weight (BW): _____ lbs

B. Current Percent Fat (%F): _____ %

C. Fat Weight (FW) = BW × %F* = _____ × _____ = _____ lbs

D. Lean Body Mass (LBM) = BW − FW = _____ − _____ = _____ lbs

E. Age: _____

F. Recommended Fat Percent (RFP) Range (see Table 2.12):

Low End of Recommended Fat Percent Range (LRFP): _____ % (Physical Fitness Standard)

High End of Recommended Fat Percent Range (HRFP): _____ % (Health Fitness Standard)

G. Recommended Body Weight Range:

Low End of Recommended Body Weight Range (LRBW) = LBM ÷ (1.0 − LRFP*)

LRBW = _____ ÷ (1.0 − _____) = _____ lbs

High End of Recommended Body Weight Range (HRBW) = LBM ÷ (1.0 − HRFP*)

HRBW = _____ ÷ (1.0 − _____) = _____ lbs

Recommended Body Weight Range: _____ to _____ lbs

*Express percentages in decimal form (e.g., 25% = .25)

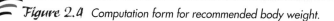

Figure 2.4 *Computation form for recommended body weight.*

According to the BMI, the lowest risk for chronic disease is in the 22 to 25 range (see Table 2.14). Individuals are classified as overweight between 25 and 30. BMIs above 30 are defined as obesity and below 20 as underweight.

BMI is a useful tool to screen the general population, but, similar to height/weight charts, it fails to differentiate fat from lean body mass or where most of the fat is located (see waist-to-hip ratio, below). Using BMI, strength-trained individuals and athletes with a large amount of muscle mass (such as body builders and football players) easily can fall in the moderate or even high-risk categories. Therefore, body composition and waist-to-hip ratios are better procedures to determine health risk and recommended body weight.

Body Mass Index*

Date: _____   _____

Weight (lbs):   _____   _____

Height (inches):   _____   _____

BMI:*   _____   _____

Disease risk: _____   _____

*BMI = [Weight in lbs. $\times$ 705 $\div$ (Height in inches)^2]
    *BMI = [Weight in kgs $\div$ (Height in meters)^2]

Waist-to-Hip Ratio

Date: _____   _____

Waist (inches):   _____   _____

Hip (inches):   _____   _____

Ratio (waist 3 hip): _____   _____

Disease risk: _____   _____

Figure 2.5. Computation form: Body Mass Index (BMI) and waist-to-hip ratio.

Waist-to-Hip Ratio

Scientific evidence suggests that the way people store fat may affect the risk for disease. Some individuals tend to store high amounts of fat in the abdominal area, and others store it primarily around the hips and thighs (gluteal femoral fat).

Data indicate that obese individuals with high abdominal fat are clearly at higher risk for coronary heart disease, congestive heart failure, hypertension, strokes, and diabetes than are obese people with similar amounts of total body fat that is stored primarily in the hips and thighs. Evidence also indicates that among individuals with high abdominal fat, those whose fat deposits are around internal organs (visceral fat) are at even greater risk for disease than those whose abdominal fat is primarily beneath the skin (subcutaneous fat).

Because of the increased risk for disease in individuals who tend to store large amounts of fat in the abdominal area, as opposed to the hips and thighs, the waist-to-hip ratio test was designed by a panel of scientists appointed by the National Academy of Sciences and the Dietary Guidelines Advisory Council for the U.S. Department of Agriculture and U.S. Department of Health and Human Services. The panel recommends that men need to lose weight if the waist-to-hip ratio is 1.0 or higher. Women need to lose weight if the ratio is .85 or higher. The waist-to-hip ratio for a man with a 40" waist and a 38" hip is 1.05 (40 $\div$ 38). That ratio may indicate increased risk for disease. Using a simple tape measure, you may determine your own waist-to-hip ratio. Record the results in Figure 2.5.

key terms

Body Mass Index (BMI) An index that incorporates height and weight to estimate critical fat values at which risk for disease increases.

Table 2.13   Body Mass Index

Height \ Weight	110	115	120	125	130	135	140	145	150	155	160	165	170	175	180	185	190	195	200	205	210	215	220	225	230	235	240	245	250
5'0"	21	22	23	24	25	26	27	28	29	30	31	32	33	34	35	36	37	38	39	40	41	42	43	44	45	46	47	48	49
5'1"	21	22	23	24	25	26	26	27	28	29	30	31	32	33	34	35	36	37	38	39	40	41	42	43	43	44	45	46	47
5'2"	20	21	22	23	24	25	26	27	27	28	29	30	31	32	33	34	35	36	37	37	38	39	40	41	42	43	44	45	46
5'3"	19	20	21	22	23	24	25	26	27	27	28	29	30	31	32	33	34	35	35	36	37	38	39	40	41	42	43	43	44
5'4"	19	20	21	21	22	23	24	25	26	27	27	28	29	30	31	32	33	33	34	35	36	37	38	39	39	40	41	42	43
5'5"	18	19	20	21	22	22	23	24	25	26	27	27	28	29	30	31	32	32	33	34	35	36	37	37	38	39	40	41	42
5'6"	18	19	19	20	21	22	23	23	24	25	26	27	27	28	29	30	31	31	32	33	34	35	36	36	37	38	39	40	40
5'7"	17	18	19	20	20	21	22	23	23	24	25	26	27	27	28	29	30	31	31	32	33	34	34	35	36	37	38	38	39
5'8"	17	17	18	19	20	21	21	22	23	24	24	25	26	27	27	28	29	30	30	31	32	33	33	34	35	36	36	37	38
5'9"	16	17	18	18	19	20	21	21	22	23	24	24	25	26	27	27	28	29	30	30	31	32	32	33	34	35	35	36	37
5'10"	16	16	17	18	19	19	20	21	22	22	23	24	24	25	26	27	27	28	29	29	30	31	32	32	33	34	34	35	36
5'11"	15	16	17	17	18	19	20	20	21	22	22	23	24	24	25	26	26	27	28	29	29	30	31	31	32	33	33	34	35
6'0"	15	16	16	17	18	18	19	20	20	21	22	22	23	24	24	25	26	26	27	28	28	29	30	31	31	32	33	33	34
6'1"	15	15	16	16	17	18	18	19	20	20	21	22	22	23	24	24	25	26	26	27	28	28	29	30	30	31	32	32	33
6'2"	14	15	15	16	17	17	18	19	19	20	21	21	22	22	23	24	24	25	26	26	27	28	28	29	30	30	31	31	32
6'3"	14	14	15	16	16	17	17	18	19	19	20	21	21	22	22	23	24	24	25	26	26	27	27	28	29	29	30	31	31
6'4"	13	14	15	15	16	16	17	18	18	19	19	20	21	21	22	23	23	24	24	25	26	26	27	27	28	29	29	30	30

Determine your BMI by looking up the number where your weight and height intersect on the table.

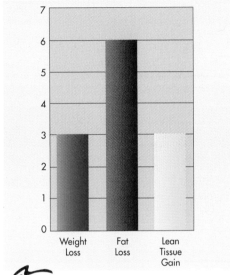

Table 2.14 *Disease Risk According to Body Mass Index (BMI)*

BMI	Disease Risk
<20.00	Moderate to Very High
20.00 to 21.99	Low
22.00 to 24.99	Very Low
25.00 to 29.99	Low
30.00 to 34.99	Moderate
35.00 to 39.99	High
≥40.00	Very High

Effects of Exercise and Diet on Body Composition

If you engage in a diet and exercise program, you should repeat body composition measurements about once a month to monitor changes in lean and fat tissue. This is important because lean body mass is affected by weight reduction programs as well as physical activity. A negative caloric balance does lead to a decrease in lean body mass. These effects will be explained in detail in Chapter 6. As lean body mass changes, so will your recommended body weight.

Changes in body composition resulting from a weight control/exercise program are illustrated by a co-ed aerobics course taught during a 6-week summer term. Students participated in aerobic dance routines four times a week, 60 minutes each time. On the first and the last day of class, several physiological parameters, including body composition, were assessed. Students also were given information on diet and nutrition and basically followed their own weight-control program. At the end of the 6 weeks, the average weight loss for the entire class was only 3 pounds. When body composition was assessed, however, class members were surprised to find that the average fat loss was actually 6 pounds, accompanied by a 3-pound increase in lean body mass (see Figure 2.6).

Figure 2.6. *Effects of a 6-week aerobics program on body composition.*

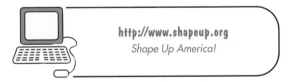

http://www.shapeup.org
Shape Up America!

Notes

1. American College of Sports Medicine, *Guidelines for Exercise Testing and Prescription* (Baltimore: Williams & Wilkins, 1995).

2. W. J. Evans, "Exercise, Nutrition, and Aging," *Journal of Nutrition*, 122(1992), 786–801.

3. W. W. Campbell, M. C. Crim, V. R. Young, and W. J. Evans, "Increased Energy Requirements and Changes in Body Composition with Resistance Training in Older Adults," *American Journal of Clinical Nutrition*, 60(1994), 167–175.

4. R. A. Faulkner, E. J. Sprigings, A. McQuarrie, and R. D. Bell, "A Partial Curl–Up Protocol for Adults Based on Analysis of Two Procedures," *Canadian Journal of Sports Science*, 14(1989), 135–141.

5. P. A. Macfarlane, "Out with the Sit–Up, in with the Curl–Up!," *Journal of Physical Exercise, Recreation and Dance*, 64(1993), 62–66.

6. D. Knudson and D. Johnston, "Validity and Reliability of a Bench Trunk–Curl Up Test of Abdominal Endurance," *Journal of Strength and Conditioning Research*, 9(1995), 165–169.

7. R. Kjorstad. *Validity of Two Field Tests of Abdominal Strength and Muscular Endurance*, unpublished master's thesis, Boise State University, 1997.

8. T. McNeill, D. Warwick, G. Anderson, and A. Schultz, "Trunk Strengths in Attempted Flexion, Extension, and Lateral Bending in Healthy Subjects and Patients with Low–Back Pain Disorders," *Spine*, 5(1980), 529–536.

9. L. D. Robertson and H. Magnusdottir, "Evaluation of Criteria Associated with Abdominal Fitness Testing," *Research Quarterly for Exercise and Sport*, 58 (1987), 355–359.

10. Macfarlane.

11. Kjorstad.

12. G. L. Hall, R. K. Hetzler, D. Perrin, and A. Weltman, " Relationship of Timed Sit–Up Tests to Isokinetic Abdominal Strength," *Research Quarterly for Exercise and Sport*, 63(1992), 80–84.

13. J. H. Wilmore. *Exercise and Weight Control: Myths, Misconceptions, Gadgets, Gimmicks, and Quackery*, lecture given at annual meeting of American College of Sports Medicine, Indianapolis, June 1994.

Exercise Prescription

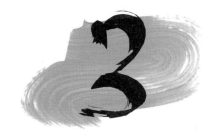

Exercise is the closest thing we'll ever get to the miracle pill that everyone is seeking. It brings weight loss, appetite control, improved mood and self-esteem, an energy kick, and longer life by decreasing the risk of heart disease, diabetes, stroke, osteoporosis, and chronic disabilities.[1]

An inspiring story illustrating what fitness can do for a person's health and well-being is that of George Snell from Sandy, Utah. At age 45 Snell weighed approximately 400

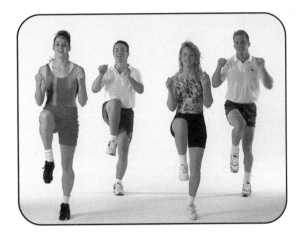

Objectives

- Determine readiness to start an exercise program.
- Learn the factors that govern cardiorespiratory exercise prescription: intensity, mode, duration, and frequency.
- Understand the variables that govern development of muscular strength and muscular endurance: mode, resistance, sets, and frequency.
- Recognize the factors that contribute to the development of muscular flexibility: mode, intensity, repetitions, and frequency.
- Learn to write personalized cardiorespiratory, strength, and flexibility exercise programs.
- Learn some ways to enhance adherence to exercise.
- Be able to write fitness goals.

pounds, his blood pressure was 220/180, he was blind because of diabetes he did not know he had, and his blood glucose (sugar) level was 487. Determined to do something about his physical and medical condition, Snell started a walking/jogging program. After about 8 months of conditioning, he had lost almost 200 pounds, his eyesight had returned, his glucose level was down to 67, and he was taken off medication. Two months later — less than 10 months after initiating his personal exercise program — he completed his first marathon, a running course of 26.2 miles!

Research results have established that participating in a lifetime exercise program contributes

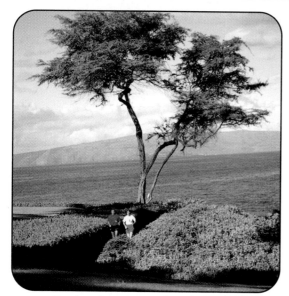

Good cardiorespiratory fitness is essential to enjoy a good quality of life.

greatly to good health.[2,3,4,5,6] Nonetheless, too many individuals who exercise regularly are surprised to find, when they take a battery of fitness tests, that they are not as conditioned as they thought they were. Although these people may be exercising regularly, they most likely are not following the basic principles of exercise prescription. Therefore, they do not reap significant benefits.

To obtain optimal results, all programs must be individualized. Our bodies are not all alike, and fitness levels and needs vary among individuals. The information presented in this chapter provides you with the necessary guidelines to write a personalized cardiorespiratory, strength, and flexibility exercise program to promote and maintain physical fitness and wellness. Information on weight control to achieve recommended body composition (the fourth component of physical fitness) is given in Chapter 6.

Readiness For Exercise

According to the U.S. Surgeon General, more than 60% of adults in the United States do not achieve the recommended amount of physical activity.[7] Only about 20% of the people who exercise are able to achieve a high physical fitness standard. More than half of those who start exercising drop out during the first 6 months of the program. Sports psychologists are trying to find out why some people exercise habitually and many do not. All of the benefits of exercise cannot help unless people commit to a lifetime program of physical activity (see Behavior Modification in Chapter 1).

If you are not exercising now, are you willing to give exercise a try? The first step is to decide positively that you will try. To help you make this decision, look at Figure 3.1. Make a list of the advantages and disadvantages of incorporating exercise into your lifestyle.

Your list of advantages may include things such as:

It will make me feel better.

My self-esteem will improve.

I will lose weight.

I will have more energy.

It will lower my risk for chronic diseases.

Your list of disadvantages may include:

I don't want to take the time.

I'm too out of shape.

There's no good place to exercise.

I don't have the willpower to do it.

When the reasons for exercise outweigh the reasons for not exercising, it will become easier to try.

A second questionnaire that may provide answers about your readiness to start an exercise program is provided in Figure 3.2. Read each statement carefully and circle the number that best describes your feelings. Be completely honest in your answers. You are evaluated in four categories: mastery (self-control), attitude, health, and commitment. The higher you score in any category — mastery, for example — the more important that reason is for you to exercise.

Scores can vary from 4 to 16. A score of 12 and above is a strong indicator that that factor is important to you, whereas 8 and below is low. If you score 12 or more points in each category, your chances of initiating and sticking to an exercise program are good. If you do not score at least 12 points in three categories, your chances of succeeding at exercise may be slim. You need to be better informed about the benefits of exercise, and a retraining process may be helpful. Tips on how to enhance commitment to exercise are provided later in the chapter.

Cardiorespiratory Endurance

A sound cardiorespiratory endurance program contributes greatly to enhancing and maintaining good health. Of the four health-related physical fitness components, cardiorespiratory endurance is the single most important — except during older age, when strength seems to be more critical. Even though certain amounts of muscular

Name: _____   Date: _____

Advantages of starting an exercise program

1. _____
2. _____
3. _____
4. _____
5. _____
6. _____
7. _____
8. _____

Disadvantages of starting an exercise program

1. _____
2. _____
3. _____
4. _____
5. _____
6. _____
7. _____
8. _____

Figure 3.1 Advantages and disadvantages of adding exercise to your lifestyle.

Name: _____ Date: _____

Carefully read each statement and circle the number that best describes your feelings in each statement. Please be completely honest with your answers.

	Strongly Agree	Mildly Agree	Mildly Disagree	Strongly Disagree
1. I can walk, ride a bike (or a wheelchair), swim, or walk in a shallow pool.	4	3	2	1
2. I enjoy exercise.	4	3	2	1
3. I believe exercise can help decrease the risk for disease and premature mortality.	4	3	2	1
4. I believe exercise contributes to better health.	4	3	2	1
5. I have previously participated in an exercise program.	4	3	2	1
6. I have experienced the feeling of being physically fit.	4	3	2	1
7. I can envision myself exercising.	4	3	2	1
8. I am contemplating an exercise program.	4	3	2	1
9. I am willing to stop contemplating and give exercise a try for a few weeks.	4	3	2	1
10. I am willing to set aside time at least three times a week for exercise.	4	3	2	1
11. I can find a place to exercise (the streets, a park, a YMCA, a health club).	4	3	2	1
12. I can find other people who would like to exercise with me.	4	3	2	1
13. I will exercise when I am moody, fatigued, and even when the weather is bad.	4	3	2	1
14. I am willing to spend a small amount of money for adequate exercise clothing (shoes, shorts, leotards, or swimsuit).	4	3	2	1
15. If I have any doubts about my present state of health, I will see a physician before beginning an exercise program.	4	3	2	1
16. Exercise will make me feel better and improve my quality of life.	4	3	2	1

Scoring Your Test:

This questionnaire allows you to examine your readiness for exercise. You have been evaluated in four categories: mastery (self-control), attitude, health, and commitment. Mastery indicates that you can be in control of your exercise program. Attitude examines your mental disposition toward exercise. Health provides evidence of the wellness benefits of exercise. Commitment shows dedication and resolution to carry out the exercise program. Write the number you circled after each statement in the corresponding spaces below. Add the scores on each line to get your totals. Scores can vary from 4 to 16. A score of 12 and above is a strong indicator that that factor is important to you, and 8 and below is low. If you score 12 or more points in each category, your chances of initiating and adhering to an exercise program are good. If you fail to score at least 12 points in three categories, your chances of succeeding at exercise may be slim. You need to be better informed about the benefits of exercise, and a retraining process may be required.

Mastery: 1. _____ + 5. _____ + 6. _____ + 9. _____ = _____

Attitude: 2. _____ + 7. _____ + 8. _____ + 13. _____ = _____

Health: 3. _____ + 4. _____ + 15. _____ + 16. _____ = _____

Commitment: 10. _____ + 11. _____ + 12. _____ + 14. _____ = _____

Figure 3.2 Exercise readiness questionnaire.

strength and flexibility are necessary to perform activities of daily living, a person can get by without a lot of strength and flexibility. A person cannot do without a good cardiorespiratory system, though.

Cardiorespiratory Exercise Prescription

The objective of aerobic exercise is to improve the capacity of the cardiorespiratory system. To accomplish this, the heart muscle has to be overloaded like any other muscle in the human body. Just as the biceps muscle in the upper arm is developed through strength training, the heart muscle is exercised to increase in size, strength, and efficiency. To better understand how the cardiorespiratory system can be developed, we have to be familiar with four factors involved in aerobic exercise: intensity, mode, duration, and frequency of exercise.

The American College of Sports Medicine (ACSM) recommends that a medical exam and a diagnostic exercise stress test be administered prior to vigorous exercise by apparently healthy men over age 40 and women over 50.[8] ACSM has defined "vigorous exercise" as an exercise intensity that provides a "substantial challenge" to the participant or one that cannot be maintained for 20 continuous minutes.

Intensity of Exercise

Muscles have to be overloaded for them to develop. Whereas the training stimulus to develop the biceps muscle can be accomplished with curl-up exercises, the stimulus for the cardiorespiratory system is provided by making the heart pump at a higher rate for a certain period of time.

Cardiorespiratory development occurs when the heart is working between 40/50% and 85% of **heart rate reserve**.[9] The 40% to 49% training intensity should be used by individuals who are quite unfit. Increases in maximal oxygen uptake (VO_{2max}), however, are accelerated when the heart is working closer to 85% of heart rate reserve. For this reason, many experts prescribe exercise between 60% and 85%. **Intensity of exercise** can be calculated easily, and training can be monitored by checking your pulse. To determine the intensity of exercise or **cardiorespiratory training zone,** follow these steps:

1. Estimate your maximal heart rate (MHR) according to the following formula: MHR = 220 minus age (220 − age)

2. Check your resting heart rate (RHR) some time after you have been sitting quietly for 15 to 20 minutes. You may take your pulse for 30 seconds and multiply by 2, or take it for a full minute. As explained in Chapter 2, you can check your pulse on the wrist by

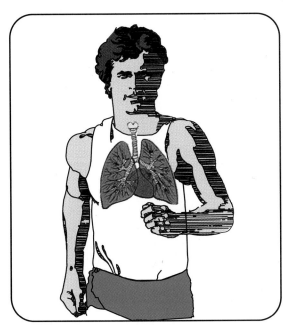

Cardiorespiratory endurance is the ability of the heart, lungs, and blood vessels to deliver adequate amounts of oxygen to the cells to meet the demands of prolonged physical activity.

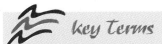

key Terms

Heart rate reserve The difference between the maximal heart rate (MHR) and resting heart rate (RHR).

Intensity of exercise How hard a person has to exercise to improve cardiorespiratory endurance.

Cardiorespiratory training zone The range of intensity at which a person should exercise to develop the cardiorespiratory system.

placing two or three fingers over the radial artery or over the carotid artery in the neck.

3. Determine the heart rate reserve (HRR) by subtracting the resting heart rate from the maximal heart rate (HRR = MHR − RHR).

4. Calculate the training intensities (TI) at 40%, 50%, 60%, and 85%. Multiply the heart rate reserve by the respective 40, 50, 60, and 85 percentages, and then add the resting heart rate to all four of these figures (for example, 85% TI = HRR × .85 + RHR).

Example. The 40%, 50%, 60%, and 85% training intensities for a 20-year-old with a resting heart rate of 68 beats per minute (bpm) would be:

MHR: 220 − 20 = 200 bpm
RHR: = 68 bpm
HRR: 200 − 68 = 132 beats
40% TI = (132 × .40) + 68 = 121 bpm
50% TI = (132 × .50) + 68 = 134 bpm
60% TI = (132 × .60) + 68 = 147 bpm
85% TI = (132 × .85) + 68 = 180 bpm

Low-intensity cardiorespiratory training zone: 121 to 134 bpm

Optimal cardiorespiratory training zone: 147 to 180 bpm

When you exercise to improve the cardiorespiratory system, you should maintain the heart rate between the 60% and 85% training intensities to obtain adequate development. If you have been physically inactive, you should train around the 40% to 50% intensity during the first 6 to 8 weeks of the exercise program. After the first few weeks, you should exercise between 60% and 85% training intensity.

When determining the training intensity for your own program, you need to consider your personal fitness goals. Individuals who exercise around the 50% training intensity will reap significant health benefits — in particular, improvements in the metabolic profile (see Physical Fitness Assessment in Chapter 2). Training at this lower percentage, however, may place you

only in the "average" or moderately fit category (see Table 2.2 in Chapter 2). Exercising at this lower intensity lowers the risk for cardiovascular mortality (health fitness) but will not allow you to achieve a "good" or "excellent" cardiorespiratory fitness rating (the physical fitness standard). The latter ratings are obtained by exercising closer to the 85% threshold.

Following a few weeks of training, you may have a considerably lower resting heart rate (10 to 20 beats fewer in 8 to 12 weeks). Therefore, you should recompute your target zone periodically. You can compute your own cardiorespiratory training zone by using the form in Figure 3.3. Once you have reached an ideal level of cardiorespiratory endurance, training in the 60% to 85% range will allow you to maintain your fitness level.

During the first few weeks of an exercise program, you should monitor your exercise heart rate regularly to make sure you are training in the proper zone. Wait until you are about 5 minutes into your exercise session before taking your first rate. When you check your heart rate, count your pulse for 10 seconds and then multiply by 6 to get the per-minute pulse rate. Exercise heart rate will remain at the same level for about 15 seconds following exercise. After 15 seconds, your heart rate will drop rapidly. Do not hesitate to stop during your exercise bout to check your pulse. If the rate is too low, increase the intensity of exercise. If the rate is too high, slow down.

To develop the cardiorespiratory system, you do not have to exercise above the 85% rate. From a fitness standpoint, training above this percentage will not give extra benefits and actually may be unsafe for some individuals. For unconditioned people and older adults, cardiorespiratory training should be conducted around the 50% rate to discourage potential problems associated with high-intensity exercise.

Mode of Exercise

The **mode of exercise** that develops the cardiorespiratory system has to be aerobic in nature.

Aerobic exercise has to involve the major muscle groups of the body, and it has to be rhythmic and continuous. As the amount of muscle mass involved during exercise increases, so does the effectiveness of the activity in providing cardiorespiratory development.

Once you have established your cardiorespiratory training zone, any activity or combination of activities that will get your heart rate up to that training zone and keep it there for as long as you exercise will give you adequate development. Examples of these activities are walking, jogging, swimming, water aerobics,

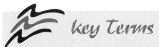

key terms

Mode of exercise Form of exercise (e.g., aerobic).
Aerobic exercise Activity that requires oxygen to produce the necessary energy to carry out the activity.

Intensity of Exercise

1. Estimate your own maximal heart rate (MHR)

 MHR = 220 minus age (220 − age)

 MHR = [ ] − [ ] = [ ] bpm

2. Resting heart rate (RHR) = [ ] bpm

3. Heart rate reserve (HRR) = MHR − RHR

 HRR = [ ] − [ ] = [ ] beats

4. Training intensity (TI) = HRR × % TI + RHR

 40% TI = [ ] × .40 + [ ] = [ ] bpm

 50% TI = [ ] × .50 + [ ] = [ ] bpm

 60% TI = [ ] × .60 + [ ] = [ ] bpm

 85% TI = [ ] × .85 + [ ] = [ ] bpm

5. Cardiorespiratory training zone. The recommended cardiorespiratory training zone is found between the 60% and 85% training intensities. Older adults, individuals who have been physically inactive or are in the poor or fair cardiorespiratory fitness categories, however, should follow a 40% to 50% training intensity during the first few weeks of the exercise program.

 Cardiorespiratory training zone: [ ] (60% TI) to [ ] (85% TI)

Mode of Exercise: List any activity or combination of aerobic activities that you will use in your cardiorespiratory training program:

_____

Duration of Exercise: Indicate the length of your exercise sessions: _____ minutes

Frequency of Exercise: Indicate the days you will exercise: _____

Student's Name: _____ Date: _____

Signature: _____

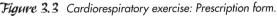

Figure 3.3 Cardiorespiratory exercise: Prescription form.

cross-country skiing, rope skipping, cycling, racquetball, stair climbing, and stationary running or cycling.

The activity you choose should be based on your personal preferences — what you enjoy doing most — and your physical limitations. Choose low-impact activities, as they greatly decrease the risk for injuries. Most injuries to beginners are related to high-impact activities. For individuals who have been inactive, general strength conditioning (discussed later in this chapter) also is recommended prior to initiating an aerobic exercise program. Strength conditioning will reduce the incidence of injuries significantly.

The amount of strength or flexibility you develop through various activities differs, but in terms of cardiorespiratory development, the heart doesn't know whether you are walking, swimming, or cycling. All the heart knows is that it has to pump at a certain rate, and as long as that rate is in the desired range, your cardiorespiratory fitness will improve.

From a health fitness point of view, training in the lower end of the cardiorespiratory zone will yield optimal health benefits. The closer the heart rate is to the higher end of the cardiorespiratory training zone, however, the greater will be the improvements in VO_{2max} (high physical fitness).

Duration of Exercise

In terms of **duration of exercise**, the general recommendation is that a person train between 20 and 60 minutes per session. The duration is based on how intensely a person trains. If the training is done around 85%, 20 minutes are sufficient. At 40/50% intensity the person should train at least 30 minutes. As mentioned in the discussion of intensity of exercise, unconditioned people and older adults should train at lower percentages; therefore, the activity should be carried out over a longer time.

Although most experts recommend 20 to 60 minutes of continuous aerobic exercise per session, recent evidence suggests that accumulating 30 minutes or more of moderate-intensity physical activity can provide substantial health bene-

fits.[10] Research further indicates that three 10-minute exercise sessions per day (separated by at least 4 hours), at approximately 70% of maximal heart rate, also produce fitness benefits.[11] Although the increases in VO_{2max} with this program were not as large (57%) as those in a group performing one continuous 30-minute bout of exercise per day, the researchers concluded that moderate-intensity exercise training, conducted for 10 minutes three times per day, benefits the cardiorespiratory system significantly.

Results of this study are meaningful because people often mention lack of time as the reason for not taking part in an exercise program. Many think they have to exercise at least 20 continuous minutes to get any benefits at all. Even though 20 to 60 minutes are recommended, short, intermittent exercise bouts also are helpful to the cardiorespiratory system.

Exercise sessions always should be preceded by a 5-minute **warm-up** and followed by a 5-minute **cool-down**. The warm-up should consist of general calisthenics, stretching exercises, or exercising at a lower intensity level than the target zone. The cool-down entails decreasing the intensity of exercise gradually. Stopping exercise abruptly causes blood to pool in the exercised body parts, diminishing the return of blood to the heart. Less blood return can cause dizziness and faintness or even bring on cardiac abnormalities.

Frequency of Exercise

At the beginning, a **frequency of exercise** of three to five 20- to 60-minute training sessions per week is the recommendation to improve VO_{2max}. When training is conducted more than 5 days a week, further improvements are minimal.

For individuals on a weight-loss program, 45- to 60-minute exercise sessions of low to moderate intensity, conducted 5 or 6 days per week, are recommended. Longer exercise sessions increase caloric expenditure for faster weight reduction (see Chapter 6).

Research also indicates that as few as three 20- to 30-minute training sessions per week, on nonconsecutive days, will maintain cardiorespiratory fitness (VO_{2max}) as long as the heart rate is in the appropriate target zone (60% to 85%).

Even though three exercise sessions per week will maintain cardiorespiratory fitness, the evidence of regular daily physical activity in preventing disease and enhancing quality of life cannot be ignored. In 1993, the American College of Sports Medicine, the U.S. Centers for Disease Control and Prevention, and the President's Council on Physical Fitness and Sports released a general recommendation stating that every American is encouraged to accumulate at least 30 minutes of moderate-intensity physical activity almost daily.[12] Examples of moderate-intensity activities include walking, pushing a stroller, cycling, volleyball, swimming, dancing fast, raking leaves, washing the car, doing household chores, and gardening.

This recommendation subsequently was upheld in the 1995 Dietary Guidelines for Americans[13] and later by the U.S. Surgeon General in its 1996 Report on Physical Activity and Health.[14] In the latter report the Surgeon General states that Americans can improve their health and quality of life substantially by including moderate amounts of physical activity on most, preferably all, days of the week. Furthermore, it states that no one, including older adults, is too old to enjoy the benefits of regular physical activity.

To enjoy better health and fitness, physical activity must be pursued regularly. According to Dr. William Haskell, from Stanford University: "Physical activity should be viewed as medication, and, therefore, should be taken on a daily basis."[15] Many of the benefits of exercise and activity diminish within 2 weeks of substantially decreased physical activity. These benefits are completely lost within 2 to 8 months of inactivity.[16]

ACSM Guidelines

A summary of the cardiorespiratory exercise prescription guidelines according to the American College of Sports Medicine is provided in Figure 3.4. Ideally, to reap both the high-fitness

Activity:	Aerobic (examples: walking, jogging, cycling, swimming, aerobics, racquetball, soccer, stair climbing)
Intensity:	40/50%–85% of heart rate reserve
Duration:	20–60 minutes of continuous aerobic activity
Frequency:	3 to 5 days per week

Based on the recommended quantity and quality of exercise for developing and maintaining cardiorespiratory and muscular fitness in healthy adults by the American College of Sports Medicine, Medical Science Sports Exercise, 30(1998):975–991.

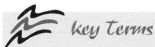

Figure 3.4 *Cardiorespiratory exercise prescription guidelines.*

and the health-fitness benefits of exercise, a person needs to exercise a minimum of three times per week in the appropriate target zone for high-fitness maintenance, and three to four additional times per week in moderate-intensity activities to enjoy the full benefits of health fitness. All exercise/activity sessions should last about 30 minutes. The form in Figure 3.10 at the end of this chapter is provided to help you keep a daily log of your aerobic activities.

Muscular Strength and Endurance

The capacity of muscle cells to exert force increases and decreases according to demands placed upon the muscular system. If specific

key Terms

Duration of exercise Time exercising per session.
Warm-up A period preceding exercise when exercise begins slowly.
Cool-down A period at the end of an exercise session when exercise is tapered off.
Frequency of exercise How often a person engages in an exercise session.

muscle cells are overloaded beyond their normal use, such as in strength-training programs, the cells increase in size (hypertrophy), strength, or endurance, or some combination of these. If the demands on the muscle cells decrease, such as in sedentary living or required rest because of illness or injury, the cells decrease in size (atrophy) and lose strength.

Overload Principle

The **overload principle** states that, for strength or endurance to improve, demands placed on the muscle must be increased over time, and the resistance (weight lifted) must be of a magnitude significant enough to produce development. In simpler terms, just like all other organs and systems of the human body, muscles have to be taxed beyond their accustomed loads to increase in physical capacity.

Specificity of Training

Muscular strength is the ability to exert maximum force against resistance. Muscular endurance (also referred to as localized muscular endurance) is the ability of a muscle to exert submaximal force repeatedly over time. Both of these components require **specificity of training.**

As discussed later in this section, a person attempting to increase muscular strength needs a program of few repetitions and near maximum resistance. To increase muscular endurance, the strength-training program consists primarily of many repetitions at a lower resistance.

In like manner, to increase isometric (static) versus dynamic strength (see Mode of Training, below) an individual must use the corresponding static or dynamic training procedures to achieve the appropriate results. In like manner, if a person is trying to improve a specific movement or skill through strength gains, the selected strength-training exercises must resemble the actual movement or skill as closely as possible.

Strength-Training Prescription

Similar to the prescription of cardiorespiratory exercise, several factors or variables have to be taken into account to improve muscular strength and endurance. These are mode, resistance, sets, and frequency of training.

Mode of Training

Two basic training methods are used to improve strength: isometric and dynamic. **Isometric exercise** involves pushing or pulling against immovable objects. **Dynamic exercise** requires movement with the muscle contraction, such as extending the knees with resistance (weight) on the ankles.

Isometric training was used commonly several years ago, but its popularity has waned. Because strength gains with isometric training are specific to the angle of muscle contraction, this type of training remains beneficial in sports such as gymnastics that require regular static contractions during routines.

Dynamic training programs can be conducted without weights or with free weights (barbells and dumbbells), fixed-resistance machines, variable-resistance machines, and isokinetic equipment. When performing dynamic exercises without weights (for example, pull-ups, push-ups), with free weights, or with fixed-resistance machines, a constant resistance (weight) is moved through a joint's full range of motion. The greatest resistance that can be lifted equals the maximum weight that can be moved

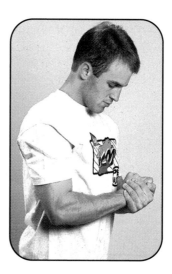

Isometric strength training.

at the weakest angle of the joint, because of changes in muscle length and angle of pull as the joint moves through its range of motion.

As strength training became more popular, new strength-training machines were developed. This technology brought about isokinetic and **variable-resistance training**. These training programs require special machines equipped with mechanical devices that provide differing amounts of resistance, with the intent of overloading the muscle group maximally through the entire range of motion. A distinction of **isokinetic exercise** is that the speed of the muscle contraction is kept constant because the machine provides resistance to match the user's force through the range of motion. Because of the expense of the equipment needed for isokinetic training, this type of program usually is reserved for clinical settings (physical therapy), research laboratories, and certain professional sports.

The mode of training depends mainly on the type of equipment available and the specific objective of the training program. Dynamic training is the most popular mode for strength training. Its primary advantage is that strength is gained through the full range of motion. Most daily activities are dynamic in nature. We constantly lift, push, and pull objects, which requires strength through a complete range of motion. Another advantage of dynamic exercise is that improvements are measured easily by the amount lifted.

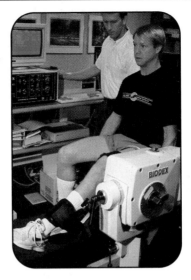

Isokinetic strength training.

Courtesy of Idaho Sports Medicine Institute, Boise, Idaho.

The benefits of isokinetic and variable-resistance training are similar to those of the other dynamic training methods. Theoretically, strength gains should be better because maximum resistance is applied through the entire range of motion. Research, however, has not shown this type of training to be more effective than other modes of dynamic training. A possible advantage is that specific speeds in various sport skills can be duplicated more closely with

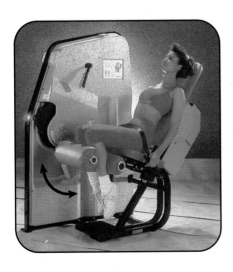

Dynamic strength training.

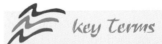

key Terms

Overload principle Training concept holding that the demands placed on a body system must be increased systematically and progressively over time to cause physiologic adaptation.

Specificity of training A principle holding that, for a muscle to increase in strength or endurance, the training program must be specific to obtain the desired effects.

Isometric exercise Strength training that entails muscle contraction producing little or no movement.

Dynamic exercise Strength training that involves a muscle contraction with movement.

Variable-resistance training Exercise that utilizes special equipment with mechanical devices that provide differing amounts of resistance through the range of motion.

Isokinetic exercise Strength training in which the equipment accommodates resistance to match the user's force through the full range of motion.

isokinetic strength training, which may enhance performance (specificity of training). A disadvantage is that the equipment is not readily available to everyone.

Resistance

Resistance in strength training is the equivalent of intensity in cardiorespiratory exercise prescription. The **resistance** depends on whether the person is trying to develop muscular strength or muscular endurance.

To stimulate strength development, a resistance of approximately 80% of the maximum capacity is recommended. For example, a person whose one repetition maximum (1 RM) for a given exercise is 150 pounds should work with at least 120 pounds (150 × .80). Using less than 80% will foster muscular endurance rather than strength. The time factor involved in constantly determining the 1 RM on each lift to ensure working above 80% is prohibitive. Therefore, a rule of thumb widely accepted by many authors and coaches is that individuals should perform between 3 and 12 repetitions maximum (3 RM to 12 RM) for adequate strength gains.

For example, if a person is training with a resistance of 120 pounds and cannot lift it more than 12 times, the training stimulus is adequate for strength development. Once the person can lift this resistance more than 12 times, the resistance should be increased by 5 to 10 pounds and the person again should build up to 12 RM. Training with more than 12 repetitions develops muscular endurance primarily. A person training with 20 maximum or near maximum repetitions, for example, will experience incremental increases in muscular endurance localized to the specific muscle groups involved in the exercise.

Research on strength indicates that the closer a person trains to the 1 RM, the greater are the strength gains. A disadvantage of working constantly at or near the 1 RM is that it increases the risk for injury. Highly trained athletes seeking maximum strength development do 1 RM to 6 RM. Working around 10 RM seems to produce the best results in terms of muscular hypertrophy.

Body builders tend to work with moderate levels of resistance (60% to 85% of the 1 RM) and perform 8 to 20 repetitions to near fatigue. A foremost objective of body building is to increase muscle size. Moderate resistance promotes blood flow to the muscles, "pumping up" the muscles (also known as "the pump") and making them look much larger than they are in a relaxed state.

From a health-fitness point of view, 6 RM to 12 RM is the recommended range. We live in a "dynamic world" in which muscular strength and endurance both are required to lead an enjoyable life. Therefore, working near a 10 RM threshold seems best to improve overall performance. For older and more frail individuals (50–60 years of age and above), 10 to 15 repetitions to near fatigue may be more appropriate.

We must mention here that a certain resistance (for example, 50 pounds) is seldom the same on two different weight machines, or between free weights and weight machines. The industry has no standard calibration procedure for strength equipment. Consequently, if you lift a certain weight with free weights or a given machine, you may or may not be able to lift the same amount on a different piece of equipment.

Sets

Strength training is done in **sets**. For example, a person lifting 120 pounds eight times performs one set of eight repetitions (1 × 8 × 120). When working with 8 to 12 repetitions maximum, three sets per exercise is the recommendation. Because of the characteristics of muscle fiber, only a limited number of sets can be done. As the number of sets increases, so does the extent of muscle fatigue and subsequent recovery time. Strength gains may be lessened by performing too many sets.

A suggested program for beginners in their first year of training is three heavy sets, up to the maximum number of repetitions, preceded by one or two light warm-up sets using about 50% of the 1 RM (no warm-up sets are necessary for subsequent exercises that use the same muscle group). Because of the lower resistances used in body building, four to eight sets can be done for each exercise.

To make the exercise program more time-effective, two or three exercises that require different muscle groups may be alternated. In this way, a person will not have to wait 2 to 3 minutes before proceeding to a new set on a different exercise. For example, the bench press, leg extension, and abdominal crunch exercises may be combined so the person can go almost directly from one set to the next. Body builders should rest no more than a minute to maximize the "pumping" effect.

To avoid muscle soreness and stiffness, new participants ought to build up gradually to the three sets of maximal repetitions. This can be done by performing only one set of each exercise with a lighter resistance on the first day. During the second session, two sets of each exercise can be done, one light and the second with the regular resistance. During the third session, three sets could be performed, one light and two heavy ones. After that, a person should be able to do all three heavy sets.

Frequency of Training

Strength training should be done either with a total body workout two to three times per week, or more frequently if using a split-body routine (upper body one day and lower body the next). After a maximum-strength workout, the muscles should be rested for about 48 hours to allow adequate recovery. If not recovered completely in 2 or 3 days, the person most likely is overtraining and therefore not reaping the full benefits of the program. In that case, a decrease in the total number of sets or exercises, or both, performed during the previous workout is recommended. A summary of strength-training guidelines for health-fitness purposes is provided in Figure 3.5.

Significant strength gains require a minimum of 8 weeks of consecutive training. After achieving the recommended strength level, one training session per week will be sufficient to maintain the new strength level.

Frequency of strength training for body builders varies from person to person. Because

Mode:	8 to 10 dynamic strength-training exercises involving the body's major muscle groups
Resistance:	Enough resistance to perform 8 to 12 repetitions to near fatigue (10 to 15 repetitions for older and more frail individuals)
Sets:	A minimum of 1 set
Frequency:	At least two times per week

Based on the recommended quantity and quality of exercise for developing and maintaining cardiorespiratory and muscular fitness in healthy adults by the American College of Sports Medicine, Medical Science Sports Exercise, 30, (1998), 975–991.

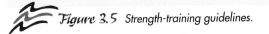 *Figure 3.5* Strength-training guidelines.

they use moderate resistances, daily or even two-a-day workouts are common. The frequency depends on the amount of resistance, number of sets performed per session, and the person's ability to recover from the previous exercise bout (see Table 3.1). The latter often is dictated by level of conditioning.

Designing Your Own Strength-Training Program

Two strength-training programs, presented in Appendix B, have been developed to provide a complete body workout. Only a minimum of equipment is required for the first program, "Strength-Training Exercises Without Weights" (Exercises 1 through 12). This program can be conducted within the walls of your own home. Your body weight is used as the primary resistance for most exercises. A few exercises call for

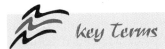 *key Terms*

Resistance Amount of weight lifted.
Set The number of repetitions performed for a given exercise.

Table 3.1 Guidelines for Various Strength Training Programs

Strength Training Program	Resistance	Sets	Rest Between Sets*	Frequency (workouts per week)**
Health fitness	8–12 reps max	3	2 min	2–3
Maximal strength	1–6 reps max	3–6	3 min	2–3
Muscular endurance	10–30 reps	3–6	2 min	3–6
Body building	8–20 reps near max	3–8	0–1 min	4–12

* Recovery between sets can be decreased by alternating exercises that use different muscle groups.

** Weekly training sessions can be increased by using a split body routine.

a friend's help or basic implements from around your home to provide greater resistance. The second program, "Strength-Training Exercises With Weights" (Exercises 13 through 22), requires machines such as those shown in the various photographs. Some of these exercises also can be performed with free weights.

Depending on the facilities available to you, choose one of the two training programs outlined in Appendix B. The resistance and the number of repetitions you use should be based on whether you want to increase muscular strength or muscular endurance. Do up to 12 RM for strength gains and more than 12 for muscular endurance. As pointed out, three training sessions per week on nonconsecutive days is an ideal arrangement for proper development. Because both strength and endurance are required in daily activities, 3 sets of about 12 RM for each exercise are recommended. In doing this, you will obtain good strength gains and yet be close to the endurance threshold.

Perhaps the only exercise that calls for more than 12 repetitions is the abdominal group of exercises. The abdominal muscles are considered primarily antigravity or postural muscles. Hence, a little more endurance may be required. When doing abdominal work, about 20 repetitions per set is the recommendation. Once you begin your strength-training program, you may use the form provided in Figure 3.11 at the end of this chapter to keep a record of your training sessions.

If time is a concern in completing your strength-training program, the American College of Sports Medicine recommends a minimum of one set of 8 to 12 repetitions performed to near fatigue, using 8 to 10 exercises that involve the major muscle groups of the body[17] (see Figure 3.12 at the end of this chapter). Training sessions should be conducted twice a week (see Figure 3.5). The recommendation is based on research showing that this training generates 70% to 80% of the improvements reported in other programs using three sets of about 10 RM.

Muscular Flexibility

Improving and maintaining good joint range of motion throughout life is important in enhancing health and quality of life. Nevertheless, health-care professionals and practitioners generally have underestimated and overlooked flexibility fitness.

The most significant detriments to flexibility are sedentary living and lack of physical activity. As physical activity decreases, muscles lose elasticity and tendons and ligaments tighten and shorten. Aging also reduces the extensibility of soft tissue, decreasing flexibility.

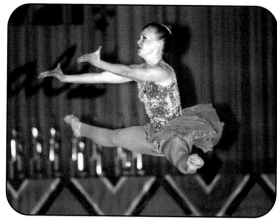

Complex motor skills improve with good flexibility.

Generally, flexibility exercises to improve range of motion around the joints are conducted following an aerobic workout. Stretching exercises seem to be most effective when a person is warmed up properly. Cool muscle temperatures decrease joint range of motion. Changes in muscle temperature can increase or decrease flexibility by as much as 20%. Because of the effects of muscular temperature on flexibility, many people prefer to do their stretching exercises after the aerobic phase of their workout.

Muscular Flexibility Prescription

The overload and specificity of training principles apply to development of muscular flexibility. To increase the total range of motion of a joint, the specific muscles surrounding that joint have to be stretched progressively beyond their accustomed length. The factors of mode, intensity, repetitions, and frequency of exercise also can be applied to flexibility programs.

Mode of Exercise

Three modes of stretching exercises promote flexibility:

1. Ballistic stretching.
2. Slow-sustained stretching.
3. Proprioceptive neuromuscular facilitation stretching.

Although all three types of stretching are effective in developing better flexibility, each has certain advantages.

Ballistic (or **dynamic**) **stretching** exercises provide the necessary force to lengthen the muscles. Although this type of stretching helps to develop flexibility, the ballistic actions may cause muscle soreness and injury as a result of small tears to the soft tissue.

Precautions must be taken not to overstretch ligaments, because they undergo plastic (permanent) elongation. If the stretching force cannot be controlled, as in fast, jerky movements, ligaments can be overstretched easily. This, in turn, leads to excessively loose joints, increasing the risk for injuries, including joint dislocation and subluxation (partial dislocation). Slow ballistic

stretching (instead of jerky, rapid, and bouncy movements) is quite effective in developing flexibility, and most people can perform this form of stretching.

Slow-sustained stretching causes the muscles to relax so greater length can be achieved. This type of stretch causes little pain and has a low risk of injury. Slow-sustained stretching exercises are the most frequently used and recommended for flexibility development programs.

Proprioceptive neuromuscular facilitation (PNF) stretching has become more popular in the last few years. This technique, based on a "contract-and-relax" method, requires the assistance of another person. The procedure is as follows:

1. The person assisting with the exercise provides initial force by pushing slowly in the direction of the desired stretch. The initial stretch does not cover the entire range of motion.

2. The person being stretched then applies force in the opposite direction of the stretch, against the assistant, who tries to hold the initial degree of stretch as closely as possible. An isometric contraction is being performed at that angle.

3. After 6 seconds of isometric contraction, the muscles being stretched are relaxed completely. The assistant then increases the degree of stretch slowly to a greater angle.

4. The isometric contraction is repeated for another 6 seconds, following which the muscle(s) is relaxed again. The assistant

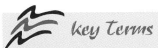

key Terms

Ballistic (or dynamic) stretching Exercises performed using jerky, rapid, and bouncy movements.

Slow-sustained stretching Technique whereby the muscles are lengthened gradually through a joint's complete range of motion and the final position is held for a few seconds.

Proprioceptive neuromuscular facilitation (PNF) A stretching technique in which muscles are stretched out progressively with intermittent isometric contractions.

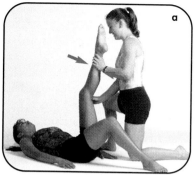

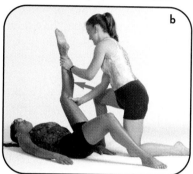

Proprioceptive neuromuscular facilitation stretching techniques: (a) isometric phase, (b) stretching phase.

then can increase the degree of stretch slowly one more time.

Steps 1 through 4 are repeated two to five times, until the exerciser feels mild discomfort. On the last trial, the final stretched position should be held for 10 to 30 seconds.

Theoretically, with the PNF technique the isometric contraction helps relax the muscle(s) being stretched, which results in longer muscles. Some fitness leaders believe PNF is more effective than slow-sustained stretching. Another benefit of PNF is an increase in strength of the muscle(s) being stretched. Recent research showed an approximate 17% and 35% increase in absolute strength and muscular endurance, respectively, in the hamstring muscle group through 12 weeks of PNF stretching.[18] The results were consistent in both men and women. These increases are attributed to the isometric contractions performed during PNF. The disadvantages are more pain with PNF, a second person is required to assist, and more time is needed to conduct each session.

Intensity of Exercise

When doing flexibility exercises, the **intensity** of the stretch should be only to a point of mild discomfort. Excessive pain is an indication that the load is too high and may lead to injury.

All stretching should be done to slightly below the pain threshold. As participants reach this point, they should try to relax the muscle being stretched as much as possible. After completing the stretch, the body part is brought back gradually to the starting point.

The time required for an exercise session for development of flexibility is based on the number of **repetitions** performed and the length of time each repetition (final stretched position) is held. The general recommendation is that each exercise be done at least four times, holding the final position each time for 10 to 30 seconds.

As flexibility increases, a person may gradually increase the time each repetition is held, to a maximum of 1 minute. Individuals who are susceptible to flexibility injuries should limit each stretch to 20 seconds.

Frequency of Exercise

Flexibility exercises should be conducted five to six times a week in the early stages of the program. After a minimum of 6 to 8 weeks of almost daily stretching, flexibility levels can be maintained with only two or three sessions per week, using about three repetitions of 10 to 15 seconds each. Figure 3.6 provides a summary of flexibility development guidelines.

When To Stretch?

Many people do not differentiate a warm-up from stretching. Warming up means starting a workout slowly with walking, slow jogging, or light calisthenics. Stretching implies movement of joints through their range of motion.

Before performing flexibility exercises, the muscles should be warmed up properly. Failing to warm up increases the risk for muscle pulls and tears. Surveys have shown that individuals

Mode:	Static or dynamic (slow ballistic or proprioceptive neuromuscular facilitation) stretching to include every major joint of the body
Intensity:	Stretch to the point of mild discomfort
Repetitions:	Repeat each exercise at least 4 times and hold the final stretched position for 10 to 30 seconds
Frequency:	2–3 days per week

Based on the recommended quantity and quality of exercise for developing and maintaining cardiorespiratory and muscular fitness in healthy adults by the American College of Sports Medicine, Medical Science Sports Exercise, 30, (1998), 975–991.

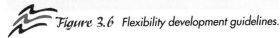

Figure 3.6   Flexibility development guidelines.

who stretch before workouts without an adequate warm-up have a higher rate of injuries than those who do not stretch at all.

A good time to do flexibility exercises is after aerobic workouts. Higher body temperature in itself helps to increase joint range of motion. Muscles also are fatigued following exercise. A fatigued muscle tends to shorten, which can lead to soreness and spasms. Stretching exercises help fatigued muscles reestablish their normal resting length and prevent unnecessary pain.

Designing a Flexibility Program

To improve body flexibility, each major muscle group should be subjected to at least one stretching exercise. A complete set of exercises for developing muscular flexibility is presented in Appendix C. You may not be able to hold a final stretched position with some of these exercises (such as lateral head tilts and arm circles), but you still should perform the exercise through the joint's full range of motion. Depending on the number and the length of repetitions, a complete workout will last between 15 and 30 minutes.

Prevention and Rehabilitation of Low-Back Pain

Few people make it through life without having low-back pain at some point. An estimated 60% to 90% of all Americans will suffer from chronic back pain in their lives.[19] About 80% of the time, backache is preventable and is caused by some combination of: (a) physical inactivity, (b) poor postural habits and body mechanics, and (c) excessive body weight.

Lack of physical activity is the most common contributor to chronic low-back pain. Deterioration or weakening of the abdominal and gluteal muscles, along with tightening of the lower back (erector spine) muscles, brings about an unnatural forward tilt of the pelvis (see Figure 3.7). This tilt puts extra pressure on the spinal vertebrae, causing pain in the lower back. Accumulation of fat around the midsection of the body contributes to the forward tilt of the pelvis, which further aggravates the condition.

Low-back pain frequently is associated with faulty posture and improper body mechanics in all of life's daily activities, including sleeping, sitting, standing, walking, driving, working, and exercising. Incorrect posture and poor mechanics, as explained in Figure 3.8, increase strain not only on the lower back but on many other bones, joints, muscles, and ligaments as well.

The incidence and frequency of low-back pain can be reduced greatly by including some specific stretching and strengthening exercises in the regular fitness program. In most cases, back pain is present only with movement and physical activity. If back pain is severe and persists even at rest, the first step is to consult a physician, who can rule out any disc damage and most likely will prescribe proper bed rest using several

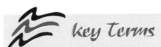

key terms

Intensity (in flexibility exercise) Degree of stretch.
Repetitions The number of times a movement is performed.

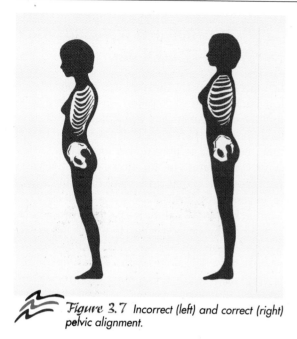

Figure 3.7 Incorrect (left) and correct (right) pelvic alignment.

pillows under the knees for leg support (see Figure 3.8). This position helps release muscle spasms by stretching the muscles involved. In addition, a physician may prescribe a muscle relaxant or anti-inflammatory medication, or both, and some type of physical therapy.

Once the individual is pain-free in the resting state, he or she needs to start correcting the muscular imbalance by stretching the tight muscles and strengthening the weak ones. Stretching exercises always are done first.

Several exercises for preventing backache and rehabilitating the back are given in Appendix D. These exercises can be done twice or more daily when a person has back pain. Under normal circumstances, three to four times a week is sufficient to prevent its occurrence.

Tips to Enhance Adherence to Exercise

Introducing new behaviors into one's daily routine takes most people months to accomplish. A fitness program is no exception. Adding exercise to a person's lifestyle may require retraining (behavior modification).

Different things motivate different people to start and remain in a fitness program. Regardless of the initial reason for initiating an exercise program, you now need to plan for ways to make your workout fun. The psychology behind it is simple: If you enjoy an activity, you will continue to do it. If you don't, you will quit. Some of the following suggestions may help:

1. Start slowly. One of the most common mistakes people make with exercise is doing too much too quickly. This increases the risk for injuries and often leads to discouragement and dropping out. Keep in mind that the body's conditioning process takes months.

2. Select aerobic activities you enjoy doing. Picking an activity you don't enjoy makes you less likely to keep exercising.

3. Combine various activities. Train by doing two or three different activities the same week. This makes exercising less monotonous than repeating the same activity again and again.

4. Find a friend or a group of friends to exercise with. Social interaction will make exercise more fulfilling. Besides, it's harder to skip if someone is waiting for you.

5. Set aside a regular time for exercise. If you don't plan ahead, it's a lot easier to skip. Holding your exercise hour "sacred" will help you adhere to the program.

6. Obtain the proper equipment for exercise. A poor pair of shoes, for instance, can increase the risk for injury, discouraging you from the very beginning.

7. Don't become a chronic exerciser. Learn to listen to your body. Overexercising can lead to chronic fatigue and injuries. Exercise should be enjoyable, and in the process you will need to "stop and smell the roses."

8. Exercise in different places and facilities to add variety to your workouts.

9. Conduct periodic assessments. Improving to a higher fitness category is a reward in itself.

HOW TO STAY ON YOUR FEET WITHOUT TIRING YOUR BACK

To prevent strain and pain in everyday activities, it is restful to change from one task to another before fatigue sets in. Housewives can lie down between chores; others should check body position frequently, drawing in the abdomen, flattening the back, bending the knees slightly.

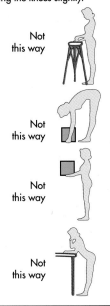

Not this way

Not this way

Not this way

Not this way

Use of a footrest relieves swayback.

Bend the knees and hips, not the waist.

Hold heavy objects close to you.

Never bend over without bending the knees.

HOW TO PUT YOUR BACK TO BED

For proper bed posture, a firm mattress is essential. Bedboards, sold commercially, or devised at home, may be used with soft mattresses. Bedboards, preferably, should be made of 3/4 inch plywood. Faulty sleeping positions intensify swayback and result not only in backache but in numbness, tingling, and pain in arms and legs.

Incorrect:
Lying flat on back makes swayback worse.

Use of high pillow strains neck, arms, shoulders.

Sleeping face down exaggerates swayback, strains neck and shoulders.

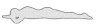

Bending one hip and knee does not relieve swayback.

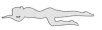

Correct:
Lying on side with knees bent effectively flattens the back. Flat pillow may be used to support neck, especially when shoulders are broad.

Sleeping on back is restful and correct when knees are properly supported.

Raise the foot of the mattress eight inches to discourage sleeping on the abdomen.

Proper arrangement of pillows for resting or reading in bed.

HOW TO SIT CORRECTLY

A back's best friend is a straight, hard chair. If you can't get the chair you prefer, learn to sit properly on whatever chair you get. <u>To correct sitting position from forward slump:</u> Throw head well back, then bend it forward to pull in the chin. This will straighten the back. Now tighten abdominal muscles to raise the chest. Check position frequently.

Relieve strain by sitting well forward, flatten back by tightening abdominal muscles, and cross knees.

Use of footrest relieves swayback. Aim is to have knees higher than hips.

Correct way to sit while driving, close to pedals. Use seatbelt or hard backrest, available commercially.

TV slump leads to "dowager's hump," strains neck and shoulders.

If chair is too high, swayback is increased.

Keep neck and back in as straight a line as possible with the spine. Bend forward from hips.

Driver's seat too far from pedals emphasizes curve in lower back.

Strained reading position. Forward thrusting strains muscles of neck and head.

Reproduced by permission of Schering Corporation. Copyright © Schering Corporation, Kenilworth, NJ.

Figure 3.8 Your back and how to care for it.

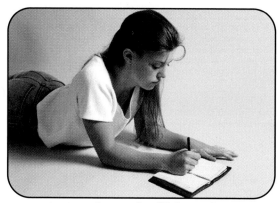

Setting realistic goals will help you design and guide your fitness program.

10. Keep a regular record of your activities. This allows you to monitor your progress and compare it with previous months and years. Use forms similar to those in Figures 3.10 and 3.11 to monitor your aerobic and strength-training programs.

11. If a health problem arises, see a physician. When in doubt, it's "better safe than sorry."

12. Set goals and share them with others. Quitting is tougher when someone knows what you are trying to accomplish. When you reach a specific goal, reward yourself with a new pair of shoes or a jogging suit or something similar that you want.

Setting Fitness Goals

Before you leave this chapter, you must consider your fitness goals. In the last few decades we have become accustomed to "quick fixes" with everything from super fast foods to one-hour dry cleaning. Fitness, however, has no quick fix. Fitness takes time and dedication, and only those who are committed and persistent will reap the rewards. As described in Chapter 1, setting realistic fitness goals will guide your program. Figure 3.9 offers a goal-setting chart that will help you determine your fitness goals. Take the time, either by yourself or with your instructor's help, to fill it out.

As you prepare to write realistic fitness goals, base these goals on the results of your initial fitness test (pre-test). For instance, if your cardiorespiratory fitness category was "poor" on the pre-test, you should not expect to improve to the "excellent" category in a little more than 3 months.

Whenever possible, your fitness goals should be measurable. A goal that simply states "to improve cardiorespiratory endurance" is not as measurable as a goal that states "to improve to the 'good' fitness category in cardiorespiratory endurance" or "to run the 1.5-mile course in less than 11 minutes."

After determining each goal, you also will need to write measurable objectives to accomplish that goal. These objectives will be the actual plan of action to accomplish your goal. A sample of objectives to accomplish the previously stated goal for cardiorespiratory endurance development could be:

1. Use jogging as the mode of exercise.

2. Jog at 10:00 a.m. five times per week.

3. Jog around the track in the fieldhouse.

4. Jog for 30 minutes each exercise session.

5. Monitor heart rate regularly during exercise.

6. Take the 1.5-Mile Run test once a month.

You will not always meet your specific objectives. If so, your goal may be out of reach. Reevaluate your objectives and make adjustments accordingly. If you set unrealistic goals at the beginning of your exercise program, be flexible with yourself and reconsider your plan of action but do not quit. Reconsidering your plan of action does not mean that you have failed. Failure comes only to those who stop trying, and success comes to those who are committed and persistent.

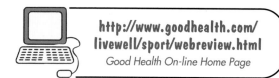

http://www.goodhealth.com/livewell/sport/webreview.html
Good Health On-line Home Page

Indicate below two or three general goals that you will work on during the next few weeks, and write the specific objectives you will use to accomplish each goal.

Cardiorespiratory endurance goal: _____

_____

Specific objectives:

1. _____

2. _____

3. _____

4. _____

5. _____

6. _____

_____   _____
My signature   Witness signature

_____   _____
Today's date   Date of completion

Muscular strength/endurance goal: _____

_____

Specific objectives:

1. _____

2. _____

3. _____

4. _____

5. _____

6. _____

_____   _____
My signature   Witness signature

_____   _____
Today's date   Date of completion

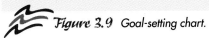 *Figure 3.9* Goal-setting chart.

Muscular flexibility goal: _____

_____

Specific objectives:

1. _____
2. _____
3. _____
4. _____
5. _____
6. _____

_____   _____
My signature   Witness signature

_____   _____
Today's date   Date of completion

Body composition goal: _____

_____

Specific objectives:

1. _____
2. _____
3. _____
4. _____
5. _____
6. _____

_____   _____
My signature   Witness signature

_____   _____
Today's date   Date of completion

Figure 3.9 Goal-setting chart (continued).

Aerobics Record Form

Date	Body Weight	Exercise Heart Rate	Type of Exercise	Distance in Miles	Time Hrs./Min.
1					
2					
3					
4					
5					
6					
7					
8					
9					
10					
11					
12					
13					
14					
15					
16					
17					
18					
19					
20					
21					
22					
23					
24					
25					
26					
27					
28					
29					
30					
31					
			Total		

 Figure 3.10 Aerobics: Record form.

Strength Training Record Form

Name _____

Date _____

Exercise	St/Reps/Res*	St/Reps/Res*	St/Reps/Res*	St/Reps/Res*	St/Reps/Res*	St/Reps/Res*	St/Reps/Res*	St/Reps/Res*	St/Reps/Res*	St/Reps/Res*

* St/Reps/Res 4 Sets, Repetitions, and Resistance (e.g., 1/6/125 4 1 set of 6 repetitions with 125 pounds)

Figure 3.11 Strength training: Record form.

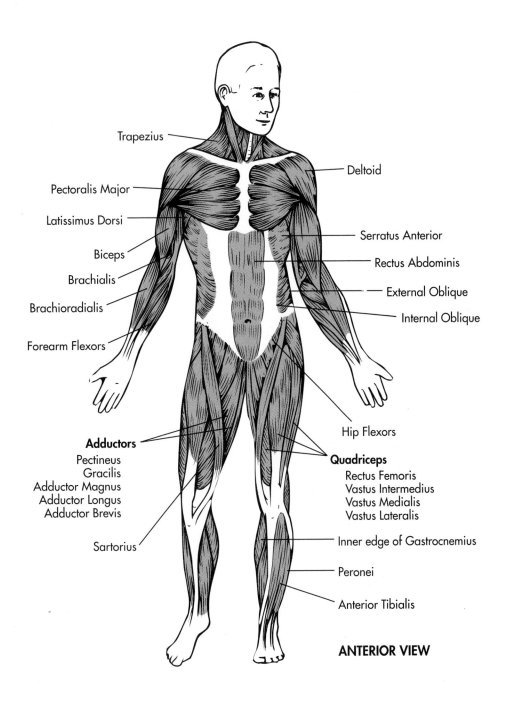

Trapezius

Pectoralis Major

Latissimus Dorsi

Biceps

Brachialis

Brachioradialis

Forearm Flexors

Deltoid

Serratus Anterior

Rectus Abdominis

External Oblique

Internal Oblique

Hip Flexors

Adductors
Pectineus
Gracilis
Adductor Magnus
Adductor Longus
Adductor Brevis

Quadriceps
Rectus Femoris
Vastus Intermedius
Vastus Medialis
Vastus Lateralis

Sartorius

Inner edge of Gastrocnemius

Peronei

Anterior Tibialis

ANTERIOR VIEW

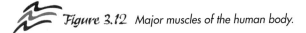

Figure 3.12   *Major muscles of the human body.*

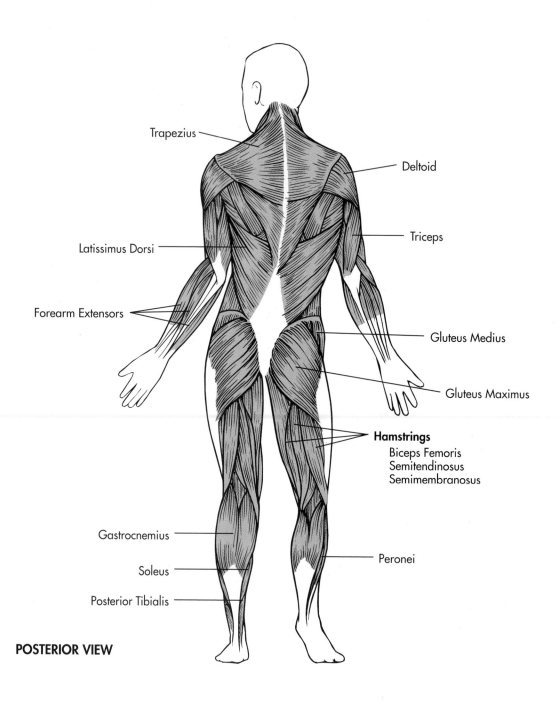

Trapezius

Deltoid

Triceps

Latissimus Dorsi

Forearm Extensors

Gluteus Medius

Gluteus Maximus

Hamstrings
Biceps Femoris
Semitendinosus
Semimembranosus

Gastrocnemius

Peronei

Soleus

Posterior Tibialis

POSTERIOR VIEW

Figure 3.12 Major muscles of the human body (continued).

Notes

1. H. Atkinson, "Exercise for Longer Life: The Physician's Perspective," *Health News*, 3:7(1997), 3.

2. R. S. Paffenbarger, Jr., R. T. Hyde, A. L. Wing, and C. H. Steinmetz, "A Natural History of Athleticism and Cardiovascular Health," *Journal of the American Medical Association*, 252(1984), 491–495.

3. S. N. Blair, H. W. Kohl III, R. S. Paffenbarger, Jr., D. G. Clark, K. H. Cooper, and L. W. Gibbons, "Physical Fitness and All-Cause Mortality: A Prospective Study of Healthy Men and Women," *Journal of the American Medical Association*, 262 (1989), 2395–2401.

4. S. N. Blair, H. W. Kohl III, C. E. Barlow, R. S. Paffenbarger, Jr., L. W. Gibbons, and C. A. Macera, "Changes in Physical Fitness and All-Cause Mortality: A Prospective Study of Healthy and Unhealthy Men," *Journal of the American Medical Association*, 273(1995), 1193–1198.

5. I. Lee, C. Hsieh, and R. S. Paffenbarger, Jr., "Exercise Intensity and Longevity in Men: The Harvard Alumni Health Study" *Journal of the American Medical Association*, 273(1995), 1179–1184.

6. J. E. Enstrom, "Health Practices and Cancer Mortality Among Active California Mormons," *Journal of the National Cancer Institute*, 81(1989) 1807–1814, 1989.

7. U. S. Department of Health and Human Services, "Physical Activity and Health: A Report of the Surgeon General" (Atlanta: U.S. Department of Health and Human Services, Centers for Disease Control and Prevention, National Center for Chronic Disease - Prevention and Health Promotion, 1996).

8. American College of Sports Medicine, *Guidelines for Exercise Testing and Prescription* (Baltimore: Williams & Wilkins, 1995).

9. American College of Sports Medicine, "The Recommended Quantity and Quality of Exercise for Developing and Maintaining Cardiorespiratory and Muscular Fitness and Flexibility in Healthy Adults," *Medicine and Science in Sports and Exercise*, 30(1998), 975–991.

10. S. N. Blair, "Surgeon General's Report on Physical Fitness: The Inside Story," *ACSM's Health & Fitness Journal*, 1(1997), 14–18.

11. R. F. DeBusk, U. Stenestrand, M. Sheehan, and W. L. Haskell, "Training Effects of Long Versus Short Bouts of Exercise in Healthy Subjects," *American Journal of Cardiology*, 65(1990), 1010–1013.

12. U. S. Centers for Disease Control and Prevention and American College of Sports Medicine, "Summary Statement: Workshop on Physical Activity and Public Health," *Sports Medicine Bulletin*, 28:4(1993), 7.

13. U.S. Department of Agriculture and U.S. Department of Health and Human Services, "Nutrition and Your Health: Dietary Guidelines for Americans," *Home and Garden Bulletin No. 232*, December 1995.

14. U.S. Department of Health and Human Services.

15. W. L. Haskell, "Scanning Sports," *Physician and Sportsmedicine*, 21:11 (1993), 34.

16. U.S. Department of Health and Human Services.

17. American College of Sports Medicine, 1998.

18. J. Kokkonen and S. Lauritzen, "Isotonic Strength and Endurance Gains Through PNF Stretching," *Medicine and Science in Sports and Exercise*, 27(1995), S22,127.

19. "Minimizing Back Pain," Tufts University Health and Nutrition Letter (New York: The Editors, May, 1998).

Evaluating Fitness Activities

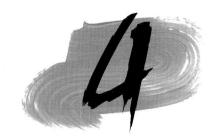

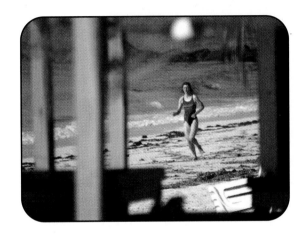

*O*ne of the fun aspects of exercise is that many different activities promoting fitness are available from which to choose. You may select one or a combination of activities for your program. The choice should be based on personal enjoyment, convenience, and availability.

Aerobic Activities

Most people who exercise pick and adhere to a single mode, such as walking, swimming, or jogging. No single activity develops total fitness. Many activities contribute to cardiorespiratory development. The extent of contribution to other fitness components is limited, though, and varies among the activities. For total fitness, aerobic activities should be supplemented with strength and flexibility exercises. **Cross-training** can add enjoyment to the program, decrease the risk of incurring injuries from overuse, and keep exercise from becoming monotonous.

Exercise sessions should be convenient. To enjoy exercise, a time should be selected when you will not be rushed. A nearby location is recommended. People do not enjoy driving across town to get to the gym, health club, track, or pool. If parking is a problem, you may get discouraged quickly and quit. All of these factors are used as excuses not to stick to an exercise program.

Walking

The most natural, easiest, safest, and least expensive form of aerobic exercise is walking. For years many fitness practitioners believed that

Objectives

🏊 Learn the benefits and advantages of selected aerobic activities.

🏊 Learn to rate the fitness benefits of aerobic activities.

🏊 Evaluate the contributions of skill-related fitness activities.

🏊 Understand the sequence of a standard aerobic workout.

🏊 Learn ways to enhance aerobic workouts.

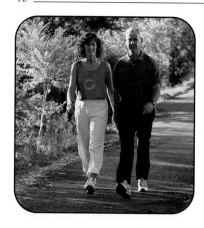

Walking is the most natural aerobic exercise.

walking was not vigorous enough to improve cardiorespiratory functioning. Now studies have established that brisk walking at speeds of 4 miles per hour or faster improves cardiorespiratory fitness. From a health-fitness viewpoint, a regular walking program can prolong life significantly (see the discussion of cardiovascular disease in Chapter 8). Although walking takes longer than jogging, the caloric cost of brisk walking is only about 10% lower than jogging the same distance.

Walking is perhaps the best activity to start a conditioning program for the cardiorespiratory system. Inactive people should start with 1-mile walks four or five times per week. Walk times can be increased gradually by 5 minutes each week. Following 3 to 4 weeks of conditioning, a person should be able to walk 2 miles at a 4-mile-per-hour pace, five times per week. Greater aerobic benefits accrue from walking longer and swinging the arms faster than normal. Light hand weights, a backpack (4 to 6 pounds), or an Aero-belt (discussed later in this chapter) also add to the intensity of walking. Because of the additional load on the cardiorespiratory system, extra weights or loads are not recommended for people who have cardiovascular disease.

Walking in water (chest-deep level) is an excellent form of aerobic activity, particularly for people with leg and back problems. Because of the buoyancy that water provides, individuals submerged in water to armpit level weigh only about 10% to 20% of their weight outside the

water. The resistance the water creates as a person walks in the pool makes the intensity quite high, providing an excellent cardiorespiratory workout.

Hiking

Hiking is an excellent activity for the entire family, especially during the summer and on summer vacations. Many people feel guilty if they are unable to continue their exercise routine during vacations. The intensity of hiking over uneven terrain is greater than walking. An 8-hour hike can burn as many calories as a 20-mile walk or jog.

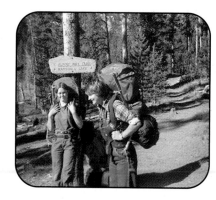

An 8-hour hike can burn as many calories as a 20-mile walk or jog.

Another benefit of hiking is the relaxing effects of beautiful scenery. This is an ideal activity for highly stressed people who live near woods and hills. A rough day at the office can be forgotten quickly in the peacefulness and beauty of the outdoors.

Jogging/Running

Jogging is the most popular form of aerobic exercise. Next to walking, it is one of the most accessible forms of exercise. A person can find places to jog almost everywhere. The lone requirement to prevent injuries is a good pair of jogging shoes.

The popularity of jogging in the United States started shortly after publication of Dr. Kenneth Cooper's first aerobics book in 1968. Jim Fixx's *Complete Book of Running* in the mid-1970s further contributed to the phenomenal growth of jogging as the predominant fitness activity in the United States.

Jogging three to five times a week is one of the fastest ways to improve cardiorespiratory fitness. The risk of injury, however, especially in beginners, is greater with jogging than walking. For proper conditioning, jogging programs should start with 1 to 2 weeks of walking. As fitness improves, walking and jogging can be combined, gradually increasing the jogging segment until it comprises the full 20 to 30 minutes.

Many people abuse this activity. People run too fast and too long. Some joggers think that if a little is good, more is better. Not so with cardiorespiratory endurance. As indicated under "Frequency of Exercise" in Chapter 3, the aerobic benefit of training more than 30 minutes five times per week is minimal. Furthermore, the risk of injury increases greatly as speed (running instead of jogging) and mileage go up. Jogging approximately 15 miles per week is sufficient to reach an excellent level of cardiorespiratory fitness.

A good pair of shoes is a must for joggers. Many foot, knee, and leg problems originate from improperly fitting or worn-out shoes. A good pair of shoes should offer good lateral stability and not lean to either side when placed on a flat surface. The shoe also should bend at the ball of the foot, not at midfoot. Worn-out shoes should be replaced. After 500 miles of use, jogging shoes lose about a third of their shock absorption capabilities. If you suddenly have problems, check your shoes first. It may be time for a new pair.

For safety reasons, joggers should stay away from high-speed roads, not wear headphones, and always run (or walk) against the traffic so they will be able to see all oncoming traffic. At night, reflective clothing or fluorescent material should be worn on different parts of the body. Carrying a flashlight is even better because motorists can see the light from a greater distance than they can see the reflective material.

An alternative form of jogging, especially for injured people, those with chronic back

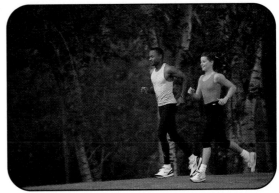

Jogging, the most popular form of aerobic exercise.

problems, and overweight individuals, is deep-water running — running in place while treading water. Deep-water running is almost as strenuous as jogging on land. In deep-water running, the running motions used on land are accentuated by pumping the arms and legs hard through a full range of motion. The participant usually wears a flotation vest to help maintain the body in an upright position. Many elite athletes train frequently in water to lessen the wear and tear on the body caused by long-distance running. These athletes have been able to maintain high oxygen uptake values through rigorous water running programs.

Aerobics

Aerobics, formerly known as **aerobic dance**, is thought to be the most common fitness activity for women in the United States. Routines consist of a combination of stepping, walking, jogging, skipping, kicking, and arm-swinging movements performed to music. It is a fun way to exercise and promote cardiorespiratory development at the same time.

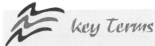

key Terms

Cross-training A combination of aerobic activities that contribute to overall fitness.

Aerobic dance A series of exercise routines performed to music.

Aerobics was developed initially in the early 1970s by Jacki Sorenson as a fitness program for Air Force wives in Puerto Rico. At first considered a fad, it now is a legitimate fitness activity with more than 20 million participants of all ages. Aerobics now are part of school curricula, health clubs, and recreational facilities.

High-impact aerobics (HIA) is the traditional form of aerobics. The movements exert a great amount of vertical force on the feet as they contact the floor. Proper leg conditioning through other forms of weight-bearing aerobic exercises (brisk walking and jogging), as well as strength training, are recommended prior to participating in high-impact aerobics.

High-impact aerobics is an intense activity, and it produces the highest rate of aerobics injuries. Shin splints, stress fractures, low-back pain, and tendinitis are all too common in HIA enthusiasts. These injuries are caused by the constant impact of the feet on firm surfaces. As a result, several alternative forms of aerobics have been developed.

In **low-impact aerobics (LIA)** the impact is less as each foot contacts the surface separately. The recommended exercise intensity has to be more difficult to maintain than HIA, though. To help elevate the exercise heart rate, all arm movements and weight-bearing actions that lower the center of gravity should be accentuated. Sustained movement throughout the program is also crucial to keep the heart rate in the target cardiorespiratory zone.

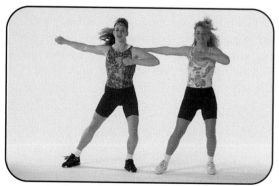

Aerobics is the most popular fitness activity for women in the United States.

A relatively new form of aerobics is **step aerobics (SA)**, in which participants step up and down from a bench. Benches range in height from 2 to 10 inches. Step aerobics adds another dimension to the aerobics program. As noted previously, variety adds enjoyment to aerobic workouts.

Step aerobics is viewed as a high-intensity but low-impact activity. The intensity of the activity can be controlled easily by the height of the bench. Aerobic benches or plates now are available commercially. The plates can be stacked together safely to adjust the height of the steps. Beginners are encouraged to use the lowest stepping height and then advance gradually to a higher bench. This will decrease the risk for injury. Even though one foot is always in contact with the floor or bench during step aerobics, this activity is not recommended for individuals with ankle, knee, or hip problems.

Other forms of aerobics include a combination of HIA and LIA, as well as moderate-impact aerobics (MIA). The latter incorporates **plyometric training**. This type of training is used frequently by jumpers (high, long, and triple jumpers) and athletes in sports that require quick jumping ability, such as basketball and gymnastics.

With moderate-impact aerobics, one foot is in contact with the ground most of the time. Participants, however, continually try to recover from all lower-body flexion actions. This is done by extending the hip, knee, and ankle joints quickly without allowing the foot (or feet) to leave the ground. These quick movements make the exercise intensity of moderate-impact aerobics quite high.

Swimming

Swimming is another excellent form of aerobic exercise. It uses almost all of the major muscle groups in the body, providing a good training stimulus for the heart and lungs. Swimming is a great exercise option for individuals who cannot jog or walk for extended periods.

Compared to other activities, the risk of injuries from swimming is low. The aquatic medium helps to support the body, taking pressure off bones and joints in the lower extremities and the back.

Maximal heart rates during swimming are approximately 10 to 13 beats per minute (bpm) lower than during running.[1] The horizontal position of the body is thought to aid blood flow distribution throughout the body, decreasing the demand on the cardiorespiratory system. Cool water temperatures and direct contact with the water seem to help dissipate body heat more efficiently, further decreasing the strain on the heart.

Some exercise specialists recommend that this difference in maximal heart rate (10 to 13 bpm) be subtracted prior to determining cardiorespiratory training intensities. For example, the estimated maximal swimming heart rate for a 20-year old would be approximately 187 bpm (220 − 20 − 13).

Studies are inconclusive as to whether this decrease in heart rate in water also occurs at submaximal intensities below 70% of maximal heart rate.[2,3,4] Further, research comparing physiologic differences between self-paced treadmill running and self-paced water aerobics exercise showed that individuals work at lower intensities in water.[5] One can argue, therefore, that apparently healthy people are able to achieve higher work capacities during land-based activities; therefore, the same exercise intensity can be given for water activities. If a lower intensity is used, training benefits may be less.

To produce better training benefits during swimming, the swimmer should minimize gliding periods such as those in the breast stroke and side stroke. Achieving proper training intensities with these strokes is difficult. The forward crawl is recommended for better aerobic results.

Overweight individuals need to swim fast enough to achieve an adequate training intensity. Excessive body fat makes the body more buoyant, and often the tendency is to just float along. This may be good for reducing stress and relaxing, but it does not greatly increase caloric

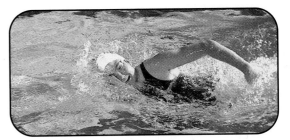

Swimming is a relatively injury-free activity.

expenditure to aid with weight loss. Walking or jogging in waist- or armpit-deep water are better choices for overweight individuals who cannot walk or jog on land for a long time.

With reference to the principle of specificity of training, swimming participants need to realize that cardiorespiratory improvements cannot be measured adequately with a walk/jog test. Most of the work with swimming is done by the upper body musculature. Although the heart's ability to pump more blood improves significantly with any type of aerobic activity, the primary increase in the cells' ability to utilize oxygen (VO_2 or oxygen uptake) with swimming occurs in the upper body and not the lower extremities. Therefore, fitness improvements with swimming are best attained by comparing changes in distances a person swims in a given time, say, 10 minutes.

Water Aerobics

Water aerobics is a relatively new form of exercise that is fun and safe for people of all ages.

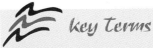

key Terms

High-impact aerobics Exercises incorporating movements in which both feet are off the ground at the same time momentarily.

Low-impact aerobics Exercises in which at least one foot is in contact with the ground or floor at all times.

Step aerobics A form of exercise that combines stepping up and down from a bench with arm movements.

Plyometric training A form of aerobic exercise that requires forceful jumps or springing off the ground immediately after landing from a previous jump.

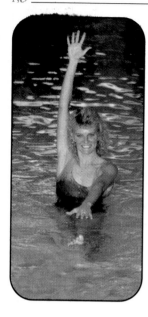

Water aerobics provides fitness, fun, and safety for people of all ages.

4. Heat dissipation in water is beneficial to obese participants, who seem to undergo a higher heat strain than average-weight individuals.

5. Water aerobics is available to swimmers and nonswimmers alike.

The exercises used during water aerobics are designed to elevate the heart rate, which contributes to cardiorespiratory development. In addition, the aquatic medium provides increased resistance for strength improvement with virtually no impact. Because of this resistance to movement, strength gains with water aerobics seem to be better than with land-based aerobic activities. Water exercises also help the joints move through their range of motion, promoting flexibility.

Another benefit is that weight can be reduced without the pain and fear of injuries that many who initiate exercise programs experience. Water aerobics provides a relatively safe environment for injury-free participation in exercise. The cushioned environment of the water allows patients recovering from leg and back injuries, individuals with joint problems, injured athletes, pregnant women, and obese people to benefit from water aerobics. In water, these people can exercise to develop and maintain cardiorespiratory endurance while limiting or eliminating the potential for further injury.

Similar to swimming, maximal heart rates achieved during water aerobics are lower than during running. The difference between water

Besides developing fitness, it provides an opportunity for socialization and fun in a comfortable and refreshing setting.

Water aerobics incorporates a combination of rhythmic arm and leg actions performed in a vertical position while submerged in waist- to armpit-deep water. The vigorous limb movements against the water's resistance during water aerobics provide the training stimuli for cardiorespiratory development.

The popularity of water aerobics as an exercise modality to develop the cardiorespiratory system has been on the rise in recent years. Its increase in popularity can be attributed to several factors:

1. Water buoyancy reduces weight-bearing stress on joints and thereby lessens the risk for injuries.

2. Water aerobics is a more feasible type of exercise for overweight individuals and those with arthritic conditions who may not be able to participate in weight-bearing activities such as walking, jogging, and aerobics.

3. Water aerobics is an excellent exercise modality to improve functional fitness in older adults (see Chapter 9).

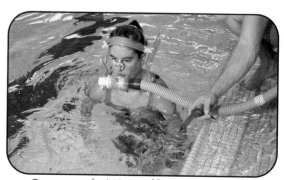

Oxygen uptake (VO_2) and heart rate assessment during water aerobics.

aerobics and running is about 10 bpm.[6] Apparently healthy people, nonetheless, can sustain land-based exercise intensities during a water aerobics workout and experience similar or greater fitness benefits than during land aerobics.[7] As with swimming, land-based exercise intensities, therefore, are recommended for water aerobics.

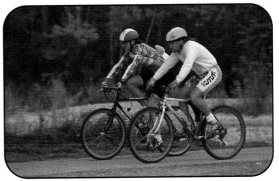

Road cycling requires skill for safety and enjoyment.

Cycling

Most people learn cycling in their youth. Because it is a non-weight-bearing activity, cycling is a good exercise modality for people with lower-body or lower-back injuries. Cycling helps to develop the cardiorespiratory system, as well as muscular strength and endurance in the lower extremities. With the advent of stationary bicycles, this activity can be performed year-round.

Raising the heart rate to the proper training intensity is more difficult with cycling. As the amount of muscle mass involved during aerobic exercise decreases, so does the demand placed on the cardiorespiratory system. The thigh muscles do most of the work in cycling, making it harder to achieve and maintain a high cardiorespiratory training intensity.

Maintaining a continuous pedaling motion and eliminating coasting periods helps the participant achieve a faster heart rate. Exercising for longer periods also helps to compensate for the lower heart rate intensity during cycling. Comparing cycling to jogging, similar aerobic benefits take roughly three times the distance at twice the speed of jogging. Cycling, however, puts less stress on muscles and joints than jogging does, making the former a good exercise modality for people who cannot walk or jog.

To increase riding efficiency, the height of the bike seat should be adjusted so the legs are almost completely extended when the heels are placed on the pedals. The body should not sway from side to side as the person rides. The cycling cadence also is important for maximal efficiency. Bike tension or gears should be set at a moderate level to be able to ride at 60 to 100 revolutions per minute.

Skill is important in road cycling. Cyclists must be in control of the bicycle at all times. They have to be able to maneuver the bike in traffic, maintain balance at slow speeds, switch gears, apply the brakes, watch for pedestrians and stoplights, and ride through congested areas. Stationary cycling, in contrast, does not require special skills. Nearly everyone can do it.

Safety is a key issue in road cycling. More than a million bicycle injuries occur each year. Proper equipment and common sense are necessary. A well designed and maintained bike is easier to maneuver. Toe clips are recommended to keep feet from sliding and to maintain equal upward and downward force on the pedals.

Bike riders must follow the same rules as motorists. Many accidents happen because cyclists run traffic lights and stop signs. Some further suggestions are:

- Use bike hand signals to let the traffic around you know of your intended actions.
- Don't ride side by side with another rider.
- Be aware of turning vehicles and cars backing out of alleys and parking lots; always yield to motorists in these situations.
- Avoid storm drains, which can cause unpleasant surprises; if you do not cross them at the proper angle, front wheels can get caught and riders may be thrown from the bike.

✎ Wear a good helmet, certified by the Snell Memorial Foundation or the American National Standards Institute. Many serious accidents and even deaths have been prevented by use of helmets. Fashion, aesthetics, comfort, or price should not be a factor when selecting and using a helmet for road cycling. Health and life are too precious to give up because of vanity and thriftiness.

✎ Wear appropriate clothes and shoes. Special clothing for cycling is not required. Clothing should be lightweight and not restrict movement. Shorts should be long enough to keep the skin from rubbing against the seat. For greater comfort, cycling shorts have extra padding sewn into the seat and crotch areas. Experienced cyclists often wear special shoes with a cleat that snaps directly onto the pedal.

The stationary bike is the most popular piece of equipment that sporting good stores sell. Before buying a stationary bike, though, be sure to try the activity for a few days. If you enjoy it, you may want to purchase one. Invest with caution. If you opt to buy a lower-priced model, you may be disappointed. Good stationary bikes have comfortable seats, are stable, and provide a smooth and uniform pedaling motion. A sticky bike that is hard to pedal leads to discouragement and ends up stored in the corner of a basement.

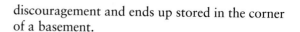

Aero-Belt Exercise

A new mode of aerobic activity is **Aero-belt** exercise. The objective of using the Aero-belt is to provide resistance to the arms during lower body physical activity, thereby increasing the person's oxygen consumption, energy expenditure, and development of upper-body strength and endurance during aerobic exercise. As in cross-country skiing, the Aero-belt provides resistance to the arms while walking, jogging, bounding, stair stepping, riding a stationary bicycle, or doing aerobics.

Using the Aero-belt actually can provide more upper-body conditioning benefits than cross-country skiing. Three different tension grades for the elastic cord are available for individual strength and fitness levels. Medium and high tension levels are mainly for strength conditioning, and low tension is for developing endurance.

The physiologic responses to Aero-belt walking (4.0 and 4.2 mph), jogging (6.0 mph), and step aerobics were investigated at Boise State University.[8,9,10] Increases in heart rate, oxygen uptake, and caloric expenditure ranged from 32% to 54% from regular walking, jogging, and step-aerobics to walking, jogging, and step-aerobics with an Aero-belt (see Figure 4.1).

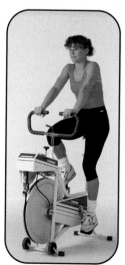

Exercising on a stationary bicycle adds variety to aerobic workouts.

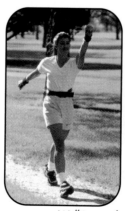
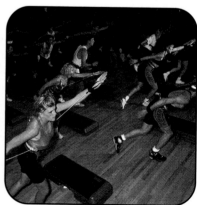

Walking and step-aerobics with an Aero-belt.

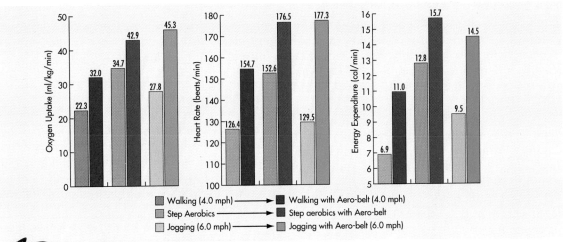

Figure 4.1 Oxygen uptake and heart rate responses to walking, jogging, and step aerobics with and without an Aero-belt.

Cross-Training

Cross-training combines two or more activities. This type of training is designed to enhance fitness, provide needed rest to tired muscles, decrease injuries, and eliminate the monotony and burnout of single-activity programs. Cross-training may combine aerobic and nonaerobic activities such as moderate jogging, speed training, and strength training.

Cross-training can produce better workouts than a single activity. For example, jogging develops the lower body and swimming builds the upper body. Rowing contributes to upper-body development and cycling builds the legs. Combining activities such as these provides good overall conditioning and at the same time helps to improve or maintain fitness. Cross-training also offers an opportunity to develop skill and have fun with different activities.

Speed training often is coupled with cross-training. Faster performance times in aerobic activities (running, cycling) are generated with speed or **interval training**. People who want to improve their running times often run shorter intervals at faster speeds than the actual racing pace. For example, a person wanting to run a

6-minute mile may run four 440-yard intervals at a speed of 1 minute and 20 seconds per interval. A 440-yard walk/jog can become a recovery interval between fast runs.

Strength training is used commonly with cross-training. It helps to condition muscles, tendons, and ligaments. Improved strength enhances overall performance in many activities and sports. For example, although road cyclists in one study who trained with weights showed no improvement in aerobic capacity, the cyclists had a 33% improvement in riding time to exhaustion when exercising at 75% of their maximal capacity.[11]

Rope Skipping

Rope skipping not only contributes to cardiorespiratory fitness, but it also helps to increase reaction time, coordination, agility, dynamic

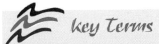

key Terms

Aero-belt® (Aerobic Endurance Resistance Overloader) A belt with an elastic band that slides freely through the belt and attaches to the wrists.

Interval training A repeated series of exercise work bouts (intervals) interspersed with low-intensity or rest intervals.

balance, and muscular strength in the lower extremities. At first, rope skipping may appear to be a highly strenuous form of aerobic exercise. Beginners often reach maximal heart rates after only 2 or 3 minutes of jumping. As skill improves, however, the energy demands decrease considerably.

Some people have claimed training benefits equal to a 30-minute jog in only 10 minutes of skipping. Although differences in strength and flexibility development are observed in different activities, 10 minutes at a certain heart rate provide similar cardiorespiratory benefits regardless of the nature of the activity. To obtain an adequate aerobic workout, the duration of exercise must be at least 20 minutes.

As with high-impact aerobics, a major concern of rope skipping is the stress placed on the lower extremities. Skipping with one foot at a time decreases the impact somewhat, but it does not eliminate the risk for injuries. Fitness experts recommend that skipping be used sparingly, and primarily as a supplement to an aerobic exercise program.

Cross-Country Skiing

Many consider cross-country skiing as the ultimate aerobic exercise because it requires vigorous lower and upper body movements. The large amount of muscle mass involved in cross-country skiing makes the intensity of the activity high, yet it places little strain on muscles and joints. One of the highest maximal oxygen uptakes ever measured (85 ml/kg/min) was found in an elite cross-country skier.

In addition to being an excellent aerobic activity, cross-country skiing is soothing. Skiing through the beauty of the snow-covered countryside can be highly enjoyable. Although the need for snow is an obvious limitation, simulating equipment for year-round cross-country training is available at many sporting goods stores.

Some skill is necessary to be proficient at cross-country skiing. Poorly skilled individuals are not able to elevate the heart rate enough to cause adequate aerobic development. Individuals contemplating this activity should seek out instruction to fully enjoy and reap the rewards of cross-country skiing.

In-Line Skating

Frequently referred to as blading, in-line skating has become a highly popular fitness activity in recent years. Suddenly millions of children and adults are trying this activity. In the early 1990s, stores could not keep up with the demand for in-line skates.

In-line skating has its origin in ice skating. Because warm-weather ice skating was not feasible, blades were replaced by wheels for summertime participation. Although four-wheel roller skates were invented in the mid 1700s, the activity did not really catch on until the late 1800s. The first in-line skate with five wheels in a row attached to the bottom of a shoe was developed in 1823. The in-line concept took hold in the United States in 1980, when hockey skates were adapted for road-skating.

In-line skating is an excellent activity to develop cardiorespiratory fitness and lower body strength. Intensity of the activity is regulated by how hard you blade. The key to effective cardiorespiratory training is to maintain a constant and rhythmic pattern, using arms and legs, and minimizing the gliding phase of blading. As a weight-bearing activity, in-line bladers also develop superior leg strength.

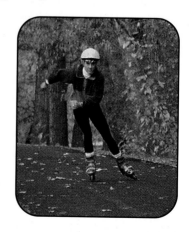

In-line skating is a low-impact fitness activity.

Instruction is necessary to achieve a minimum level of proficiency in this sport. Bladers commonly encounter hazards — potholes, cracks, rocks, gravel, sticks, oil, street curbs, and driveways. Unskilled bladers are more prone to falls and injuries.

Good equipment will make the activity safer and more enjoyable. Blades range in price from $40 to $500. Recreational participants need not purchase the more costly competitive skates. An adequate blade should provide strong ankle support; soft and flexible boots do not provide enough support. Small wheels offer more stability, and larger wheels enable greater speed. Blades should be purchased from stores that understand the sport and can provide sound advice according to skill level and needs.

Protective equipment is a must for in-line skating. Similar to road cycling, a good helmet that meets the safety standards set by the Snell Memorial Foundation or the American National Standards Institute is important to protect yourself in case of a fall. Wrist guards and knee and elbow pads also are recommended. The kneecap and the elbows are easily injured in a fall. Nighttime bladers should wear light-colored clothing and reflective tape.

Rowing

Rowing is a low-impact activity that provides a complete body workout. It mobilizes most major muscle groups including those in the arms, legs, hips, abdomen, trunk, and shoulders. Rowing is a good form of aerobic exercise and also, because of the nature of the activity (constant pushing and pulling against resistance) promotes total strength development.

To accommodate different fitness levels, workloads can be regulated on most rowing machines. Stationary rowing, however, is not among the most popular forms of aerobic exercise. Similar to stationary bicycles, people should try the activity for a few weeks before purchasing a unit.

Stair Climbing

If sustained for at least 20 minutes, stair climbing is an extremely efficient form of aerobic exercise. Precisely because of the high intensity of stair climbing, many people stay away from stairs and instead take escalators and elevators. Many people dislike living in two-story homes because they have to climb the stairs frequently.

Not too many places have enough flights of stairs to climb continuously for 20 minutes. Stair-climbing machines offer an alternative. Stair climbing has become so popular that fitness enthusiasts often wait in line at health clubs to use the machines.

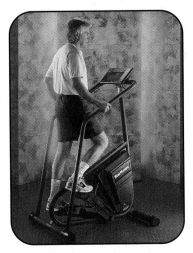

Stair climbing provides a rigorous aerobic workout.

In terms of injuries, stair climbing seems to be a relatively safe exercise modality. Because the feet never leave the climbing surface, it is considered to be a low-impact activity. Joints and ligaments are not strained during climbing. The intensity of exercise is controlled easily because most stair climbing equipment can be programmed to regulate the workload.

Racquet Sports

In racquet sports such as tennis, racquetball, squash, and badminton, the aerobic benefits are dictated by players' skill, intensity of the game,

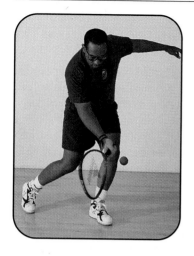

Racquet sports require rhythmic and continuous activity to provide cardiorespiratory benefits.

and how long they play the game. Skill is necessary to participate effectively in these sports and also is crucial to sustain continuous play. Frequent pauses during play do not allow people to maintain the heart rate in the appropriate target zone to stimulate cardiorespiratory development.

Many people who participate in racquet sports do so for enjoyment, social fulfillment, and relaxation. For cardiorespiratory fitness development these people supplement the sport with other forms of aerobic exercise such as jogging, cycling, or swimming.

If a racquet sport is the main form of aerobic exercise, participants need to try to run hard, fast, and as constantly as possible during play. They should not have to spend much time retrieving balls (bird or shuttlecock in badminton). Similar to low-impact aerobics, all movements should be accentuated by reaching out and bending more than usual, for better cardiorespiratory development.

Rating the Fitness Benefits of Aerobic Activities

The fitness contributions of the aerobic activities discussed in this chapter vary according to activities and individuals. As noted previously, the health-related components of physical fitness are cardiorespiratory endurance, muscular strength

and endurance, muscular flexibility, and body composition. Although an accurate assessment of the contributions to each fitness component are difficult to establish, a summary of likely benefits of these activities is provided in Table 4.1. Instead of a single rating or number, ranges are given for some of the categories because the benefits derived are based on the person's effort while participating in the activity.

Regular participation in aerobic activities provides notable health benefits, including an increase in cardiorespiratory endurance, quality of life, and longevity. The extent of cardiorespiratory development (improvement in VO_{2max}) depends on the intensity, duration, and frequency of the activity. The nature of the activity often dictates potential aerobic development. For example, jogging is much more strenuous than walking. The effort during exercise also influences the amount of physiological development. The training benefits of just going through the motions of a low-impact aerobics routine, as compared to accentuating all motions (see earlier discussion of low-impact aerobics) are of a different magnitude.

Table 4.1 includes a starting fitness level for each aerobic activity. Beginners should start with low-intensity activities that have a minimum risk for injuries. In some cases, such as in high-impact aerobics and rope skipping, the risk of injuries remains high despite adequate conditioning. These activities should be used only to supplement training and are not recommended as the sole mode of exercise.

The **MET** range for the various activities is included in Table 4.1. Physicians who work with cardiac patients frequently use METS. A 10-MET activity requires a tenfold increase in the resting energy requirement, or approximately 35 ml/kg/min. MET levels for a given activity vary

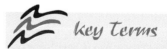

key Terms

METs (metabolic equivalent) An alternative method of prescribing exercise intensity; 1 MET represents body's energy requirement at rest, or equivalent of VO_2 of 3.5 ml/kg/min.

Table 4-1   Ratings for Various Aerobic Activities

Activity	Recommended Starting Fitness Level[1]	Injury Risk[2]	Potential Cardiovascular Endurance Development (VO_{2max})[3,5]	Upper Body Strength Development[3]	Lower Body Strength Development[3]	Upper Body Flexibility Development[3]	Lower Body Flexibility Development[3]	Weight Control[3]	MET Level[4,5,6]	Caloric Expenditure (cal/hour)[5,6]
Walking	B	L	1–2	1	2	1	1	3	4–6	300–450
Walking, Water—Chest-Deep	I	L	2–4	2	3	1	1	3	6–10	450–750
Hiking	B	L	2–4	1	3	1	1	3	6–10	450–750
Jogging	I	M	3–5	1	3	1	1	5	6–15	450–1125
Jogging, Deep Water	A	L	3–5	2	2	1	1	5	8–15	600–1125
High-Impact Aerobics	A	H	3–4	2	4	3	2	4	6–12	450–900
Low-Impact Aerobics	B	L	2–4	2	3	3	2	3	5–10	375–750
Step Aerobics	I	M	2–4	2	3–4	3	2	3–4	5–12	375–900
Moderate-Impact Aerobics	I	M	2–4	2	3	3	2	3	6–12	450–900
Swimming (front crawl)	B	L	3–5	4	2	3	1	3	6–12	450–900
Water Aerobics	B	L	2–4	3	3	3	2	3	6–12	450–900
Stationary Cycling	B	L	2–4	1	4	1	1	3	6–10	450–750
Road Cycling	I	M	2–5	1	4	1	1	3	6–12	450–900
Cross-Training	I	M	3–5	2–3	3–4	2–3	1–2	3–5	6–15	450–1125
Rope Skipping	I	H	3–5	2	4	1	2	3–5	8–15	600–1125
Cross-Country Skiing	B	M	4–5	4	4	2	2	4–5	10–16	750–1200
Aero-belt Exercise	B	M	4–5	4	4	3	2	4–5	10–16	750–1200
In-Line Skating	I	M	2–4	2	4	2	2	3	6–10	450–750
Rowing	B	L	3–5	4	2	3	1	4	8–14	600–1050
Stair Climbing	B	L	3–5	1	4	1	1	4–5	8–15	600–1125
Racquet Sports	I	M	2–4	3	3	3	2	3	6–10	450–750

[1] B = Beginner, I = Intermediate, A = Advanced
[2] L = Low, M = Moderate, H = High
[3] 1 = Low, 2 = Fair, 3 = Average, 4 = Good, 5 = Excellent
[4] One MET represents the rate of energy expenditure at rest (3.5 ml/kg/min). Each additional MET is a multiple of the resting value. For example, 5 METs represents an energy expenditure equivalent to five times the resting value or about 17.5 ml/kg/min.
[5] Varies according to the person's effort (exercise intensity) during exercise.
[6] Varies according to body weight.

according to the effort the individual expends. The harder a person exercises, the higher is the MET level.

The effectiveness of the various aerobic activities in aiding with weight management also is provided in Table 4.1. As a rule of thumb, the greater the muscle mass involved during exercise, the better are the results. Rhythmic and continuous activities that involve large amounts of muscle mass are most effective in burning calories.

Higher intensity activities burn more calories as well. Increasing exercise time will compensate for lower intensities. If carried out long enough (45 to 60 minutes five to six times per week), even walking can be an excellent exercise mode for weight loss. Additional information on a comprehensive weight management program is given in Chapter 6.

Skill-Related Fitness

Skill-related fitness is needed for success in athletics and effective performance of lifetime sports and activities. The components of skill-related fitness, defined in Chapter 1, are agility, balance, coordination, power, speed, and reaction time. All of these are important, to varying degrees, in sports and athletics.

For example, outstanding gymnasts must achieve good skill-related fitness in all components. A significant amount of *agility* is necessary to perform a double back somersault with a full twist — a skill during which the athlete must rotate simultaneously around one axis and twist around a different one. *Static balance* is essential for maintaining a handstand or a scale. *Dynamic balance* is needed to perform many of the gymnastics routines (e.g., balance beam, parallel bars, pommel horse). *Coordination* is important to successfully integrate various skills requiring varying degrees of difficulty into one routine. *Power* and *speed* are needed to propel the body into the air, such as when tumbling or vaulting. *Reaction time* is necessary in determining when to end rotation upon a visual clue, such as spotting the floor on a dismount.

As with the health-related fitness components, the principle of specificity of training also applies to skill-related components. According to this principle, the training program must be specific to the type of skill the individual is trying to achieve.

Development of agility, balance, coordination, and reaction time is highly task-specific. To attain a certain skill, the individual must practice the same task many times. It seems to have little crossover learning effect.

For instance, proper practice of a handstand (balance) eventually will lead to successful performance of the skill, but complete mastery of this skill does not ensure that the person will have immediate success when attempting to perform other static balance positions in gymnastics. Power and speed may be improved with a specific strength-training program or frequent repetition of the specific task to be improved, or both.

The rate of learning in skill-related fitness varies from person to person, mainly because these components seem to be determined to a large extent by hereditary factors. Individuals with good skill-related fitness tend to do better and learn faster when performing a wide variety of skills. Nevertheless, few individuals enjoy complete success in all skill-related components. Furthermore, though skill-related fitness can be enhanced with practice, improvements in reaction time and speed are limited and seem to be related primarily to genetic endowment.

Although we do not know how much skill-related fitness is desirable, everyone should attempt to develop and maintain a better than average level. This type of fitness is not only crucial for athletes, but it also is important in leading a better and happier life. Improving skill-related fitness not only affords an individual more enjoyment and success in lifetime sports (for instance, basketball, tennis, and racquetball), but it also can help a person cope more effectively in emergency situations. For example:

1. Good reaction time, balance, coordination, and agility can help you avoid a fall or break a fall and thereby minimize injury.

2. The ability to generate maximum force in a short time (power) may be crucial to ameliorate injury or even preserve life in a situation in which you may be called upon to lift a heavy object that has fallen on another person or even on yourself.

3. In our society, with an expanding average lifespan, maintaining speed can be especially important for older adults. Many of them and, for that matter, many unfit and overweight young people no longer have the speed they need to cross an intersection safely before the light changes for oncoming traffic.

Regular participation in a health-related fitness program can heighten performance of skill-related components, and vice versa. For example, significantly overweight people do not have good agility or speed. Because participating in aerobic and strength-training programs helps take off body fat, an overweight individual who loses weight through an exercise program can improve agility and speed.

A sound flexibility program decreases resistance to motion around body joints, which may increase agility, balance, and overall coordination. Improvements in strength definitely help develop power.

Similar to the fitness benefits of the aerobic activities discussed previously in this chapter and given in Table 4.1, the contributions of skill-related activities also vary among activities and individuals. The extent to which an activity helps develop each skill-related component varies not only by the effort the individual makes but, most important, by proper execution (technique) of the skill (correct coaching is highly recommended) and the individual's potential based on genetic endowment. As with aerobic activities, a summary of potential contributions to skill fitness for selected activities is provided in Table 4.2.

Team Sports

Choosing activities that you enjoy will greatly enhance your adherence to exercise. People tend to repeat things they enjoy doing. Enjoyment by itself is a reward. In this regard, combining individual activities (such as jogging or swimming) with team sports is fitting.

People with good skill-related fitness usually participate in lifetime sports and games, which in turn helps develop health-related fitness. Individuals who enjoyed basketball or soccer in their youth tend to stick to those activities later in life. Joining teams and community leagues may be all that is needed to stop contemplating and start participating.

The social aspect of team sports provides added incentive to participate. Team sports offer

Table 4-2 Contributions of Selected Activities to Skill-related Components

Activity	Agility	Balance	Coordination	Power	Reaction Time	Speed
Alpine Skiing	4	5	4	2	3	2
Archery	1	2	4	2	3	1
Badminton	4	3	4	2	4	3
Baseball	3	2	4	4	5	4
Basketball	4	3	4	3	4	3
Bowling	2	2	4	1	1	1
Cross-country Skiing	3	4	3	2	2	1
Football	4	4	4	4	4	3
Golf	1	2	5	3	1	3
Gymnastics	5	5	5	4	3	3
Ice Skating	5	5	5	3	3	3
In-line Skating	4	4	4	3	2	4
Judo/Karate	5	5	5	4	5	4
Racquetball	5	4	4	4	5	4
Soccer	5	3	5	5	3	4
Table Tennis	5	3	5	3	5	3
Tennis	4	3	5	3	5	3
Volleyball	4	3	5	4	5	3
Water Skiing	3	4	3	2	2	1
Wrestling	5	5	5	4	5	4

* 1 = Low, 2 = Fair, 3 = Average, 4 = Good, 5 = Excellent

an opportunity to interact with people who share a common interest with you. Being a member of a team creates responsibility — another incentive to exercise because you are expected to be there. Furthermore, team sports foster lifetime friendships, strengthening the social and emotional dimensions of wellness.

For those who were not able to participate in youth sports, it's never too late to start (see the discussion of behavior modification and motivation in Chapter 1). Don't be afraid to select a new activity, even if that means learning new skills. The fitness and social rewards will be ample.

Tips to Enhance Your Aerobic Workout

A typical aerobic workout is divided into three parts (see Figure 4.2):

1. A 5-minute warm-up phase during which the heart rate is increased gradually to the target zone.

2. The actual aerobic workout, during which the heart rate is maintained in the target zone for 20 to 60 minutes.

3. A 5- to 10-minute aerobic cool-down, when the heart rate is lowered gradually toward the resting level.

To monitor the target training zone, you will need to check your exercise heart rate. As described in Chapter 2, the pulse can be checked on the radial or the carotid artery. When you check the heart rate, begin with zero and count the number of beats in a 10-second period, then multiply by 6 to get the per-minute pulse rate. You should take your exercise heart rate for 10 seconds rather than a full minute because the heart rate begins to slow down 15 seconds after you stop exercising.

Feeling the pulse while exercising is difficult. Participants should stop during exercise to check the pulse. If the heart rate is too low, increase the intensity of the exercise. If the rate is too high, slow down. You may want to practice

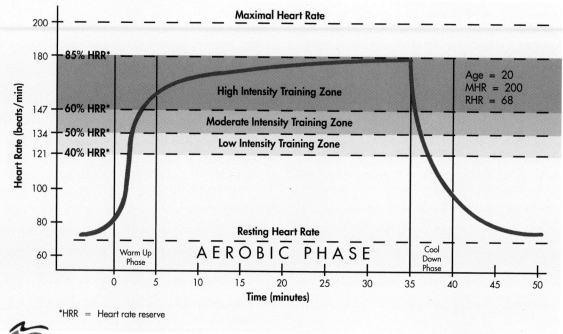

*HRR = Heart rate reserve

Figure 4.2 Typical aerobic workout pattern.

taking your pulse several times during the day to become familiar with the technique.

For the first few weeks of your program, you should monitor your heart rate several times during the exercise session. As you become familiar with your body's response to exercise, you may have to monitor the heart rate only twice — once at 5 to 7 minutes into the exercise session and a second time near the end of the workout.

Another technique sometimes used to determine your exercise intensity is simply to talk during exercise and then take the pulse immediately after that. Learning to associate the amount of difficulty when talking with the actual exercise heart rate will allow you to develop a sense of how hard you are working. Generally, if you can talk easily, you are not working hard enough. If you can talk but are slightly breathless, you should be close to the target range. If you cannot talk at all, you are working too hard.

If you have difficulty keeping up with your exercise program, you may need to reconsider your objectives and start much more slowly. Behavior modification is a process. From a physiological and psychological point of view, you may

not be able to carry out an exercise session for a full 20 to 30 minutes. For the first 2 to 3 weeks, therefore, you may just want to take a few 5-minute daily walks. As your body adapts physically and mentally, you then may increase the length and intensity of the exercise sessions gradually.

You should learn to listen to your body. At times you will feel unusually fatigued or have much discomfort. Pain is the body's way of letting you know something is wrong. If you have pain or undue discomfort during or after exercise, you need to slow down or discontinue your exercise program and notify the course instructor. The instructor may be able to pinpoint the reason for the discomfort or recommend that you consult your physician. You also are going to be able to prevent potential injuries by paying attention to pain signals and making adjustments accordingly.

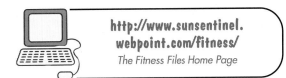

http://www.sunsentinel.
webpoint.com/fitness/
The Fitness Files Home Page

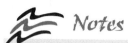

Notes

1. W. D. McArdle, F. I. Katch, and V. L. Katch, *Essentials of Exercise Physiology* (Philadelphia: Lea & Febiger, 1994).

2. J. L. Christi, L. M. Sheldahl, F. E. Tristani, L. S. Wann, K. B. Sagar, S. G. Levandoski, M. J. Ptacin, K. A. Sobocinski, and R. D. Morris, "Cardiovascular Regulation During Head-out Water Immersion Exercise," *Journal of Applied Physiology*, 69(1990), 657–664.

3. L. M. Sheldahl, F. E. Tristani, P. S. Clifford, C. V. Hughes, K. A. Sobocinski, and R. D. Morris, "Effect of Head-out Water Immersion on Cardiorespiratory Response to Dynamic Exercise," *Journal of American College of Cardiology*, 10(1987), 1254–1258.

4. J. Svedenhang and J. Seger, "Running on Land and in Water: Comparative Exercise Physiology," *Medicine and Science in Sports and Exercise*, 24(1992), 1155–1160.

5. W. W. K. Hoeger, "Is Water Aerobics Aerobic?" *Fitness Management*, 11(April 1995), 29–30, 43.

6. W. Hoeger, D. Hopkins, and D. Barber, "Physiologic Responses to Maximal Treadmill Running and Water Aerobic Exercise," *National Aquatics Journal*, 11(1995), 4–7.

7. W. W. K. Hoeger, T. S. Gibson, J. Moore, and D. R. Hopkins, "A Comparison of Selected Training Responses to Low Impact Aerobics and Water Aerobics," *National Aquatics Journal*, 9(1993), 13–16.

8. W. W. K. Hoeger, M. L. Chupurdia, W. J. Nurge, and D. E. Van Zee, "Physiologic Responses to Step Aerobics and Aero-belt Step Aerobics," *Medicine and Science in Sports and Exercise*, 26(1994) S43, 246.

9. D. R. Hopkins, W. W. K. Hoeger, D. E. Van Zee, and W. J. Nurge, "Physiologic Responses to Aero-belt Walking." *Medicine and Science in Sports and Exercise*, 26(1994) S43, 245.

10. W. J. Nurge, D. E. Van Zee, and W. W. K. Hoeger, "Physiologic Responses to Aero-belt Walking and Jogging," *Medicine and Science in Sports and Exercise*, 26(1994) S43, 247.

11. E. J. Marcinick, J. Potts, G. Schlabach, S. Will, P. Dawson, and B. F. Hurley, "Effects of Strength Training on Lactate Threshold and Endurance Performance," *Medicine and Science in Sports and Exercise*, 23(1991), 739–743.

Nutrition for Wellness

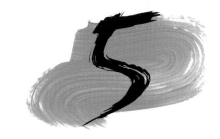

Scientific evidence has long linked good **nutrition** to overall health and well-being. Proper nutrition means that a person's diet is supplying all the essential nutrients to carry out normal tissue growth, repair, and maintenance. It also implies that the diet will provide enough substrates to produce the energy necessary for work, physical activity, and relaxation.

The typical American diet is too high in calories, sugar, fat, saturated fat, and sodium and not high enough in fiber. These factors all undermine good health. Over-consumption now is a major concern for many people in developed countries.

Diet and nutrition often play a crucial role in the development and progression of chronic diseases. A diet high in saturated fat and cholesterol increases the risk for atherosclerosis and coronary heart disease. In sodium-sensitive individuals, high salt intake has been linked to high blood pressure.

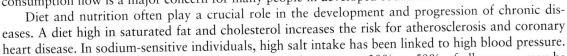

As many as 30% to 50% of all cancers may be diet-related. Obesity, diabetes mellitus, and osteoporosis also have been associated with faulty nutrition.

Objectives

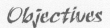

- Define nutrition and describe its relationship to health and well-being.
- Learn the functions of nutrients in the human body.
- Become familiar with the various food groups and learn how to achieve a balanced diet.
- Understand the role of antioxidants in preventing disease.
- Become familiar with eating disorders, their associated medical problems, and behavior patterns.
- Identify myths and fallacies regarding nutrition.

Essential Nutrients

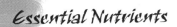

The essential nutrients the human body requires are carbohydrates, fats, protein, vitamins, minerals, and water. Carbohydrates, fats, proteins, and water are termed *macronutrients* because proportionately large amounts are needed daily. Nutritionists refer to vitamins and minerals as *micronutrients* because the body requires them in only small amounts.

Depending on the amount of nutrients and calories they contain, foods can be classified as

93

high-nutrient density or low-nutrient density. High-nutrient density foods contain a low or moderate amount of calories but are packed with nutrients. Foods that are high in calories but contain few nutrients are of low-nutrient density and are commonly called "junk food."

Carbohydrates

Carbohydrates are the major source of calories the body uses to provide energy for work, cell maintenance, and heat. They also help regulate fat and metabolize protein. Each gram of carbohydrates provides the human body with 4 calories. The major sources of carbohydrates are breads, cereals, fruits, vegetables, and milk and other dairy products. Carbohydrates are divided into simple carbohydrates and complex carbohydrates.

Simple Carbohydrates

Simple carbohydrates (such as candy, soda, and cakes) frequently are denoted as sugars and have little nutritive value. These carbohydrates are divided into monosaccharides (glucose, fructose, and galactose) and disaccharides (sucrose, lactose, and maltose). Simple carbohydrates often take the place of more nutritive foods in the diet.

Complex Carbohydrates

Complex carbohydrates are formed when simple carbohydrate molecules are linked together. Two types of complex carbohydrates are starches and dextrins. *Starches* are found commonly in seeds, corn, nuts, grains, roots, potatoes, and legumes. *Dextrins* are formed from the breakdown of large starch molecules exposed to dry heat, such as when bread is baked or cold cereals are produced. Complex carbohydrates provide many valuable nutrients and also are an excellent source of fiber or roughage.

Fiber

Another form of complex carbohydrate is **fiber**. A high-fiber diet gives a person a feeling of fullness without added calories. Fiber is present mainly in leaves, skins, roots, and seeds.

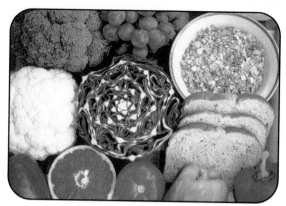

High-fiber foods are essential in a healthy diet.

Processing and refining foods removes almost all of the natural fiber. In our diet the main sources of fiber are whole-grain cereals and breads, fruits, vegetables, and legumes. Fiber is important in the diet because it helps decrease the risk for cardiovascular disease and cancer. Other health disorders that have been tied to low fiber intake are constipation, diverticulitis, hemorrhoids, gallbladder disease, and obesity.

The recommended amount of fiber intake is about 25 to 30 grams per day. Because most Americans eat only 10 to 12 grams per day, they

Fiber Content of Selected Foods

Food	Portion	Fiber (grams)
Apple with skin	1 medium	3
Beans, baked	1/2 cup	6
Beans, red/kidney	1/2 cup	10
Bread, whole wheat	1 slice	2
Bread, white	1 slice	1
Broccoli (cooked)	1/2 cup	2
Carrot, raw	1 medium	2
Cereal, Raisin Bran	1 cup	8
Cereal, All Bran	1 cup	10
Cereal, Quaker Oats	1 cup	8
Cereal, Cheerios	1 cup	3
Lentils	1/2 cup	4
Orange	1 medium	3
Potato	1 medium	4
Strawberries	1 cup	4

are at increased risk for disease. Fiber intake can be increased by eating more fruits, vegetables, legumes, grains, and cereals. A 6-year follow-up study provided further evidence linking increased fiber intake of 30 grams per day to a significant reduction in heart attacks, cancer of the colon, breast cancer, diabetes, and diverticulitis.[1]

Fibers typically are classified according to their solubility in water. Soluble fiber dissolves in water and forms a gel-like substance that encloses food particles. This property allows soluble fiber to bind and excrete fats from the body. This type of fiber has been shown to decrease blood cholesterol and blood sugar levels.

Tips to Increase Fiber in the Diet

- Eat more vegetables, either raw or steamed until crunchy
- Eat daily salads that include a wide variety of vegetables
- Eat more fruit, including the skin
- Choose whole-wheat and whole-grain products
- Choose breakfast cereals with more than 3 grams of fiber per serving
- Sprinkle a teaspoon or two of unprocessed bran or 100% bran cereal on your favorite breakfast cereal
- Add high-fiber cereals to casseroles and desserts
- Add beans to soups, salads, and stews
- Add vegetables to sandwiches: sprouts, green and red pepper strips, diced carrots, sliced cucumbers, red cabbage, onions
- Add vegetables to spaghetti: broccoli, cauliflower, sliced carrots, mushrooms.
- Experiment with unfamiliar fruits and vegetables — collards, kale, broccoflower, asparagus, papaya, mango, kiwi, starfruit.
- Blend fruit juice with small pieces of fruit and crushed ice.
- When increasing fiber in your diet, drink plenty of fluids.

Soluble fibers are found primarily in oats, fruits, barley, and legumes.

Insoluble fiber is not easily dissolved in water, and the body cannot digest it. This fiber is important because it binds water causing a softer and bulkier stool that increases peristalsis (involuntary muscle contractions of intestinal walls, forcing the stool onward) and allows food residues to pass through the intestinal tract more quickly. Speeding up passage of food residues through the intestines seems to lower the risk for colon cancer, mainly because cancer-causing agents are not in contact as long with the intestinal wall. Insoluble fiber also is thought to bind with carcinogens (cancer-producing substances), and more water in the stool may dilute the cancer-causing agents, lessening their potency. Sources of insoluble fiber include wheat, cereals, vegetables, and skins of fruits.

Fats

Fats, or **lipids**, are the most concentrated source of energy. Each gram of fat supplies 9 calories to the body. Fats also are part of the cell structure, used as stored energy and as an insulator to preserve body heat. They absorb shock, supply essential fatty acids, and carry the fat-soluble vitamins A, D, E, and K. The main sources of dietary fat are milk and other dairy products, and meats and alternates. Fats are classified into simple, compound, and derived fats.

Simple fats consist of a glyceride molecule linked to one, two, or three units of fatty acids. According to the number of fatty acids attached, simple fats are divided into *monoglycerides* (one

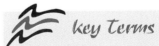 key Terms

Nutrition A science that studies the relationship of foods to optimal health and performance.

Carbohydrates Compounds composed of carbon, hydrogen, and oxygen used by the body as its major source of energy.

Fiber A general term used to denote plant material that cannot be digested by human digestive enzymes.

Fats (lipids) A class of nutrients used by the body as a source of energy.

fatty acid), *diglycerides* (two fatty acids), and *triglycerides* (three fatty acids). More than 90% of the weight of fat in foods and more than 95% of the stored fat in the human body are in the form of triglycerides.

The length of the carbon atom chain and the amount of hydrogen saturation in fatty acids vary. Based on the extent of saturation, fatty acids are said to be *saturated* or *unsaturated*. Unsaturated fatty acids are classified further into *monounsaturated* and *polyunsaturated* fats. Saturated fatty acids are mainly of animal origin. Unsaturated fats are found mostly in plant products.

In *saturated fatty acids* the carbon atoms are fully saturated with hydrogens; only single bonds link the carbon atoms on the chain. These saturated fatty acids often are called saturated fats. Examples of foods high in saturated fatty acids are meats, meat fat, lard, whole milk, cream, butter, cheese, ice cream, hydrogenated oils (a process that makes oils saturated), coconut oil, and palm oils.

In unsaturated fatty acids (unsaturated fats) double bonds form between the unsaturated carbons. In monounsaturated fatty acids (MUFA) only one double bond is found along the chain. Examples are olive, canola, rapeseed, peanut, and sesame oils. Polyunsaturated fatty acids (PUFA) contain two or more double bonds between unsaturated carbon atoms along the chain. Corn, cottonseed, safflower, walnut, sunflower, and soybean oils are high in polyunsaturated fatty acids.

Saturated fats tend to be solids that typically do not melt at room temperature. Unsaturated fats usually are liquid at room temperature. Coconut and palm oils are exceptions; they are liquids that are high in saturated fats. Shorter fatty acid chains also tend to be liquid at room temperature. In general, saturated fats raise the blood cholesterol level, whereas polyunsaturated and monounsaturated fats tend to lower blood cholesterol (the role of cholesterol in health and disease is discussed in Chapter 8).

Compound fats are a combination of simple fats and other chemicals. Examples are phospholipids, glucolipids, and lipoproteins.

Derived fats combine simple and compound fats. Sterols are an example. Although sterols contain no fatty acids, they are considered lipids because they do not dissolve in water. The most often mentioned sterol is cholesterol, which is found in many foods or can be manufactured from saturated fats in the body.

Proteins

Proteins are used to build and repair tissues including muscles, blood, internal organs, skin, hair, nails, and bones. They are a part of hormones, enzymes, and antibodies, and help maintain normal body fluid balance. Proteins also can be used as a source of energy, but only if not enough carbohydrates are available. The primary sources are meats and alternates and milk and other dairy products.

They are composed of **amino acids.** Amino acids contain nitrogen, carbon, hydrogen, and oxygen. Nine of the 20 amino acids are called *essential amino acids* because the body cannot produce them. The other 11, termed *nonessential amino acids*, can be manufactured in the body if food proteins in the diet provide enough nitrogen. For normal body function all amino acids must be present at the same time.

Protein deficiency is not a problem in the usual North American diet. Two glasses of skim milk combined with about 4 ounces of poultry or fish meet the daily protein requirement. Protein deficiency, however, could be a concern in some vegetarian diets. Vegetarians rely primarily on foods from the bread and cereal and fruit and vegetable groups and avoid most foods from the animal sources found in the milk and meat groups. Vegetarian diets can be balanced, but this is a complicated issue that cannot be covered in a few paragraphs. Those who are interested in vegetarian diets should consult other resources.

Vitamins

Vitamins function as antioxidants; as coenzymes (primarily the B complex), which regulate the work of enzymes; and vitamin D even functions as a hormone. Based on their solubility, **vitamins** are classified into two types: *fat-soluble vitamins* (A, D, E, and K) and *water-soluble vitamins* (B complex and C). The body cannot manufacture vitamins; they can be obtained only through a well balanced diet. Additional information on the importance of vitamins is presented later in this chapter.

Minerals

Minerals serve several important functions. They are constituents of all cells, especially those in hard parts of the body (bones, nails, teeth). They are crucial in maintaining water balance and the acid-base balance. They are essential components of respiratory pigments, enzymes, and enzyme systems, and they regulate muscular and nervous tissue excitability.

Water

Water is the most important nutrient, involved in almost every vital body process. Water is used in digesting and absorbing food, in the circulatory process, in removing waste products, in building and rebuilding cells, and in transporting other nutrients. Water is contained in almost all foods but primarily in liquid foods, fruits, and vegetables. In addition to the natural water content consumed in foods, every person should drink eight to ten glasses of fluids a day.

A Balanced Diet

Most people would like to live life to its fullest, have good health, and lead a productive life. One of the ways to do this is through a well balanced diet. As illustrated in Figure 5.1, the recommended guidelines state that daily caloric intake should be distributed so about 58% of the total calories come from carbohydrates (48% complex carbohydrates and 10% sugar), less than 30% of the total calories from fat (equally divided, 10% each, among saturated, monounsaturated, and polyunsaturated fats), and 12% of the total calories from protein (0.8 grams of protein per kilogram, or 2.2 pounds, of body weight). The diet also must include all the essential vitamins, minerals, and water.

One of the most detrimental health habits facing people today is the large amount of fat in

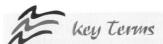

key Terms

Proteins A nutrient classification used by the body to build and repair body tissues.

Amino acids The basic building blocks of protein.

Vitamins Organic substances essential for normal bodily metabolism, growth, and development.

Minerals Inorganic elements needed by the body.

Current

Complex 24%	Simple 27%	Mono-unsaturated 12%	Poly-unsaturated 12%	Saturated 13%	Protein 12%

◄——— Carbohydrates: 51% ———► ◄——— Fat: 37% ———►

Recommended

Complex 48%	Simple 10%	Mono-unsaturated 10%	Poly-unsaturated 10%	Saturated 10%	Protein 12%

◄——— Carbohydrates: 58% ———► ◄——— Fat: 30% ———►

Figure 5.1 *Current and recommended caloric distribution of fat, carbohydrate, and protein intake (expressed in percentages of total daily caloric intake.*

the diet. Fat consumption in the average diet is about 37% of the total caloric intake; 30% or lower is recommended. To decrease the risk for disease, particularly cardiovascular disease and cancer, people must make a deliberate effort to decrease total fat intake. Being able to identify sources of fat in the diet is imperative to decrease fat intake.

As illustrated in Figure 5.2, each gram of carbohydrates and protein supplies the body with 4 calories, and fat provides 9 calories per gram consumed (alcohol yields 7 calories per gram). In this regard, just looking at the total amount of grams consumed for each type of food can be misleading.

For example, a person who consumes 160 grams of carbohydrates, 100 grams of fat, and 70 grams of protein has a total intake of 330 grams of food. This indicates that 33% of the total grams of food is in the form of fat (100 grams of fat ÷ 330 grams of total food × 100).

Almost half of this diet consists of fat calories. In the diet, 640 calories are derived from carbohydrates (160 grams × 4 calories/gram), 280 calories from protein (70 grams × 4 calories/gram), and 900 calories from fat (100 grams × 9 calories/gram), for a total of 1,820 calories. If 900 calories are derived from fat, you can see that almost half of the total caloric intake is in the form of fat (900 ÷ 1,820 × 100 = 49.5%).

Realizing that each gram of fat equals 9 calories is a useful guideline when figuring the fat content of individual foods. As shown in Figure 5.3, all you need to do is multiply the grams of fat by 9 and divide by the total calories in that specific food. Multiply that number by 100 to get the percentage. For example, if a food label lists a total of 100 calories and 7 grams of fat, the fat content is 63% of total calories. This simple guideline can help you decrease fat in your diet.

Recommended Dietary Allowances and Daily Values

Every 10 years or so the National Academy of Sciences issues new **Recommended Dietary Allowances (RDA)** based on a review of the most current research. The RDAs usually are set high enough to encompass 97.5% of the healthy population in the United States.

Based on 1993 regulations by the Food and Drug Administration (FDA), food labels now provide consumers with **Daily Values (DVs)**. The DVs are based on a 2,000-calorie diet and may require adjustments depending on an individual's daily caloric needs.

The food label (Figure 5.4) is a better guide for planning a daily diet. For example, if the DV for carbohydrates in a given meal adds up to only 35%, you know that several additional high-carbohydrate food items are required throughout that day to reach the 100% DV. Further, if the DV for fat from another food item is 60% or 70%, you should limit your fat intake during the rest of that day.

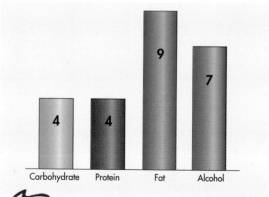

Figure 5.2 Caloric value (calories) per gram of food.

Servings = 120 calories   Fat = 5 g

Percent Fat Calories = (g of fat × 9) ÷ calories per serving × 100

5 g of fat × 9 calories per g of fat = 45 calories from fat

45 calories from fat ÷ 120 calories per serving × 100 = 38% fat

Figure 5.3 Determining percent calories from fat in food.

Both the RDA and the DVs apply only to healthy people. They are not intended for people who are ill and may require additional nutrients or dietary adjustments.

Nutrient Analysis

Achieving and maintaining a balanced diet is not as difficult as most people think. The Food Guide Pyramid contained in Figure 5.5, published by the U.S. Department of Agriculture, provides simple and sound instructions for nutrition. The pyramid contains five major food groups, along with fats, oils, and sugar, which are to be used sparingly. The daily recommended number of servings of the five major food groups are:

1. 6 to 11 servings of the bread, cereal, rice, and pasta group
2. 3 to 5 servings of the vegetable group
3. 2 to 4 servings of the fruit group
4. 2 or 3 servings of the milk, yogurt, and cheese group
5. 2 or 3 servings of the meat, poultry, fish, dry beans, eggs, and nuts group

As illustrated in the Food Guide Pyramid, grains, vegetables, and fruits provide the nutritional foundation for a healthy diet. Fruits and vegetables should include as a daily minimum one good source of vitamin A (apricots, cantaloupe, broccoli, carrots, pumpkin, dark green leafy vegetables) and one good source of vitamin C (citrus fruit, kiwi, cantaloupe, strawberries, broccoli, cabbage, cauliflower, green pepper).

An entirely new field of research with promising results in disease prevention, especially in the fight against cancer, is in the area of **phytochemicals**[2] ("phyto" comes from the Greek word for plant). The main function of phytochemicals in plants is to protect them from sunlight. In humans, however, they seem to have a powerful ability to block the formation of cancerous tumors. Their actions are so diverse that, at almost every stage of cancer, phytochemicals

---

Nutrition Facts

Serving Size 1 cup (240 ml)
Servings Per Container 4

Amount Per Serving

Calories 120   Calories from Fat 45

	% Daily Value*
Total Fat 5g	8%
Saturated Fat 3g	15%
Cholesterol 20mg	7%
Sodium 120mg	5%
Total Carbohydrate 12g	4%
Dietary Fiber 0g	0%
Sugars 12g	
Protein 8g	

Vitamin A	10%	Vitamin C	4%
Calcium	30%	Iron	0%

* Percent Daily Values are based on a 2,000 calorie diet. Your daily values may be higher or lower depending on your calorie needs:

		Calories	2,000	2,500
Total Fat	Less than		65g	80g
Sat Fat	Less than		20g	25g
Cholesterol	Less than		300mg	300mg
Sodium	Less than		2,400mg	2,400mg
Total Carbohydrate			300g	375g
Fiber			25g	30g

Calories per gram:
Fat 9 • Carbohydrate 4 • Protein 4

Figure 5.4 Current food label using Daily Values (DVs).

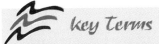

key Terms

Recommended Dietary Allowances (RDAs) Daily nutrient intakes suggested for healthy people.

Daily Values (DVs) The percentage of recommended daily amounts of vitamins, minerals, total fat, saturated fat, cholesterol, sodium, carbohydrates, fiber, and sugar.

Phytochemicals Compounds found in vegetables and fruits with cancer-fighting properties.

KEY
● Fat (naturally occurring and added)
▼ Sugars (added)

These symbols show fats, oils, and added sugars in foods.

Fats, Oils, & Sweets
USE SPARINGLY

Meat, Poultry, Fish, Dry Beans, Eggs, & Nuts Group
2-3 SERVINGS

Milk, Yogurt, & Cheese Group
2-3 SERVINGS

Vegetable Group
3-5 SERVINGS

Fruit Group
2-4 SERVINGS

Bread, Cereal, Rice, & Pasta Group
6-11 SERVINGS

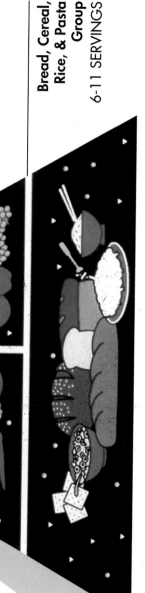
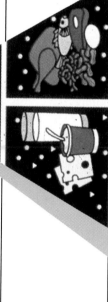
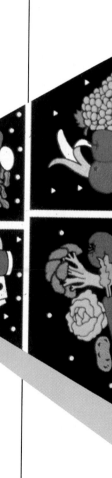

What counts as one serving?

Breads, Cereals, Rice, and Pasta
1 slice of bread
1/2 cup of cooked rice or pasta
1/2 cup of cooked cereal
1 ounce of ready-to-eat cereal

Vegetables
1/2 cup of chopped raw or cooked vegetables
1 cup of leafy raw vegetables

Fruits
1 piece of fruit or melon wedge
3/4 cup of juice
1/2 cup of canned fruit
1/4 cup of dried fruit

Milk, Yogurt, and Cheese
1 cup of milk or yogurt
1½ to 2 ounces of cheese

Meat, Poultry, Fish, Dry Beans, Eggs, and Nuts
2-½ to 3 ounces of cooked lean meat, poultry, or fish
Count 1/2 cup of cooked beans, or 1 egg, or 2 tablespoons of peanut butter as 1 ounce of lean meat (about 1/3 serving)

Fats, Oils, and Sweets
LIMIT CALORIES FROM THESE especially if you need to lose weight

The amount you eat may be more than one serving. For example, a dinner portion of spaghetti would count as two or three servings of pasta.

How many servings do you need each day?

	Women & some older adults	Children, teen girls, active women, most men	Teen boys & active men
Calorie level*	about 1,600	about 2,200	about 2,800
Bread group	6	9	11
Vegetable group	3	4	5
Fruit group	2	3	4
Milk group	2–3**	2–3**	**2–3
Meat group	2, for a total of 5 ounces	2, for a total of 6 ounces	3, for a total of 7 ounces

* These are the calorie levels if you choose lowfat, lean foods from the 5 major food groups and use foods from the fats, oils, and sweets group sparingly.

** Women who are pregnant or breastfeeding, teenagers, and young adults to age 24 need 3 servings.

A Closer Look at Fat and Added Sugars

The small tip of the Pyramid shows fats, oils, and sweets. These are foods such as salad dressings, cream, butter, margarine, sugars, soft drinks, candies, and sweet desserts. Alcoholic beverages are also part of this group. These foods provide calories but few vitamins and minerals. Most people should go easy on foods from this group.

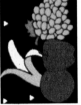
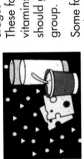

Some fat or sugar symbols are shown in the other food groups. That's to remind you that some foods in these groups can also be high in fat and added sugars, such as cheese or ice cream from the milk group, or french fries from the vegetable group. When choosing foods for a healthful diet, consider the fat and added sugars in your choices from all the food groups, not just fats, oils, and sweets from the Pyramid tip.

*Developed by the U.S. Department of Agriculture to promote a healthy diet for people in the United States.

Figure 5.5   *Food Guide Pyramid: A guide to daily food choices.*

have the ability to block, disrupt, slow down, or even reverse the process (also see Chapter 8).

These compounds are not found in pills. The message here is to eat a diet with ample fruits and vegetables. The recommendation of five to nine servings of fruits and vegetables daily has absolutely no substitute. People can't expect to eat a poor diet, pop a few pills, and derive the same benefits.

Milk, poultry, fish, and meats are to be consumed in moderation. Skim milk and low-fat milk products are recommended. Daily, 3 ounces of poultry, fish, or meat are advised, and no more than 6 ounces per day. All visible fat and skin should be trimmed off meats and poultry before cooking.

The difficult part for most people is retraining themselves to adopt a lifetime healthy nutrition plan. You can achieve a balanced diet if you (a) avoid excessive fats, oils, sweets, sodium, and alcohol, (b) increase your fiber intake, and (c) eat the minimum number of servings recommended for each of the five major groups in the Food Guide Pyramid.

To aid you in balancing your diet, a form is given in Figure 5.6 for you to record your daily food intake. First, make as many copies as the number of days you wish to analyze. Whenever you eat something, record the food and amount eaten. Doing this immediately after each meal will enable you to keep track of your actual food intake more easily.

At the end of each day, consult the list of foods in Appendix E and record the code and number of calories for all foods consumed. Referring to Figure 5.6, record the number of servings under the respective food groups. If you eat twice the amount of a standard serving, double the calories and the number of servings.

You can evaluate your diet by checking whether you ate the minimum required servings for each food group. If you meet the minimum required servings at the end of each day, you are doing quite well in balancing your diet.

In addition to meeting the daily serving guidelines, a complete nutrient analysis is recommended to rate your diet accurately. A nutrient analysis can pinpoint potential problem areas in your diet, such as too much fat, saturated fat, cholesterol, sodium, and the like. A complete nutrient analysis can be an educational experience because most people do not realize how detrimental and non-nutritious many common foods are.

You may want to do the analysis with the aid of computer software.* Use the information you have recorded already on the form provided in Figure 5.6. Before running the software, fill out the information at the top of this form (age, weight, sex, activity rating, and number of days to be analyzed), and make sure the foods are recorded by the code and standard amounts given in the list of selected foods in Appendix E. The software accommodates up to 7 days of analysis. It covers calories, carbohydrates, fats, cholesterol, and sodium, as well as eight crucial nutrients: protein, calcium, iron, vitamin A, thiamin, riboflavin, niacin, and vitamin C. If the diet has enough of these eight nutrients, the foods (in natural form) consumed to provide these nutrients typically contain all the other nutrients the human body needs. The computer-generated printout also includes the average daily nutrient intake and the RDA comparison for all the above nutrients.

Nutrient Supplementation

Approximately half of all adults in the United States take daily nutrient supplements. RDA vitamin and mineral requirements for the body normally can be met by consuming as few as 1,200 calories per day, as long as the diet contains the recommended servings from the five food groups.

For most people, excessive vitamin and mineral supplementation is unnecessary and sometimes is unsafe. Iron deficiency (determined through blood testing) is an exception for women who have heavy menstrual flow. Some

---

*Your instructor may have a copy of the Nutrient Analysis software available from Morton Publishing Company, Englewood, Colorado.

Date: _____

Name: _____ Age: _____ Weight: _____ lbs.

Sex: _____ M _____ F   (Pregnant – P, Lactating – L, Neither – N)

Activity Rating: Sedentary (limited physical activity)   = 1
                Moderate physical activity   = 2
                Hard labor (strenuous physical activity)   = 3

Number of days to be analyzed: _____   Day: _____ (1, 2 . . .)

No.	Code*	Food	Amount	Calories	Bread, Cereal, Rice & Pasta	Vegetable	Fruit	Milk, Yogurt & Cheese	Meat, Poultry, Fish, Dry Beans, Eggs, & Nuts
									Food Groups
1									
2									
3									
4									
5									
6									
7									
8									
9									
10									
11									
12									
13									
14									
15									
16									
17									
18									
19									
20									
21									
22									
23									
24									
25									
26									
27									
28									
29									
30									
Totals									
Recommended Servings				**	6–11	3–5	2–4	2–3	2–3
Deficiencies									

*See list of nutritive value of selected foods in Appendix E.
**See Table 5.1.

 Figure 5.6   Daily diet record form.

Date: _____

Name: _____ Age: _____ Weight: _____ lbs.

Sex: _____ M _____ F   (Pregnant – P, Lactating – L, Neither – N)

Activity Rating: Sedentary (limited physical activity)   = 1
                  Moderate physical activity   = 2
                  Hard labor (strenuous physical activity)   = 3

Number of days to be analyzed: _____   Day: _____ (1, 2 . . .)

No.	Code*	Food	Amount	Calories	Bread, Cereal, Rice & Pasta	Vegetable	Fruit	Milk, Yogurt & Cheese	Meat, Poultry, Fish, Dry Beans, Eggs, & Nuts
					Food Groups				
1									
2									
3									
4									
5									
6									
7									
8									
9									
10									
11									
12									
13									
14									
15									
16									
17									
18									
19									
20									
21									
22									
23									
24									
25									
26									
27									
28									
29									
30									
Totals									
Recommended Servings				**	6–11	3–5	2–4	2–3	2–3
Deficiencies									

*See list of nutritive value of selected foods in Appendix E.
**See Table 5.1

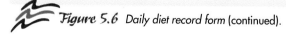

Figure 5.6   Daily diet record form (continued).

pregnant and lactating women also may need supplementation. In these instances, supplements should be taken under a physician's supervision.

Other people who may benefit from supplementation are alcoholics and street-drug users who do not eat a balanced diet, smokers, strict vegetarians, individuals on extremely low-calorie diets, elderly people who don't eat balanced meals regularly, and newborn infants (usually given a single dose of vitamin K to prevent abnormal bleeding).

Antioxidants: Free Radical Combatants

Much research currently is being done to study the effects of **antioxidants** in thwarting several chronic diseases. Vitamins C, E, beta-carotene (a precursor to vitamin A), and the mineral selenium are antioxidants (see Table 5.1). Oxygen is utilized during metabolism to change carbohydrates and fats into energy. During this process oxygen is transformed into stable forms of water and carbon dioxide. A small amount of oxygen, however, ends up in an unstable form, referred to as *oxygen free radicals.*

A free radical molecule has a normal proton nucleus with a single unpaired electron. Having only one electron makes the free radical extremely reactive, and it looks constantly to pair the electron with one from another molecule. When a free radical steals the second electron from another molecule, that other molecule in

turn becomes a free radical. This chain reaction goes on until two free radicals meet to form a stable molecule.

Free radicals attack and damage proteins and lipids, in particular cell membranes and DNA. This damage is thought to contribute to the development of conditions such as cardiovascular disease, cancer, emphysema, cataracts, Parkinson's disease, and premature aging. Solar radiation, cigarette smoke, radiation, and other environmental factors also seem to encourage the formation of free radicals. Antioxidants are thought to offer protection by absorbing free radicals before they can cause damage and also by interrupting the sequence of reactions once damage has begun, thwarting certain chronic diseases.

Antioxidants are found abundantly in food, especially in fruits and vegetables. Unfortunately, only 9% of Americans eat the minimum five daily servings of fruits and vegetables[3] (five to nine is the recommendation).

In a departure from past recommendations, in 1994 the editorial board of the University of California at Berkeley *Wellness Letter* issued the

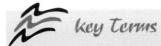

key Terms

Antioxidants Compounds that prevent oxygen from combining with other substances it might damage.

Table 5.1 Antioxidant Content of Selected Foods

Nutrient	Good Sources	Antioxidant Effect
Vitamin C	Citrus fruit, kiwi fruit, cantaloupe, strawberries, broccoli, green or red peppers, cauliflower, cabbage	Appears to inactivate oxygen free radicals
Vitamin E	Vegetable oils, yellow and green leafy vegetables, margarine, wheatgerm, oatmeal, almonds, and whole grain breads, cereals	Protects lipids from oxidation
Beta-carotene	Carrots, squash, pumpkin, sweet potatoes, broccoli, green leafy vegetables	Soaks up oxygen free radicals
Selenium	Seafood, meat, whole grains	Helps prevent damage to cell structures

following antioxidant nutrient guidelines for people who eat at least five daily servings of antioxidant-rich fruits and vegetables:[4]

🖎 250 to 500 mg of vitamin C

🖎 200 to 800 IU [International Units] of vitamin E

🖎 10,000 to 25,000 IU of beta-carotene

In a special report, the editorial board also issued the following statement:[5]

> *The editorial board of the* Wellness Letter *has been reluctant to recommend supplementary vitamins on a broad scale for healthy people eating healthy diets. But the accumulation of research in recent years has caused us to change our minds.*

Based on these recommendations, people who consume nine servings of fresh fruits and vegetables daily could get their daily beta-carotene and vitamin C requirements through the diet. To obtain the recommended guideline for vitamin E through diet alone, however, is practically impossible. As shown in Table 5.2, vitamin E is not easily found in large quantities in foods typically consumed in the diet. Thus, supplements are encouraged. When supplements (in general) are taken, they should be taken with meals and split in two to three doses per day.[6]

These antioxidant nutrients often work in conjunction with other nutrients in food that may further enhance their beneficial actions. Because vitamin E is fat-soluble, it should be taken with a meal that has some fat in it. Vitamin C is water-soluble, and the body eliminates it in about 12 hours. For best results, divide your vitamin C dose in half and take it twice a day. According to further evidence released in 1996, the daily dose of beta-carotene should come from natural sources (food) rather than supplements.[7]

Two separate clinical trials found that beta-carotene supplements offered no protection against heart disease and cancer. One of these studies actually found a higher lung cancer and mortality rate in smokers who took beta-carotene

Table 5.2 *Antioxidant Content of Selected Foods*

Beta-Carotene	IU
Apricot (1 medium)	675
Broccoli (½ cup, frozen)	1,740
Broccoli (½ cup, raw)	680
Cantaloupe (1 cup)	5,160
Carrot, (1 medium, raw)	20,255
Green peas (½ cup, frozen)	535
Mango (1 medium)	8,060
Mustard greens (½ cup, frozen)	3,350
Papaya (1 medium)	6,120
Spinach (½ cup, frozen)	7,395
Sweet potato (1 medium, baked)	24,875
Tomato (1 medium)	1,395
Turnip greens (½ cup, boiled)	3,960

Vitamin C	mg
Acerola (1 cup, raw)	1,640
Acerola juice (8 oz)	3,864
Cantaloupe (½ melon, medium)	90
Cranberry juice (8 oz)	90
Grapefruit (½, medium, white)	52
Grapefruit juice (8 oz)	92
Guava (1 medium)	165
Kiwi (1 medium)	75
Lemon juice (8 oz)	110
Orange (1 medium)	66
Orange juice (8 oz)	120
Papaya (1 medium)	85
Pepper (½ cup, red, chopped, raw)	95
Strawberries (1 cup, raw)	88

Vitamin E	IU	mg*
Almond oil (1 tbsp)		5.3
Almonds (1 oz)	10.1	
Canola oil (1 tbsp)		9.0
Cottonseed oil (1 tbsp)		5.2
Hazelnuts (1 oz)	4.4	
Kale (1 cup)	15.0	
Margarine (1 tbsp)		2.0
Peanuts (1 oz)	3.0	
Shrimp (3 oz, boiled)	3.1	
Sunflower seeds (1 oz, dry)	14.2	
Sunflower seed oil (1 tbsp)		6.9
Sweet potato (1 medium, baked)	7.2	
Wheat germ oil (1 tbsp)		20.0

* Vitamin E values for oils are commonly expressed in milligrams (mg). One mg is almost equal to 1 IU.

supplements. For former smokers and nonsmokers, these supplements do not cause any harm but offer no additional health benefits either. Therefore, it is recommended that you "skip the pill and eat the carrot." One medium raw carrot contains about 20,000 IU of beta-carotene (the recommended daily dose).

Supplements of the mineral selenium are encouraged. Research published in 1996 showed that individuals who took 200 mcg of selenium daily decreased the risk of prostate cancer by 63%, colorectal cancer by 58%, and lung cancer by 46%.[8] Other evidence suggests that taking 100 mcg of selenium supplements daily increases energy levels, decreases anxiety, and improves immune function.[9] Because selenium may interfere with the body's absorption of vitamin C, they should be taken at separate times.[10]

One unshelled Brazil nut (which you may crack yourself) provides about 100 mcg of selenium. Shelled nuts found in supermarkets average only about 20 mcg each. Toxic levels of selenium are thought to be around 2,500 mcg per day. Based on the current body of research, 100 to 200 mcg per day seem to provide the necessary amount of antioxidant for this nutrient. There is no reason to take more than 200 mcg daily.

Folate

Although it is not an antioxidant, folate (a B vitamin) also is recommended (400 mcg) for all premenopausal women.[11] Folate helps prevent certain birth defects and seems to offer protection against colon and cervical cancers.

Increasing evidence also indicates that 400 mcg of folate along with vitamins B_6 and B_{12} prevent heart attacks by reducing homocysteine levels in the blood (see Chapter 8). High concentrations of homocysteine accelerate the process of plaque formation (atherosclerosis) in the arteries.[12] Five servings of fruits and vegetables per day usually meet the needs for these nutrients. Currently, almost 9 of 10 adults in the United States do not meet the recommended 400 mcg of folate per day. Because of the critical role of folate in preventing heart disease, some experts

also recommend a daily vitamin B complex that includes 400 mcg of folate.[13]

Side Effects

Toxic effects with antioxidant supplements are rare when they are taken in the recommended amounts. Generally, up to 4000 mg of vitamin C, 3200 IU of vitamin E, and 50,000 IU of beta-carotene seem safe. If any of the following side effects arise, you should stop supplementation and check with your physician:

🐾 Vitamin E: gastrointestinal disturbances; increase in blood lipids (determined through blood tests)

How and When to Take Supplements

Knowing when and how to take nutrient supplements can enhance their potential benefits.

🐾 Take supplements with food.

🐾 Preferably, take vitamin C with other foods that contain this same nutrient.

🐾 Split vitamin C in two or more doses taken throughout the day.

🐾 Do not take vitamin C in combination with selenium. The latter can interfere with absorption of vitamin C.

🐾 Take vitamin E with meals that contain some fat.

🐾 Split vitamin E in two doses when taking more than 400 IU per day.

🐾 Take a vitamin B complex that includes 400 mcg of folate (often found in daily multi-vitamin complexes). Split the dosage in half and take it twice a day.

🐾 Take some of the vitamin C and the B complex with breakfast. Take vitamin E for breakfast if this meal has some fat in it. Take selenium a couple of hours later with a mid-morning snack. Take vitamin E with lunch if you didn't taken it with breakfast. For people taking over 500 mg, the additional vitamin C can be taken with lunch as well. Take the last dose of vitamin C, B complex, and any additional vitamin E with dinner.

🏊 Vitamin C: nausea, diarrhea, abdominal cramps, kidney stones, liver problems

🏊 Beta-carotene: although not harmful, yellow pigmentation of the skin

🏊 Selenium: nausea, vomiting, diarrhea, irritability, fatigue, flulike symptoms, lesions of the skin and nervous tissue, loss of hair and nails, respiratory failure, liver damage

Substantial supplementation of vitamin E is not recommended for individuals on anticoagulant therapy. Vitamin E is an anticoagulant in itself. Therefore, if you are on such therapy, check with your physician. Pregnant women need a physician's approval prior to beta-carotene supplementation. It also may be unsafe if taken with alcohol and by people who drink more than 4 ounces of pure alcohol per day (the equivalent of eight beers).

A few researchers are expressing concern for people who participate regularly in high-intensity exercise (above 70% of heart rate reserve — see Chapter 3) or prolonged exercise (more than 5 hours per week). Overtraining increases the production of free radicals and well may exceed the body's antioxidant defense mechanism. This high amount of free radicals may increase the risk for chronic diseases, including cancer.[14]

As a result of these findings, scientists are examining a possible link between "heavy" exercise and disease in people who otherwise lead a healthy lifestyle. Although the research is sparse, Dr. Kenneth Cooper, in his book *Antioxidant Revolution*, recommends higher doses of antioxidants for athletes and heavy exercisers: 3000 mg of vitamin C, 1200 IU of vitamin E, and 50,000 IU of beta-carotene.[15] Awareness of side effects is important if these higher amounts are taken.

Benefits of Foods

While supplements are encouraged, fruits and vegetables are the richest sources of antioxidants and phytochemicals. In 1996, researchers at the U.S. Department of Agriculture compared the antioxidant effects of vitamins C and E with those of various common fruits and vegetables.[16] The results indicated that 3/4 cup of cooked kale neutralized as many free radicals as approximately 800 IU of vitamin E or 600 mg of vitamin C. Three-fourths cup of cooked kale contains only 11 IU of vitamin E and 76 mg of vitamin C. Other excellent sources investigated by these researchers included blueberries, strawberries, spinach, Brussels sprouts, plums, broccoli, beets, oranges, and grapes. More good sources are red bell peppers, pink grapefruit, onions, white grapes, corn, eggplant, cauliflower, potatoes, cabbage, leaf lettuce, bananas, apples, green beans, carrots, tomatoes, and pears.

Many people who regularly eat foods high in fat content or too many sweets think they need supplementation to balance their diet. This is another fallacy about nutrition. The problem here is not necessarily a lack of vitamins and minerals but, instead, a diet too high in calories, fat, and sodium. Vitamin, mineral, and fiber supplements do not supply all of the nutrients and other beneficial substances present in food and needed for good health. Supplements will provide added health benefits, but by no means are they substitutes for a well-balanced diet.

Wholesome foods contain vitamins, minerals, carbohydrates, fiber, proteins, fats, phytochemicals, and other substances not yet discovered. Researchers do not know if the protective effects are caused by the antioxidants themselves, in combination with other nutrients (such as phytochemicals), or actually by some other nutrients in food that have not been investigated yet. Many nutrients work in synergy, enhancing chemical processes in the body. Supplementation will not offset poor eating habits. Pills are no substitute for common sense.

If you think your diet is not balanced, you first need to conduct a nutrient analysis to determine which nutrients you lack in sufficient amounts. Eat more of them, as well as foods that are high in antioxidants and phytochemicals.

Eating Disorders

Anorexia nervosa and bulimia nervosa are physical and emotional conditions thought to stem from individual, family, or social pressures. These disorders are characterized by an intense fear of becoming fat, which does not disappear even when losing extreme amounts of weight. Anorexia nervosa and bulimia nervosa are increasing steadily in most industrialized nations where society encourages low-calorie diets and thinness.

Anorexia Nervosa

Approximately 19 of every 20 individuals with **anorexia nervosa** are young women. An estimated 1% of the female population in the United States is anorexic. Anorexic individuals seem to fear weight gain more than death from starvation. Furthermore, they have a distorted image of their body and think of themselves as being fat even when they are emaciated.

Although a genetic predisposition may contribute, the anorexic person often comes from a mother-dominated home, with possible drug addictions in the family. The syndrome may emerge following a stressful life event and uncertainty about one's ability to cope efficiently.

Because the female role in society is changing rapidly, women seem to be especially susceptible. Life experiences such as gaining weight, starting the menstrual period, beginning college, losing a boyfriend, having poor self-esteem, being socially rejected, starting a professional career, or becoming a wife or a mother may trigger the syndrome.

These individuals typically begin a diet and at first feel in control and happy about the weight loss, even if they are not overweight. To speed up the weight loss, they frequently combine extreme dieting with exhaustive exercise and overuse of laxatives and diuretics.

Anorexics commonly develop obsessive and compulsive behaviors and emphatically deny their condition. They are preoccupied with food, meal planning, grocery shopping, and unusual eating habits. As they lose weight and their health begins to deteriorate, anorexics feel weak and tired and may realize they have a problem but will not stop the starvation and refuse to consider the behavior as abnormal.

Once they have lost a lot of weight and malnutrition sets in, physical changes become more visible. Typical changes are amenorrhea (stopping menstruation), digestive problems, extreme sensitivity to cold, hair and skin problems, fluid and electrolyte abnormalities (which may lead to an irregular heartbeat and sudden stopping of the heart), injuries to nerves and tendons, abnormalities of immune function, anemia, growth of fine body hair, mental confusion, inability to concentrate, lethargy, depression, skin dryness, lower skin and body temperature, and osteoporosis.

Diagnostic criteria for anorexia nervosa are:[17]

- Refusal to maintain body weight over a minimal normal weight for age and height (weight loss leading to maintenance of body weight less than 85% of that expected or failure to make expected weight gain during periods of growth, leading to body weight less than 85% of that expected).

- Intense fear of gaining weight or becoming fat, even though underweight.

- Disturbance in the way in which one's body weight, size, or shape is perceived, undue influences of body weight or shape on self-evaluation, or denial of the seriousness of the current low body weight.

- In postmenarcheal females, amenorrhea (the absence of at least three consecutive menstrual cycles). (A woman is considered to have amenorrhea if her periods occur only following estrogen therapy).

Many of the changes induced by anorexia nervosa can be reversed. Treatment almost always requires professional help, and the sooner it is started, the better are the chances for reversibility and cure. Therapy consists of a combination of medical and psychological

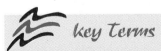

key terms

Anorexia nervosa A condition of self-imposed starvation to lose and then maintain very low body weight.

techniques to restore proper nutrition, prevent medical complications, and modify the environment or events that triggered the syndrome.

Seldom can anorexics overcome the problem by themselves. They strongly deny their condition. They are able to hide it and deceive friends and relatives. Based on their behavior, many of them meet all of the characteristics of anorexia nervosa, but it goes undetected because both thinness and dieting are socially acceptable. Only a well-trained clinician is able to diagnose anorexia nervosa.

Bulimia Nervosa

Bulimia nervosa is more prevalent than anorexia nervosa. For many years it was thought to be a variant of anorexia nervosa, but now it is identified as a separate condition. It afflicts mainly young people. As many as one in every five women on college campuses may be bulimic, according to some estimates. Bulimia nervosa also is more prevalent than anorexia nervosa in males.

Bulimics usually are healthy-looking people, well-educated, near recommended body weight. They seem to enjoy food and often socialize around it. In actuality, they are emotionally insecure, rely on others, and lack self-confidence and self-esteem. Recommended weight and food are important to them.

The binge-purge cycle usually occurs in stages. As a result of stressful life events or the simple compulsion to eat, bulimics engage periodically in binge eating that may last an hour or longer.

With some apprehension, bulimics anticipate and plan the cycle. Next they feel an urgency to begin, followed by large and uncontrollable food consumption during which they may eat several thousand calories (up to 10,000 calories in extreme cases). After a short period of relief and satisfaction, feelings of deep guilt, shame, and intense fear of gaining weight ensue. Purging seems to be an easy answer, as the binging cycle can continue without fear of gaining weight.

The diagnostic criteria for bulimia nervosa are:[18]

- Recurrent episodes of binge eating. An episode of binge eating is characterized by both of the following:
  (1) Eating, in a discrete period of time (e.g., within any 2-hour period), an amount of food that is definitely larger than most people would eat during a similar period of time and under similar circumstances.
  (2) A sense of lack of control over eating during the episode (e.g., a feeling that one cannot stop eating or control what or how much one is eating).

- Recurrent inappropriate compensatory behaviors in order to prevent weight gain, such as self-induced vomiting; misuse of laxatives, diuretics, enemas, or other medications; fasting; or excessive exercise.

- The binge eating and inappropriate compensatory behaviors both occur, on average, at least twice a week for three months.

- Self-evaluation is unduly influenced by body shape and weight.

- The disturbance does not occur exclusively during episodes of anorexia nervosa.

The most typical form of purging is self-induced vomiting. Bulimics, too, frequently ingest strong laxatives and emetics. Near-fasting diets and strenuous bouts of exercise are common. Medical problems associated with bulimia nervosa include cardiac arrhythmias, amenorrhea, kidney and bladder damage, ulcers, colitis, tearing of the esophagus or stomach, tooth erosion, gum damage, and general muscular weakness.

Unlike anorexics, bulimics realize their behavior is abnormal and feel great shame about it. Fearing social rejection, they pursue the binge-purge cycle in secrecy and at unusual hours of the day.

Bulimia nervosa can be treated successfully when the person realizes that this destructive behavior is not the solution to life's problems. A change in attitude can prevent permanent damage or death.

Treatment for anorexia nervosa and bulimia nervosa is available on most school campuses through the school's counseling center or the health center. Local hospitals also offer treatment for these conditions. Many communities have support groups, frequently led by professional personnel and usually free of charge.

Dietary Guidelines for North Americans

Based on the available scientific research on nutrition and health and current dietary habits, the Scientific Committee of the U.S. Department of Health and Human Services and the U.S. Department of Agriculture on diet and health in 1995 issued the fourth edition of the Dietary Guidelines for healthy American adults and children. These guidelines potentially can reduce the risk of developing certain chronic diseases. The committee's recommendations are:[19]

- Eat a variety of food.
- Balance the food you eat with physical activity to maintain or improve your weight.
- Choose a diet with plenty of grain products, vegetables, and fruits.
- Choose a diet low in fat, saturated fat, and cholesterol.

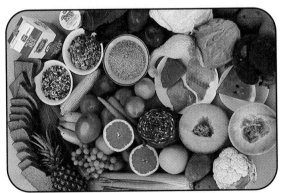

Foods from a wide variety of sources are necessary in a well-balanced diet.

- Choose a diet moderate in sugars.
- Choose a diet moderate in salt and sodium (keep total intake of salt to less than 6 grams per day).
- If you drink alcoholic beverages, do so in moderation (limit consumption to less than an ounce of pure alcohol per day or the equivalent of two cans of beer, two small glasses of wine, or two average cocktails. If pregnant, avoid alcoholic beverages altogether).

A Lifetime Commitment to Wellness

Proper nutrition, a sound exercise program, and quitting smoking (for those who smoke) are the three factors that do the most for health, longevity, and quality of life. Achieving and maintaining a balanced diet is not as difficult as most people would think. The difficult part for most people is retraining themselves to follow a lifetime healthy nutrition plan.

A well balanced diet contains a variety of foods from all five basic food groups, including wise selection of foods from animal sources. The diet should include lots of grains, legumes, fruits, vegetables, and low-fat dairy products, with moderate use of animal protein, sodium, and alcohol. Based on current nutrition data, meat (poultry and fish included) should be replaced by grains, legumes, vegetables, and fruits as main courses. Meats should be used more for flavoring than for substance. Daily consumption of beef, poultry, or fish should be limited to 3 ounces (about the size of a deck of cards) to 6 ounces.

No single food can provide all of the necessary nutrients and other beneficial substances in the amounts the body needs. For good nutrition,

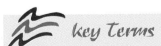

key Terms

Bulimia nervosa An eating disorder characterized by a pattern of binge eating and purging.

you should meet the recommended number of daily servings from each of the five food groups in the Food Guide Pyramid. Within each food group, choose a variety of foods. Food items vary, and each item provides different combinations of nutrients and other substances needed for good health.

In spite of the ample scientific evidence linking poor dietary habits to early disease and mortality rates, many people are not willing to change their eating patterns. Even when faced with obesity, elevated blood lipids, hypertension, and other nutrition-related conditions, many people do not change. They remain in the precontemplation stage of change (see Behavior Modification in Chapter 1). The motivating factor to change one's eating habits seems to be a major health breakdown, such as a heart attack, a stroke, or cancer. An ounce of prevention is worth a pound of cure. The sooner you implement the dietary guidelines presented in this chapter, the better will be your chances of preventing chronic diseases and reaching a higher state of wellness.

http://www.ama-assn.org/
Interactive Health Personal Nutritionist
(AMA sponsored)
(see Health and Fitness — Nutrition Link)

Notes

1. E. B. Rimm, A. Ascherio, E. Giovannucci, D. Spiegelman, M. J. Stampfer, and W. C. Willett, "Vegetable, Fruit, and Cereal Fiber Intake and Risk of Coronary Heart Disease Among Men," *Journal of the American Medical Association,* 275(1996), 447–451.

2. S. Begley. "Beyond Vitamins," *Newsweek,* April 25, 1994, pp. 45–49.

3. "Vitamin Report," University of California at Berkeley *Wellness Letter* (Palm Coast, FL: The Editors, October, 1994).

4. "Antioxidants: Never Too Late," University of California at Berkeley *Wellness Letter,* 10:8(1994), 2.

5. "Vitamin Report."

6. S. Kalish, "The Free Radical Radical: Kenneth Cooper, M.D., on Antioxidants and the Dangers of Hard Running." *Running Times,* March 1995, 16–17.

7. "Beta Carotene Pills: Should You Take Them?" University of California at Berkeley *Wellness Letter,* 12:7(1996), 1–2.

8. C. Clark et al., "Effects of Selenium Supplementation for Cancer Prevention in Patients with Carcinoma of the Skin: A Randomized Controlled Trial," *Journal of the American Medical Association,* 276(1996), 1957–1963.

9. J. Carper, "Selenium: A Cancer Knockout?" *USA Weekend,* October 2–4, 1996, p. 8.

10. A. Weil, "Dr. Andrew Weil's Surprising Secrets of Optimum Health," *Bottom Line/ Personal,* 18:13(1997), 9–10.

11. "Vitamin Report."

12. C. J. Boushey, S. A. A. Beresford, G. S. Omenn, and A. G. Motulsky, "A Quantitative Assessment of Plasma Homocysteine as a Risk Factor for Vascular Disease," *Journal of the American Medical Association,* 274(1995), 1049–1057.

13. W. Castelli, "Smart Heart Strategies: Best Ways to Beat Heart Disease," *Bottom Line/Personal,* 19:4 (1998), 1–3.

14. K. H. Cooper, *Antioxidant Revolution* (Nashville, TN: Thomas Nelson Publishers, 1994).

15. Cooper.

16. "The Antioxidant All-Stars," University of California at Berkeley *Wellness Letter* (Palm Coast, FL: The Editors, March 1997).

17. American Psychiatric Association, *Diagnostic and Statistical Manual of Mental Disorders* (Washington, DC: APA, 1994), pp. 262, 263.

18. APA.

19. U.S. Department of Agriculture and U.S. Department of Health and Human Services, "Nutrition and Your Health: Dietary Guidelines for Americans," *Home and Garden Bulletin* No. 232, December 1995.

Weight Management

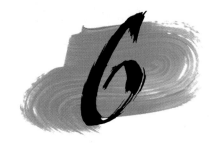

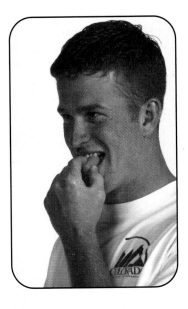

Approximately 65 million people living in the United States are either overweight or consider themselves to be overweight. Of these, 30 million are obese. About 50% of all women and 25% of all men are on diets at any given moment. People spend about $40 billion to $50 billion yearly attempting to lose weight. More than $10 billion goes to memberships in weight reduction centers and another $30 billion to diet food sales.

Achieving and maintaining ideal body weight is a major objective of a good physical fitness program. The assessment of recommended body weight was discussed in detail in Chapter 2. Next to poor cardiorespiratory fitness, excessive body weight (fat) is the most frequently encountered problem in fitness and wellness assessments.

Two terms commonly used in reference to people who weigh more than recommended are **overweight** and **obesity**. Overweight and obesity are not the same thing. Most overweight (10 to 15 pounds) people are not obese. Obesity levels are established at a point at which the excess body fat can lead to serious health problems. Obesity by itself has been associated with critical health problems and accounts for 15% to 20% of the annual mortality rate in the United States.[1] Obesity is a major risk factor for diseases of the cardiovascular system, including coronary heart disease, hypertension, congestive heart failure, high levels of blood lipids, atherosclerosis, strokes, thromboembolitic disease, diabetes, osteoarthritis, varicose veins, and intermittent claudication.

Other research points toward a possible link between obesity and cancer of the colon, rectum, prostate, gallbladder, breast, uterus, and ovaries. In addition, obesity has been associated with

Objectives

☞ Recognize myths and fallacies regarding weight management.

☞ Understand the physiology of weight control.

☞ Become familiar with the effects of diet and exercise on resting metabolic rate.

☞ Recognize the role of a lifetime exercise program in a successful weight management program.

☞ Learn to write and implement weight reduction and weight maintenance programs.

☞ Identify behavior modification techniques that help a person adhere to a lifetime weight maintenance program.

diabetes, ruptured intervertebral discs, gallstones, gout, respiratory insufficiency, and complications during pregnancy and delivery. Furthermore, it is implicated in psychological maladjustment and a higher accidental death rate.

Data from the Aerobics Research Institute in Dallas confirm that as body fat increases, so does blood cholesterol and triglycerides. The data, however, also showed that the higher the fitness level, the lower the mortality rate, regardless of body weight.[2] This finding is of significance, because obese men who were fit had a lower risk of death than unfit men of average weight and as low as fit men of average weight. Thus, at least partially, lack of physical activity and not the weight problem itself may be the cause of premature death in some obese people.

Although obese men in the study who become active decreased their risk of premature mortality regardless of whether they lost weight, few obese men in the study were fit. This pattern holds true in real life. Most obese people either don't exercise or are unable to do so because of functional limitations when attempting to participate in traditional fitness activities such as jogging, walking, and cycling. Those who do exercise tend to lose weight.

A few pounds of excess weight may not be harmful to most people. People who have a few extra pounds of weight but who are otherwise healthy and are physically active, exercise regularly, and eat a healthy diet may not be at greater risk for early death. Overweight people with diabetes and other cardiovascular risk factors (elevated blood lipids, high blood pressure, physical inactivity, and poor eating habits), however, benefit from weight loss.

Recommended body composition is a primary objective of overall physical fitness and enhanced quality of life. Individuals at recommended body weight are able to participate in a wide variety of moderate to vigorous activities without functional limitations. These people have the freedom to enjoy most of life's recreational activities to their fullest potential. Excessive body weight does not afford an individual the fitness level to enjoy vigorous lifetime activities such as basketball, soccer, racquetball, surfing, mountain cycling, and mountain climbing. Maintaining high fitness and recommended body weight gives a person a degree of independence throughout life that the majority of people in developed nations no longer enjoy.

Tolerable Weight

Many people want to lose weight so they will look better. That's a noteworthy goal. The

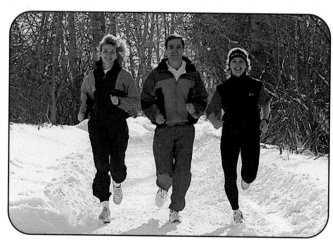
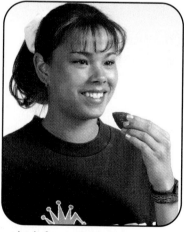

Achieving and maintaining a high physical fitness percent body fat standard requires a lifetime commitment to regular physical activity and proper nutrition.

problem, however, is that they often have a distorted image of what they would look like if they were to reduce to what they think is their ideal weight. Hereditary factors play a big role, and only a small fraction of the population has the genes for a "perfect body." **Tolerable weight** is a more realistic goal. This is a realistic standard that is not "ideal" but is "acceptable." It is likely to be closer to the health-fitness standard than the physical-fitness standard for many people.

In setting their own target weight, people should be realistic. Attaining the high physical fitness percent body fat standard in Table 2.12, Chapter 2, is extremely difficult for some people. Unless they are willing to make a commitment to a vigorous lifetime exercise program and permanent dietary changes, this standard is not realistic. Few people are willing to make this commitment. The health-fitness percent body fat category may be a more attainable goal for these people.

A question you should ask yourself is: Am I happy with my weight? Part of enjoying a better quality of life is being happy with yourself. If you are not, you either should do something about it or learn to live with it!

If you are above the health-fitness percent body fat standard (the percent body fat at which there seems to be no detriment to health), you should try to come down and stay there. If you have achieved the health-fitness standard but would like to be better, ask yourself a second question: How badly do I want it? Enough to implement lifetime exercise and dietary changes? If you are not willing to change, you should stop worrying about your weight and deem the health-fitness standard as tolerable for you.

Principles of Weight Management

In keeping with the **energy-balancing equation**, if caloric input exceeds output, the person gains weight; when caloric output is more than intake, the individual loses weight. Each pound of fat equals 3500 calories. Therefore, theoretically, to increase body fat (weight) by 1 pound, a person

would have to consume an excess of 3500 calories. Equally, to lose 1 pound, the individual would have to decrease caloric intake by 3500 calories. This principle seems straightforward, but, as you will learn later in this chapter, it is not quite that simple with the human body.

Only about 10% of all people who begin a traditional weight-loss program (without exercise) are able to lose the desired weight. Worse, less than 5% of this group is able to keep the weight off for a significant time. Traditional diets have failed because few of them incorporate lifetime changes in food selection, overall daily physical activity, and exercise as the keys to successful weight loss and maintenance.

Meanwhile, fad diets continue to deceive people. Most of these diets are low in calories and deprive the body of certain nutrients, generating a metabolic imbalance that can even cause death. Under these conditions a lot of the weight lost is in the form of water and protein, not fat. On a crash diet close to half of the weight loss is in lean (protein) tissue[3] (see Figure 6.1). When the body uses protein instead of a combination of fats and carbohydrates as a source of energy, the individual loses weight as much as 10 times faster.[4] A gram of protein produces less than half the amount of energy that fat does. In the case of muscle protein, one-fifth of protein is mixed with four-fifths of water. Each pound of muscle yields only one-tenth the amount of energy as a pound of fat. As a result, most of the weight loss is in the form of water, which on the scale, of course, looks good.

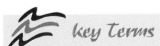 *key Terms*

Overweight Excess weight when compared to a given standard such as height or recommended percent body fat.

Obesity A chronic disease characterized by an excessively high amount of body fat (about 20% above recommended weight).

Tolerable weight A realistic body weight that is close to the health-fitness percent-body fat standard.

Energy-balancing equation A body weight formula stating that when caloric intake equals caloric output, weight remains unchanged.

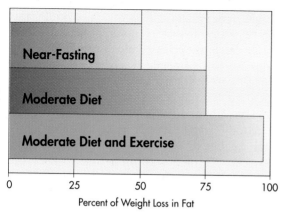

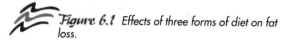

Percent of Weight Loss in Fat

Adapted from *Alive Man: The Physiology of Physical Activity,* by R. J. Shephard (Springfield, IL: Charles C Thomas, 1975), p. 484–488.

Figure 6.1 *Effects of three forms of diet on fat loss.*

Some diets allow only certain specialized foods. If people would realize that no "magic" foods provide all the necessary nutrients, that a person has to eat a variety of foods to be well nourished, the diet industry would not be as successful. Most of these diets create a nutritional deficiency, which at times is fatal. Some people eventually get tired of eating the same thing day in and day out and start eating less — which results in weight loss. If they achieve the lower weight without making permanent dietary changes, however, they gain back the weight quickly if they go back to their old eating habits.

A few diets recommend exercise along with caloric restrictions — the best method for weight reduction, of course. A lot of the weight lost is a result of the exercise, so the diet achieves its purpose. As discussed later in this chapter, exercise in itself plays a major role in how much a person weighs. If people do not change their food selection and activity level permanently, however, they gain back the weight quickly after they discontinue dieting and exercising.

Only a few years ago the principles governing a weight loss and maintenance program seemed to be fairly clear. Now we realize that the final answers are not in yet. Traditional concepts related to weight control have centered on three assumptions:

1. Balancing food intake against output allows a person to achieve recommended weight.

2. Fat people just eat too much.

3. The human body doesn't care how much (or little) fat is stored.

Although these statements contain some truth, they still are open to much debate and research. The genetic instinct to survive tells the body that fat storage is vital, and, therefore, the **setpoint** sets an acceptable fat level for each person. This setpoint remains somewhat constant or may climb gradually because of poor lifestyle habits.

Especially under strict calorie reduction (fewer than 800 calories per day), the body makes compensatory metabolic adjustments in an effort to maintain its fat storage. The **basal metabolic rate (BMR)** may drop dramatically against a consistent negative caloric balance, and the person may be on a plateau for days or even weeks without losing much weight. When the dieter goes back to the normal or even below-normal caloric intake, at which the weight may have been stable for a long time, he or she quickly regains the fat loss as the body strives to restore a comfortable fat level.

These findings were substantiated by research conducted at Rockefeller University in New York.[5] The authors showed that the body resists maintenance of altered weight. Obese and lifetime nonobese individuals were used in the investigation. Following a 10% weight loss, in an attempt to regain the lost weight, the body compensated by burning up to 15% fewer calories than expected for the new reduced weight (after accounting for the 10% loss). The effects were similar in the obese and nonobese participants. These results imply that after a 10% weight loss, a person would have to eat less or exercise more to account for the estimated deficit of about 200 to 300 daily calories.

In this same study, when the participants were allowed to increase their weight to 10% above their "normal" body weight (pre-weight loss), the body burned 10% to 15% more calories than expected. This indicates an attempt by the body to waste energy and return to the preset weight. The study provides another indication that the body is highly resistant to weight changes unless additional lifestyle changes are incorporated to ensure successful weight management. Methods to manage weight will be discussed in this chapter.

This research shows why most dieters regain the weight they lose through dietary means alone. Let's use a practical illustration: Jim would like to lose some body fat and assumes that he has reached a stable body weight at an average daily caloric intake of 2500 calories (no weight gain or loss at this daily intake). In an attempt to lose weight rapidly, he now goes on a strict low-calorie diet (or, even worse, a near-fasting diet). Immediately the body activates its survival mechanism and readjusts its metabolism to a lower caloric balance.

After a few weeks of dieting at under 400 to 600 calories per day, the body now can maintain its normal functions at 1000 calories per day. Having lost the desired weight, Jim terminates the diet but realizes the original intake of 2500 calories per day will have to be lower to maintain the new lower weight. To adjust to the new lower body weight, the intake is restricted to about 2200 calories per day. Jim is surprised to find that even at this lower daily intake (300 fewer calories), his weight comes back at a rate of about 1 pound every 1 to 2 weeks. After the diet ends, this new lowered metabolic rate may take several months to kick back up to its normal level.

From this explanation, individuals clearly should not go on very low-calorie diets. Not only will this decrease the resting metabolic rate, but it also will deprive the body of basic daily nutrients required for normal function. Under no circumstances should a person go on a diet that calls for below 1200 and 1500 calories respectively, for women and men. Weight (fat) is gained over months and years, not overnight. Equally, weight loss should be gradual, not abrupt. A daily caloric intake of 1200 to 1500

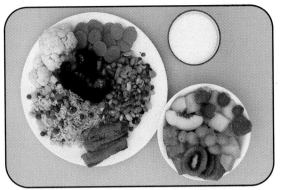

A wide variety of foods is required to maintain a well nourished body.

calories provides the necessary nutrients if properly distributed over the various food groups (meeting the minimum daily required servings from each group). Of course, the individual has to learn which foods meet the requirements and yet are low in fat, sugar, and calories.

Furthermore, when a person tries to lose weight by dietary restrictions alone, lean body mass (muscle protein, along with vital organ protein) decreases. The amount of lean body mass lost depends entirely on the caloric limitation. When people go on a near-fasting diet, up to half of the weight loss can be lean body mass and the other half, actual fat loss. If the diet is combined with exercise, close to 100% of the weight loss is in the form of fat, and lean tissue actually may increase (see Figure 6.1). Loss of lean body mass is not good because it weakens the organs and muscles and slows the metabolism.

Reduction in lean body mass is common in people on severely restricted diets. No diet with caloric intakes below 1200 to 1500 calories will prevent loss of lean body mass. Even at this intake level, some loss is inevitable unless the diet

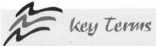

key Terms

Setpoint Body weight and body fat percentage unique to each person that is regulated by genetic and environmental factors.

Basal metabolic rate (BMR) The lowest level of caloric intake necessary to sustain life.

is combined with exercise. Although many diets claim they do not alter the lean component, the simple truth is that, regardless of what nutrients may be added to the diet, caloric restrictions always prompt a loss of lean tissue.

Too many people go on low-calorie diets again and again. Every time they do, the metabolic rate slows as more lean tissue is lost. People in their 40s or older who weigh the same as they did when they were 20 often think they are at "recommended body weight." During this span of 20 years or more, they may have dieted too many times without exercising. Shortly after terminating each diet, they regain the weight, but most of that gain is in fat. Maybe at age 20 they weighed 150 pounds, of which only 15% to 16% was fat. Now, at age 40, even though they still weigh 150 pounds, they might be 30% fat (see Figure 6.2 and also Figure 2.2 in Chapter 2). At "recommended body weight," they wonder why they are eating so little and still having trouble staying at that weight.

Further, a diet high in fats and refined carbohydrates, near-fasting diets, and perhaps even artificial sweeteners keep people from losing weight and, in reality, contribute to fat gain. The only practical and sensible way to lose fat weight is to combine exercise and a sensible diet high in complex carbohydrates and low in fat and sugar.

After studying the effects of proper food management, many nutritionists believe the source of calories should be the primary concern in a weight-control program. Most of the effort in this regard is spent in retraining eating habits, increasing the intake of complex carbohydrates and high-fiber foods, and decreasing the consumption of refined carbohydrates (sugars) and fats. For most people this change in eating habits brings about a decrease in total daily caloric intake. Because 1 gram of carbohydrates provides only 4 calories, as opposed to 9 calories per gram of fat, you could eat twice the volume of food (by weight) when substituting carbohydrates for fat.

A "diet" no longer is viewed as a temporary tool to aid in weight loss but, instead, as a permanent change in eating behaviors to ensure

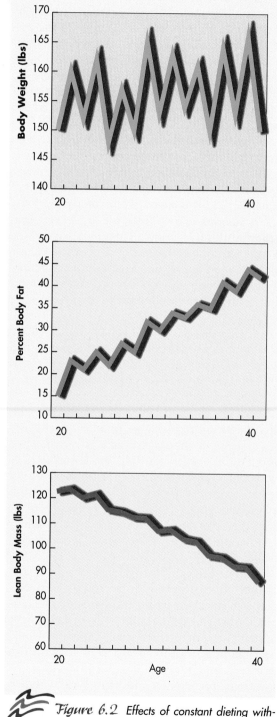

Figure 6.2 Effects of constant dieting without exercise on body weight, percent body fat, and lean body mass.

weight management and better health. The role of increased physical activity also must be considered because successful weight loss and recommended body composition seldom are attainable without a moderate reduction in caloric intake combined with a regular exercise program.

Exercise: The key to Successful Weight Management

A more effective way to tilt the energy-balancing equation in your favor is by burning calories through physical activity. Exercise also seems to exert control over how much a person weighs.

If, starting at age 25, the typical person gains 1 pound of weight per year, this represents a simple energy surplus of under 10 calories per day (10 × 365 = 3,650). In most cases the additional weight accumulated in middle age comes from people becoming less physically active and not resulting from increased caloric intake. Dr. Jack Wilmore, a leading exercise physiologist and expert weight management researcher, stated:[6]

> *Physical inactivity is certainly a major, if not the primary, cause of obesity in the United States today. A certain minimal level of activity might be necessary for us to accurately balance our caloric intake to our caloric expenditure. With too little activity, we appear to lose the fine control we normally have to maintain this incredible balance. This fine balance amounts to less than 10 calories per day, or the equivalent of one potato chip.*

If a person is trying to lose weight, a combination of aerobic and strength-training exercises works best. Because of the continuity and duration of aerobic exercise, it burns many calories. Strength training, in contrast, has a greater impact on increasing lean body mass.

The role of aerobic exercise in successful lifetime weight management cannot be underestimated. As illustrated in Figure 6.3, greater weight loss is achieved by combining a diet with an aerobic exercise program.[7] Of even greater significance, only the individuals who participated in an 18-month post-diet aerobic exercise program were able to keep the weight off. Those who discontinued exercise gained weight. Furthermore, all of the participants who initiated or resumed exercise during the 18-month follow-up were able to lose weight again. Individuals who only dieted and never exercised regained 60% and 92% of their weight loss at the 8- and 18-month follow-ups, respectively.

Weight loss can be accelerated by combining aerobic exercise with a strength-training program. Each additional pound of muscle tissue can raise the basal metabolic rate by 35 calories per day.[8] Thus, an individual who adds 5 pounds of muscle tissue as a result of strength training increases the basal metabolic rate by 175 calories per day (35 × 5), which equals 63,875 calories per year (175 × 365), or the equivalent of 18.25 pounds of fat (63,875 ÷ 3,500).

Note: Numbers in parenthesis indicate number of participants.

Source: "Exercise as an Adjunct to Weight Loss and Maintenance in Moderately Obese Subjects," K. N., Pavlou, S. Krey, and W. P. Steffe, *American Journal of Clinical Nutrition*, 49 (1989), 1115–1123.

Figure 6.3 Aerobic exercise and weight loss and maintenance in moderately obese individuals.

Because exercise promotes an increase in lean body mass, body weight often remains the same or even increases after beginning an exercise program, while inches and percent body fat decrease. More lean tissue means more functional capacity of the human body. With exercise, most of the weight loss becomes apparent after a few weeks of training, when the lean component has stabilized.

Research has revealed the fallacy of spot-reducing or losing cellulite, as some people call the fat deposits that bulge out in certain areas of the body. These deposits are nothing but enlarged fat cells from accumulated body fat. Merely doing several sets of sit-ups daily will not get rid

of fat in the midsection of the body. When fat comes off, it does so throughout the entire body, not just the exercised area. Although the greatest proportion of fat may come off the biggest fat deposits, the caloric output of a few sets of sit-ups has almost no effect on reducing total body fat. A person has to exercise much longer to really see results.

Dieting never has been fun and never will be. People who are overweight and are serious about losing weight will have to make exercise a regular part of their daily life, along with proper food management and perhaps a sensible cut in caloric intake. Some precautions are in order, as excessive body fat is a risk factor for cardiovascular disease. Depending on the extent of the weight problem, a medical examination and possibly a stress ECG may be necessary before undertaking the exercise program. A physician should be consulted in this regard.

Significantly overweight individuals also may have to choose activities in which they will not have to support their own body weight but still will be effective in burning calories. Injuries to joints and muscles are common in overweight individuals who participate in weight-bearing exercises such as walking, jogging, and aerobics. Better alternatives for overweight people are riding a bicycle (either road or stationary), water aerobics, walking in a shallow pool, or running in place in deep water (treading water). The latter three modes of exercise are gaining quickly in popularity because little skill is required to participate. These activities seem to be just as effective as other forms of aerobic activity in helping individuals lose weight without the pain and the fear of injuries.

One final benefit of exercise for weight control is that it allows fat to be burned more efficiently. Both carbohydrates and fats are sources of energy. When the glucose levels begin to drop during prolonged exercise, more fat is used as energy substrate. Equally important is that fat-burning enzymes increase with aerobic training. Fat is lost primarily by burning it in muscle. Therefore, as the concentration of the enzymes increases, so does the ability to burn fat.

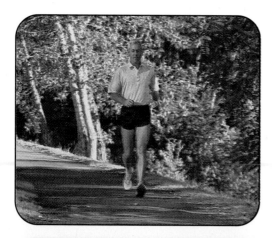

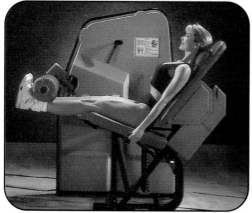

Regular participation in a combined lifetime aerobic and strength-training exercise program is the key to successful weight management.

Designing Your Own Weight-Loss Program

In addition to exercise and food management, sensible adjustments in caloric intake are recommended. Most research finds that a negative caloric balance is required to lose weight. Perhaps the only exception is with people who are eating too few calories. A nutrient analysis often reveals that "faithful" dieters are not consuming enough calories. These people actually need to increase their daily caloric intake (combined with an exercise program) to get the metabolism to kick back up to a normal level.

Estimating Your Caloric Intake

Referring to Figure 6.4 and Tables 6.1 and 6.2, you can estimate your daily caloric requirement. As this is only an estimated value, individual adjustments related to many of the factors discussed in this chapter may be necessary to establish a more precise value. Nevertheless, the estimated value does offer a beginning guideline for weight control or reduction.

The average daily caloric requirement without exercise is based on typical lifestyle patterns, total body weight, and gender. Individuals who hold jobs that require heavy manual labor burn more calories during the day than those who

Daily Caloric Requirement

A. Current body weight   _____

B. Caloric requirement per pound of body weight (use Table 6.1)   _____

C. Typical daily caloric requirement without exercise to maintain body weight (A × B)   _____

D. Selected physical activity (e.g., jogging)*   _____

E. Number of exercise sessions per week   _____

F. Duration of exercise session (in minutes)   _____

G. Total weekly exercise time in minutes (E × F)   _____

H. Average daily exercise time in minutes (G ÷ 7)   _____

I. Caloric expenditure per pound per minute (cal/lb/min) of physical activity (use Table 6.2)   _____

J. Total calories burned per minute of exercise (A × I)   _____

K. Average daily calories burned as a result of the exercise program (H × J)   _____

L. Total daily caloric requirement with exercise to maintain body weight (C + K)   _____

M. Number of calories to subtract from daily requirement to achieve a negative caloric balance (multiply current body weight by 5)**   _____

N. Target caloric intake to lose weight (L − M)   _____

---

* If more than one physical activity is selected, you will need to estimate the average daily calories burned as a result of each additional activity (steps D through K) and add all of these figures to L above.

** This figure should never be below 1,200 calories for women or 1,500 calories for men.

 Figure 6.4 Daily caloric requirement: Computation form.

Table 6.1 *Average Caloric Requirement per Pound of Body Weight*

	Calories per pound	
Activity Rating	Men	Women[1]
Sedentary — Limited physical activity	13.0	12.0
Moderate physical activity	15.0	13.5
Hard Labor — Strenuous physical effort	17.0	15.0

[1] Pregnant or lactating women: Add 3 calories to these values.

 Table 6.2 *Caloric Expenditure of Selected Physical Activities*

Activity*	Cal/lb/min**	Activity*	Cal/lb/min**	Activity*	Cal/lb/min**
Aerobelt Exercise		Dance		StairMaster	
Aero-belt Jogging/ 6 mph	0.098	Moderate	0.030	Moderate	0.070
Aero-belt Step-Aerobics/8"	0.105	Vigorous	0.055	Vigorous	0.090
		Golf	0.030	Stationary Cycling	
Aero-belt Walking/ 4 mph	0.073	Gymnastics		Moderate	0.055
Aerobics		Light	0.030	Vigorous	0.070
Moderate	0.065	Heavy	0.056	Strength Training	0.050
High Impact	0.095	Handball	0.064	Swimming (crawl)	
Step-Aerobics	0.070	Hiking	0.040	20 yds/min	0.031
Archery	0.030	Judo/Karate	0.086	25 yds/min	0.040
Badminton		Racquetball	0.065	45 yds/min	0.057
Recreation	0.038	Rope Jumping	0.060	50 yds/min	0.070
Competition	0.065	Rowing (vigorous)	0.090	Table Tennis	0.030
Baseball	0.031	Running		Tennis	
Basketball		11.0 min/mile	0.070	Moderate	0.045
Moderate	0.046	8.5 min/mile	0.090	Competition	0.064
Competition	0.063	7.0 min/mile	0.102	Volleyball	0.030
Bowling	0.030	6.0 min/mile	0.114	Walking	
Calisthenics	0.033	Deep water***	0.100	4.5 mph	0.045
Cycling (level)		Skating (moderate)	0.038	Shallow pool	0.090
5.5 mph	0.033	Skiing		Water Aerobics	
10.0 mph	0.050	Downhill	0.060	Moderate	0.050
13.0 mph	0.071	Level (5 mph)	0.078	Vigorous	0.070
		Soccer	0.059	Wrestling	0.085

*Values are only for actual time engaged in the activity.
**Cal/lb/min = calories per pound of body weight per minute of activity
***Treading water

Adapted from *Fitness for Life: An Individualized Approach*, by P. E. Allsen, J. M. Harrison, and B. Vance (Dubuque, IA: Wm. C. Brown, 1989); *Fitness for College and Life*, by C. A. Bucher, and W. E. Prentice (St. Louis: Times Mirror/Mosby College Publishing, 1989); *Physiological Measurements of Metabolic Functions in Man*, by C. F. Consolazio, R. E. Johnson, and L. J. Pecora (New York: McGraw-Hill, 1963); *Physical Fitness: The Pathway to Healthful Living*, by R. V. Hockey (St. Louis: Times Mirror/Mosby College Publishing, 1989); and research conducted at Boise State University by W. W. K. Hoeger et al, 1986–1993.

have sedentary jobs (such as working behind a desk). To find your activity level, refer to Table 6.1 and rate yourself accordingly. The number given in Table 6.1 is per pound of body weight, so you multiply your current weight by that number. For example, the typical caloric requirement to maintain body weight for a moderately active male who weighs 160 pounds is 2400 calories (160 lbs × 15 cal/lb).

The second step is to determine the average number of calories you burn daily as a result of exercise. To get this number, figure out the total number of minutes you exercise weekly, and then figure the daily average exercise time. For instance, a person cycling at 13 miles per hour five times a week, 30 minutes each time, exercises 150 minutes per week (5 × 30). The average daily exercise time is 21 minutes (150 ÷ 7, rounded off to the lowest unit).

Next, from Table 6.2, find the energy requirement for the activity (or activities) chosen for the exercise program. In the case of cycling (13 miles per hour), the requirement is .071 calories per pound of body weight per minute of activity (cal/lb/min). With a body weight of 160 pounds, this man would burn 11.4 calories each minute (body weight × .071, or 160 × .071). In 21 minutes he burns approximately 240 calories (21 × 11.4).

The third step is to obtain the estimated total caloric requirement, with exercise, needed to maintain body weight. To do this, add the typical daily requirement (without exercise) and the average calories burned through exercise. In our example it is 2640 calories (2400 + 240).

If a negative caloric balance is recommended to lose weight, this person has to consume fewer than 2640 calories daily to achieve the objective. Because of the many factors that play a role in weight control, the previous value is only an estimated daily requirement. Furthermore, to lose weight, we cannot predict that you will lose exactly 1 pound of fat in 1 week if you cut your daily intake by 500 calories (500 × 7 = 3500 calories, or the equivalent of 1 pound of fat).

The estimated daily caloric figure is only a target guideline for weight control. Periodic readjustments are necessary because individuals differ, and the estimated daily cost changes as you lose weight and modify your exercise habits.

To determine the target caloric intake to lose weight, multiply your current weight by 5 and subtract this amount from the total caloric requirement with exercise, determined previously. This final caloric intake to lose weight never should be below 1200 calories for women and 1500 for men. If distributed properly over the various food groups, these figures are the lowest caloric intakes that provide the necessary nutrients the body needs. In terms of percentages of total calories, the daily distribution should be approximately 60% carbohydrates (mostly complex carbohydrates), less than 30% fat, and about 12% protein.

The time of day when food is consumed also may play a part in weight reduction. A study conducted at the Aerobics Research Institute in Dallas, Texas, indicated that when a person is on a diet, weight is lost most effectively if he or she consumes most of the calories before 1:00 p.m. and not during the evening meal. The Institute recommends that when a person is attempting to lose weight, intake should consist of a minimum of 25% of the total daily calories for breakfast, 50% for lunch, and 25% or less at dinner.

Other experts have reported that if most of the daily calories are consumed during one meal, the body may perceive that something is wrong and will slow down the metabolism so it can store a greater amount of calories in the form of fat. Also, eating most of the calories in one meal causes a person to go hungry the rest of the day, making adherence to the diet more difficult.

Monitoring Your Diet With Daily Food Logs

To help you monitor and adhere to your diet plan, you may use the daily food logs provided in Figures 6.5 through 6.8 at the end of this chapter. Before using any of these forms, make a master copy for your files so that you can make future copies as needed. Guidelines are provided for 1200-, 1500-, 1800-, and 2000-calorie diet plans. These plans have been developed based on the Food Guide Pyramid and the Dietary Guidelines for Americans to meet the Recommended Dietary Allowances.[9,10,11] The objective is to meet (not exceed) the number of servings allowed for each diet plan. Each time you eat a serving of a particular food, record it in the appropriate box.

To lose weight, you should use the diet plan that most closely approximates your target caloric intake. Choosing low-fat/lean foods, the plan is based on the following caloric allowances for each food group:

🖝 Bread, cereal, rice, and pasta group: 80 calories per serving.

🖝 Fruit group: 60 calories per serving.

🖝 Vegetable group: 25 calories per serving.

🖝 Milk, yogurt, and cheese group (use low-fat products): 120 calories per serving.

🖝 Meat, poultry, fish, dry beans, eggs, and nuts group: Use 300-calorie low-fat frozen entrees per serving or an equivalent amount if you prepare your own main dish (see discussion below).

As you start your diet-plan, pay particular attention to food serving size. Refer to the Food Guide Pyramid (see Figure 5.5 in Chapter 5) to find out what counts as one serving. Exercise care with cup and glass sizes. A standard cup is 8 ounces, and most glasses nowadays contain between 12 and 16 ounces. If you drink 12 ounces of fruit juice, in essence you are getting two servings of fruit because a standard serving is 3/4 cup of juice.

Read labels carefully to compare the caloric value of the serving listed on the label with the caloric guidelines provided above. Here are some examples:

1. One slice of standard white bread has about 80 calories. A plain bagel may have 200 to 350 calories. Although it is low in fat, if you eat a 350-calorie bagel, you are getting almost 4½ servings in the bread, cereal, rice, and pasta group.

2. The standard serving size listed on the food label for most cereals is 1 cup. As you read the nutrition information, however, you find that for the same 1 cup of cereal, a certain type of cereal has 120 calories whereas another cereal has 200 calories. Because a standard serving in the bread, cereal, rice and pasta group is 80 calories, the first cereal would be 1½ servings and the second one 2½ servings.

3. In looking at fruit sizes, a medium size fruit usually is considered to be one serving. Large fruits could provide as many as 3 servings.

4. In the milk, yogurt, and cheese groups 1 serving represents 120 calories. A cup of whole milk has about 160 calories, while a cup of skim milk contains 88 calories. A cup of whole milk, therefore, would provide 1⅓ servings in this food group.

To be more accurate with caloric intake and to simplify meal preparation, use commercially prepared low-fat frozen entrees as the main dish for lunch and dinner meals (only one entree for the 1,200-calorie diet plan — see Figure 6.5). Look for entrees that provide about 300 calories and no more than 6 grams of fat per entree. These two entrees can be used as the meat, poultry, fish, dry beans, eggs, and nuts group selections and will provide most of the daily protein requirement for the body. Along with each entree, supplement the meal with some of your servings from the other food groups. This diet plan has been used successfully in weight-loss research programs.[12,13] If you choose not to use these low-fat entrees, prepare a similar meal using 3 ounces (cooked) of lean meat, poultry, or fish with additional vegetables, rice, or pasta that will provide 300 calories with fewer than 6 grams of fat per dish.

As you record your food choices in your daily logs, be sure to record the precise amount in each serving. If you choose to do so, you can then run a computerized nutrient analysis to verify your caloric intake and food distribution pattern (percent of total calories from carbohydrate, fat, and protein).

Tips For Behavior Modification and Adherence To a Lifetime Weight Management Program

Achieving and maintaining recommended body composition is by no means impossible, but it does require desire and commitment. If adequate weight management is to become a reality, some retraining of behavior is crucial for success. Modifying old habits and developing new, positive behaviors take time. Individuals have applied the following management techniques to change detrimental behavior successfully and adhere to a positive lifetime weight control program. In developing a retraining program, people are not expected to use all of the strategies listed but should pick the ones that apply to them.

Tips for Healthy Eating

🖎 Make a commitment to change. The first necessary ingredient to modify behavior is the desire to do so. The reasons for change must be more compelling than those for continuing present lifestyle patterns. You must accept that you have a problem and decide by yourself whether you really want to change. If you are sincerely committed, the chances for success are enhanced already.

🖎 Set realistic goals. Most people with a weight problem would like to lose weight in a relatively short time but fail to realize that the weight problem developed over a span of several years. A sound weight reduction and maintenance program can be accomplished only by establishing new lifetime eating and exercise habits, both of which take time to develop.

In setting a realistic long-term goal, short-term objectives also should be planned.

The long-term goal may be to decrease body fat to 20% of total body weight. The short-term objective may be a 1% decrease in body fat each month. Objectives like these allow for regular evaluation and help maintain motivation and renewed commitment to attain the long-term goal.

🖎 Incorporate exercise into the program. Choosing enjoyable activities, places, times, equipment, and people to work with helps a person adhere to an exercise program. Details on developing a complete exercise program are given in Chapter 3.

🖎 Differentiate hunger from appetite. Hunger is the actual physical need for food. Appetite is a desire for food, usually triggered by factors such as stress, habit, boredom, depression, food availability, or just the thought of food itself. People should eat only when they have a physical need. In this regard, developing and sticking to a regular meal pattern help control hunger.

🖎 Pay attention to calories. Some people think that because a certain food is low in fat, they can eat as much as they want. Entire boxes of fat-free cookies and bags of pretzels have been consumed under this pretense. A homemade chocolate-chip cookie may have 100 calories, whereas a low-fat one may have 50. Simple math will tell you that eating one homemade cookie is better than eating a half dozen low-fat ones.

🖎 Eat less fat. Each gram of fat provides 9 calories, and protein and carbohydrates provide only 4. In essence, you can eat more food on a low-fat diet because you consume fewer calories with each meal.

🖎 Add foods to your diet that reduce cravings.[14] Many people suffer from a biological imbalance of insulin. Insulin helps the body use and conserve energy. Some people produce so much insulin that their bodies can't use it all. This imbalance leads to an overpowering craving for carbohydrates. As more carbohydrates are eaten, even more insulin is released. Foods that reduce cravings include eggs, red meat, fish, poultry, cheese, tofu, oils, fats, and non-starchy vegetables such as lettuce, green beans, peppers, asparagus, broccoli, mushrooms, and Brussels sprouts. If you watch your portion sizes, eating foods that reduce cravings at regular meals and for snacks helps to decrease the intense desire for carbohydrates, prevent overeating, and aid with weight loss.

🏃 Avoid automatic eating. Many people associate certain daily activities with eating. For example, people may eat while cooking, watching television, or reading. Most of the time the foods consumed in these situations lack nutritional value or are high in sugar and fat.

🏃 Stay busy. People tend to eat more when they sit around and do nothing. Occupying the mind and body with activities not associated with eating helps take away the desire to eat. Some options are walking, cycling, playing sports, gardening, sewing, or visiting a library, a museum, a park. To break the routine of life, you might develop other skills and interests or try something new and exciting.

🏃 Plan meals ahead of time. Sensible shopping is necessary to accomplish this objective. (By the way, shop on a full stomach, because hungry shoppers tend to buy unhealthy foods impulsively — and then snack on the way home). The shopping list should include whole-grain breads and cereals, fruits and vegetables, low-fat milk and dairy products, lean meats, fish, and poultry.

🏃 Cook wisely.

— Use less fat and refined foods in food preparation.

— Trim all visible fat from meats and remove skin from poultry before cooking.

— Skim the fat off gravies and soups.

— Bake, broil, boil, and steam instead of frying.

— Sparingly use butter, cream, mayonnaise, and salad dressings.

— Avoid coconut oil, palm oil, and cocoa butter.

— Prepare plenty of bulky foods — those containing fiber.

— Include whole-grain breads and cereals, vegetables, and legumes in most meals.

— Eat fruits for dessert.

— Beware of soda pop, fruit juices, and fruit-flavored drinks.

— In addition to sugar, cut down on other refined carbohydrates such as corn syrup, malt sugar, dextrose, and fructose.

— Drink plenty of water — at least six glasses a day.

🏃 Do not serve more food than you should eat. Measure the food in portions, and keep serving dishes away from the table. In this way you will eat less, have a harder time getting seconds, and have less appetite because the food is not visible. People should not be forced to eat when they are satisfied (including children after they already have had a healthy, nutritious serving).

🏃 Try "junior size" instead of "super size." Use smaller plates, bowls, cups, and glasses. Over the years the sizes of dishes and glasses have gotten bigger. Consequently, people serve and eat a lot more food than they need. If you use a smaller plate, it will look like more food and you'll tend to eat less. Watch for portion sizes at restaurants as well. Plate and portion sizes at restaurants now are so large that people overeat and still end up with leftovers to take home.

🏃 Eat slowly and at the table only. Eating is one of the pleasures of life, and we need to take time to enjoy it. Eating on the run is not good because the body doesn't have enough time to "register" nutritive and caloric consumption and people overeat before the body perceives the fullness signal. Eating at the table also forces people to take time out to eat, and it deters snacking between meals, primarily because of the extra time and effort required to sit down and eat. When people are done eating, they should not sit around the table but, rather, clean up and put away the food to keep from unnecessary snacking.

✍ Avoid social binges. Social gatherings tend to entice self-defeating behavior. Visual imagery might help before attending social gatherings. Plan ahead and visualize yourself there. Do not feel pressured to eat or drink, and don't rationalize in these situations. Choose low-calorie foods, and entertain yourself with other activities such as dancing and talking.

✍ Do not raid the refrigerator and the cookie jar. In these tempting situations take control. Stop and think. Do not bring high-calorie, high-sugar, or high-fat foods into the house. If they are there already, store them where they are hard to get to or see. If they are out of sight or not readily available, the temptation is less. Keeping food in places such as the garage and basement tends to discourage people from taking the time and effort to get them. By no means should you have to eliminate treats entirely, but all things should be done in moderation.

✍ Avoid evening food raids. Most people with weight problems do really well during the day but then lose it at nighttime. Excessive snacking following the evening meal is a common pitfall. Stay busy after your evening meal. Go for a short walk, and get to bed earlier. In most cases the intense desire for food that you get during the evening hours disappears following a good night's rest.

✍ Practice stress-management techniques (more on stress in Chapter 7). Many people snack and increase food consumption in stressful situations. Eating is not a stress-releasing activity and, instead, can aggravate the problem if weight control is an issue.

✍ Monitor changes and reward accomplishments. Feedback on fat loss and lean tissue gain is a reward in itself. Awareness of changes in body composition also helps reinforce new behaviors. Being able to exercise without interruption for 15, 20, 30, 60 minutes, swimming a certain distance, running a mile — all these accomplishments deserve recognition. Meeting objectives calls for rewards that are not related to eating: new clothing, a tennis racquet, a bicycle, exercise shoes, or something else that is special and you would not have acquired otherwise.

✍ Think positive. Avoid negative thoughts about how difficult changing past behaviors might be. Instead, think of the benefits you will reap, such as feeling, looking, and functioning better, plus enjoying better health and improving the quality of life. Avoid negative environments and people who will not be supportive.

In Conclusion

Taking off excessive body fat and keeping it off for good has no simple solution. Weight management is accomplished through lifetime commitment to physical activity and proper food selection. When taking part in a weight reduction program, people have to decrease their caloric intake moderately and implement strategies to modify unhealthy eating behaviors.

Relapses into past negative behaviors are almost inevitable. Making mistakes is human and does not mean failure. Failure comes to those who give up and do not use previous experiences to build upon and, instead, develop skills that will prevent self-defeating behaviors in the future. "Where there's a will, there's a way," and those who persist will reap the rewards.

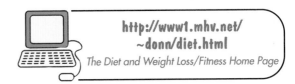
http://www1.mhv.net/
~donn/diet.html
The Diet and Weight Loss/Fitness Home Page

Notes

1. J. H. McGinnis and W. H. Foege, "Actual Causes of Death in the United States," *Journal of the American Medical Association* 270(1993), 2207–2212.

2. C. E. Barlow, H. W. Kohl, III, L. W. Gibbons, and S. N. Blair, "Physical Fitness, Mortality, and Obesity," *International Journal of Obesity*, 19(1996), S41–44.

3. R. J. Shepard, *Alive Man: The Physiology of Physical Activity* (Springfield, IL: Charles C Thomas, 1975), pp. 484–488.

4. D. Remington, A. G. Fisher, and E. A. Parent, *How to Lower Your Fat Thermostat* (Provo, UT: Vitality House International, 1983).

5. R. L. Leibel, M. Rosenbaum, and J. Hirsh, "Changes in Energy Expenditure Resulting from Altered Body Weight," *New England Journal of Medicine*, 332(1995), 621–628.

6. J. H. Wilmore. "Exercise, Obesity, and Weight Control," *Physical Activity and Fitness Research Digest* (Washington DC: President's Council on Physical Fitness & Sports, 1994).

7. K. N. Pavlou, S. Krey, and W. P. Steffe, "Exercise as an Adjunct to Weight Loss and Maintenance in Moderately Obese Subjects," *American Journal of Clinical Nutrition*, 49(1989), 1115–1123.

8. W. W. Campbell, M. C. Crim, V. R. Young, and W. J. Evans, "Increased Energy Requirements and Changes in Body Composition with Resistance Training in Older Adults," *American Journal of Clinical Nutrition*, 60(1994), 167–75.

9. U.S. Department of Agriculture and U.S. Department of Health and Human Services, "Nutrition and Your Health: Dietary Guidelines for Americans," *Home and Garden Bulletin No. 232*, December 1995.

10. U.S. Department of Agriculture, Human Nutrition Information Service, "The Food Guide Pyramid," *Home and Garden Bulletin No. 252*, December 1992.

11. National Academy Press, Food and Nutrition Board, *Recommended Dietary Allowances* (Washington D.C.: NAP, 1989).

12. W. W. K. Hoeger. et al., "Effects of the Dietary Supplement Chroma Slim® CT200 on Body Composition," *Medicine and Science in Sports and Exercise*, 30(1998), S62, 350.

13. C. Harris et al., "Twenty Five Days of Dietary Supplementation with Chroma Slim® Augments Body Fat Reduction," *Medicine and Science in Sports and Exercise*, 30(1998), S62, 351.

14. R. Heller and R. Heller, "How The Weight-Loss Scientists Lost Their Weight: You Can, Too," *Bottom Line/Personal*, 18:11(1997), 9–10.

Name:_____ Date: _____

Instructions:

The objective of the diet plan is to meet (not exceed) the number of servings allowed for the food groups listed. Each time that you eat a particular food, record it in the space provided for each group along with the appropriate serving size. Refer to the Food Guide Pyramid to find out what counts as one serving for each group listed (see Figure 5.5 in Chapter 5). Instead of the meat, poultry, fish, dry beans, eggs, and nuts group, you are allowed to have a commercially available low-fat frozen entree for your main meal (this entree should provide no more that 300 calories and less than 6 grams of fat). You can make additional copies of this form as needed.

Bread, Cereal, Rice, Pasta Group (80 calories/serving): 6 servings

1 _____
2 _____
3 _____
4 _____
5 _____
6 _____

Vegetable Group (25 calories/serving): 3 servings

1 _____
2 _____
3 _____

Fruit Group (60 calories/serving): 2 servings

1 _____
2 _____

Milk Group (120 calories/serving, use low-fat milk and low-fat milk products): 2 servings

1 _____
2 _____

Low-fat Frozen Entree (300 calories and less than 6 grams of fat): 1 serving

1 _____

 Figure 6.5 *Daily Food Intake Record: 1,200 Calorie-Diet Plan.*

Name:_____ Date: _____

Instructions:

The objective of the diet plan is to meet (not exceed) the number of servings allowed for the food groups listed. Each time that you eat a particular food, record it in the space provided for each group along with the appropriate serving size. Refer to the Food Guide Pyramid to find out what counts as one serving for each group listed (see Figure 5.5 in Chapter 5). Instead of the meat, poultry, fish, dry beans, eggs, and nuts group, you are allowed to have two commercially available low-fat frozen entrees for two of your meals (these entrees should provide no more that 300 calories and less than 6 grams of fat). You can make additional copies of this form as needed.

Bread, Cereal, Rice, Pasta Group (80 calories/serving): 6 servings

1 _____
2 _____
3 _____
4 _____
5 _____
6 _____

Vegetable Group (25 calories/serving): 3 servings

1 _____
2 _____
3 _____

Fruit Group (60 calories/serving): 2 servings

1 _____
2 _____

Milk Group (120 calories/serving, use low-fat milk and low-fat milk products): 2 servings

1 _____
2 _____

Two Low-fat Frozen Entrees (300 calories and less than 6 grams of fat): 2 servings

1 _____
2 _____

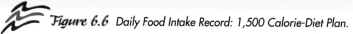

Figure 6.6 Daily Food Intake Record: 1,500 Calorie-Diet Plan.

Name:_____ Date: _____

Instructions:

The objective of the diet plan is to meet (not exceed) the number of servings allowed for the food groups listed. Each time that you eat a particular food, record it in the space provided for each group along with the appropriate serving size. Refer to the Food Guide Pyramid to find out what counts as one serving for each group listed (see Figure 5.5 in Chapter 5). Instead of the meat, poultry, fish, dry beans, eggs, and nuts group, you are allowed to have two commercially available low-fat frozen entrees for two of your meals (these entrees should provide no more that 300 calories and less than 6 grams of fat). You can make additional copies of this form as needed.

Bread, Cereal, Rice, Pasta Group (80 calories/serving): 8 servings

1 _____	5 _____
2 _____	6 _____
3 _____	7 _____
4 _____	8 _____

Vegetable Group (25 calories/serving): 5 servings

1 _____
2 _____
3 _____
4 _____
5 _____

Fruit Group (60 calories/serving): 3 servings

1 _____
2 _____
3 _____

Milk Group (120 calories/serving, use low-fat milk and low-fat milk products): 2 servings

1 _____
2 _____

Two Low-fat Frozen Entrees (300 calories and less than 6 grams of fat): 2 servings

1 _____
2 _____

 Figure 6.7 *Daily Food Intake Record: 1,800 Calorie-Diet Plan.*

Name:_____ Date: _____

Instructions:

The objective of the diet plan is to meet (not exceed) the number of servings allowed for the food groups listed. Each time that you eat a particular food, record it in the space provided for each group along with the appropriate serving size. Refer to the Food Guide Pyramid to find out what counts as one serving for each group listed (see Figure 5.5 in Chapter 5). Instead of the meat, poultry, fish, dry beans, eggs, and nuts group, you are allowed to have two commercially available low-fat frozen entrees for two of your meals (these entrees should provide no more that 300 calories and less than 6 grams of fat). You can make additional copies of this form as needed.

Bread, Cereal, Rice, Pasta Group (80 calories/serving): 10 servings

1	_____	6	_____
2	_____	7	_____
3	_____	8	_____
4	_____	9	_____
5	_____	10	_____

Vegetable Group (25 calories/serving): 5 servings

1 _____

2 _____

3 _____

4 _____

5 _____

Fruit Group (60 calories/serving): 4 servings

1 _____

2 _____

3 _____

4 _____

Milk Group (120 calories/serving, use low-fat milk and low-fat milk products): 2 servings

1 _____

2 _____

Two Low-fat Frozen Entrees (300 calories and less than 6 grams of fat): 2 servings

1 _____

2 _____

 Figure 6.8 Daily Food Intake Record: 1,800 Calorie-Diet Plan.

Stress Management and Assessment

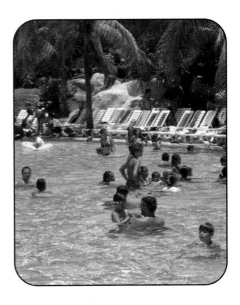

*L*earning to live and get ahead today is not possible without stress. To succeed in an unpredictable world that changes with every new day, working under pressure has become the rule rather than the exception for most people. As a result, stress has become one of the most common problems we face. Current estimates indicate that the annual cost of stress and stress-related diseases in the United States exceeds $100 billion, a direct result of health-care costs, lost productivity, and absenteeism.

Stress is a fact of modern life. Every person actually has an optimal level of stress that is most conducive to adequate health and performance. When stress levels reach mental, emotional, and physiological limits, however, stress becomes distress and the person no longer functions effectively.

The body's response to stress has been the same ever since humans were first put on the earth. Stress prepares the organism to react to the stress-causing event, called the **stressor**. The problem, is the way in which we react to stress. Many people thrive under stress. Others under similar circumstances are unable to handle it. An individual's reaction to a stress-causing agent determines whether stress is positive or negative.

Chronic distress raises the risk for many health disorders, including coronary heart disease, hypertension, eating disorders, ulcers, diabetes, asthma, depression, migraine headaches, sleep disorders, and chronic fatigue and may even play a role in the development of certain types of cancer. Recognizing when stress becomes distress and overcoming the problem quickly and efficiently are crucial in maintaining emotional and physiological stability.

The good news is that stress can be self-controlled. Most people have accepted stress as

Objectives

- Define stress, eustress, and distress.
- Explain how stress affects health and optimal performance.
- Define the two major types of behavior patterns or personality types.
- Learn to lower your vulnerability to stress.
- Develop time-management skills.
- Identify the major sources of stress in your life.
- Define the role of physical exercise in reducing stress.
- Learn to use various stress-management techniques.

a normal part of daily life, and even though everyone has to deal with it, few seem to understand it and know how to cope effectively. Stress should not be avoided entirely, as a certain amount is necessary for optimum health, performance, and well-being. It is difficult to succeed and have fun in life without "hits, runs, and errors."

The Body's Reaction to Stress

Dr. Hans Selye, one of the foremost authorities on **stress**, defined it as "the nonspecific response of the human organism to any demand that is placed upon it."[1] "Nonspecific" indicates that the body reacts in a similar way regardless of the nature of the event that leads to the stress response. In simpler terms, stress is the body's mental, emotional, and physiological response to any situation that is new, threatening, frightening, or exciting.

The body responds to stress with a rapid-fire sequence of physical changes known as **fight-or-flight.** The hypothalamus activates the sympathetic nervous system, and the pituitary gland triggers the release of catecholamines (hormones) from the adrenal glands. These hormonal changes increase heart rate, blood pressure, blood flow to active muscles and the brain, glucose levels, oxygen consumption, and strength — all necessary for the body to *either* fight or flee. In both cases of fight or flight the body relaxes and stress dissipates. If the person is unable to take action, however, the muscles tense up and tighten (see Figure 7.1).

Stress isn't necessarily bad. Dr. Selye further defined stress as either **eustress** or **distress.** In both cases, the nonspecific response is almost the same. In the case of eustress, health and performance continue to improve even as stress increases. With distress, health and performance begin to deteriorate.

Behavior Patterns

Common life events are not the only source of stress in life. All too often individuals bring on stress as a result of their characteristic behavior patterns. The two main types of behavior patterns are Type A and Type B. Each type is based on several characteristics that are used to classify people into one of these behavioral patterns.

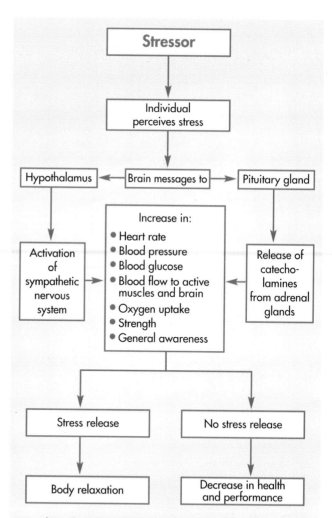

From *Lifetime Physical Fitness & Wellness,* by W. W. K. Hoeger and S. A. Hoeger (Englewood, CO: Morton Publishing, 1998), p. 286.

Figure 7.1 Physiological response to stress: fight or flight mechanism.

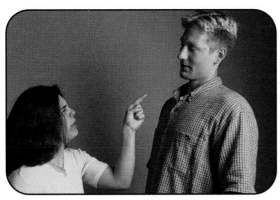

Anger and hostility can be a health risk factor.

Type A behavior characterizes a primarily hard-driving, overambitious, aggressive, at times hostile and overly competitive person. Type A individuals often set their own goals, are self-motivated, try to accomplish many tasks at the same time, are excessively achievement-oriented, and have a high degree of time urgency. In contrast, **Type B** behavior is characteristic of calm, casual, relaxed, easy-going individuals. Type B people take one thing at a time, do not feel pressured or hurried, and seldom set their own deadlines.

Over the years, experts have indicated that individuals classified as Type A have a significantly higher incidence for disease, especially cardiovascular conditions.[2] More recent evidence indicates that not all typical Type A people are at higher risk for disease. Type A individuals who have chronic anger and hostility are at higher risk.[3] The questionnaire provided in Figure 7.2 can help you determine whether you have a hostile personality.

Some experts believe that emotional stress is far more likely than physical stress to trigger a heart attack. People who are impatient and readily annoyed when they have to wait for someone or something — an employee, a traffic light, in a restaurant line — are especially vulnerable. Research also is focusing on individuals who have anxiety, depression, and feelings of helplessness when they encounter setbacks and failures in life. People who lose control of their lives, those who give up on their dreams in life, knowing

that they could and should be doing better, may be more likely to have heart attacks than hard-driving people who enjoy their work.

Many of the Type A characteristics are learned behaviors. Consequently, if people can learn to identify the sources of stress, they can change their behavioral responses. The main assessment tool to determine behavioral type is the *Structured Interview*, in which the interviewee is asked to reply to several questions that describe Type A and Type B behavior patterns. The interviewer notes not only the responses to the questions but also mental, emotional, and physical behaviors the individual exhibits as he or she replies to each question. Based on the answers and the associated behaviors, the interviewer rates the person along a continuum ranging from Type A to Type B.

Vulnerability to Stress

Researchers have identified a number of factors that can affect the way in which people handle stress. How people deal with these factors actually can increase or decrease vulnerability to stress. The questionnaire provided in Figure 7.3 lists these factors so you can determine your vulnerability rating. Many of the items on this

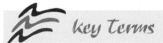

key terms

Stress The mental, emotional, and physiological response of the body to any situation that is new, threatening, frightening, or exciting.

Stressor Stress-causing agent.

Fight or flight A series of physical responses activated automatically in response to environmental stressors.

Eustress Positive stress.

Distress Negative or harmful stress under which health and performance begin to deteriorate.

Type A Behavior pattern characteristic of a hard-driving, overambitious, aggressive, at times hostile, and overly competitive person.

Type B Behavior pattern characteristic of a calm, casual, relaxed, and easy-going individual.

Hostility Could Harm Your Heart

Experts now conclude that feelings of hostility increase your risk of heart disease. Dr. Redford Williams, Duke University Medical Center, has designed a questionnaire to help you determine whether you have a hostile personality. Circle the answer that most closely fits how you would respond to the given situation:

1. **A teenager drives by my yard blasting the car stereo:**
   A. I begin to understand why teenagers can't hear.
   B. I can feel my blood pressure starting to rise.

2. **A boyfriend/girlfriend calls at the last minute "too tired to go out tonight." I'm stuck with two $15 tickets:**
   A. I find someone else to go with.
   B. I tell my friend how inconsiderate he/she is.

3. **Waiting in the express checkout line at the supermarket where a sign says "No More Than 10 Items Please":**
   A. I pick up a magazine and pass the time.
   B. I glance to see if anyone has more than 10 items.

4. **Most homeless people in large cities:**
   A. Are down and out because they lack ambition.
   B. Are victims of illness or some other misfortune.

5. **At times when I've been very angry with someone:**
   A. I was able to stop short of hitting him/her.
   B. I have, on occasion, hit or shoved him/her.

6. **When I am stuck in a traffic jam:**
   A. I am usually not particularly upset.
   B. I quickly start to feel irritated and annoyed.

7. **When there's a really important job to be done:**
   A. I prefer to do it myself.
   B. I am apt to call on my friends to help.

8. **The cars ahead of me start to slow and stop as they approach a curve:**
   A. I assume there is a construction site ahead.
   B. I assume someone ahead had a fender-bender.

9. **An elevator stops too long above where I'm waiting:**
   A. I soon start to feel irritated and annoyed.
   B. I start planning the rest of my day.

10. **When a friend or co-worker disagrees with me:**
    A. I try to explain my position more clearly.
    B. I am apt to get into an argument with him or her.

11. **At times when I was really angry in the past:**
    A. I have never thrown things or slammed a door.
    B. I've sometimes thrown things or slammed a door.

12. **Someone bumps into me in a store:**
    A. I pass it off as an accident.
    B. I feel irritated at their clumsiness.

13. **When my spouse (significant other) is fixing a meal:**
    A. I keep an eye out to make sure nothing burns.
    B. I talk about my day or read the paper.

14. **Someone is hogging the conversation at a party:**
    A. I look for an opportunity to put him/her down.
    B. I soon move to another group.

15. **In most arguments:**
    A. I am the angrier one.
    B. The other person is angrier than I am.

Score one point for each of these answers: 1. B, 2. B, 3. B, 4. A, 5. B, 6. B, 7. A, 8. B, 9. A, 10. B, 11. B, 12. B, 13. A, 14. A, 15. A. If you scored 4 or more points you may be hostile. Questions 1, 6, 9, 12 and 15 reflect anger. Questions 2, 5, 10, 11, 14, reflect aggression. Questions 3, 4, 7, 8, 13 reflect cynicism. If you scored 2 points in any category, you should work on that area of your personality.

From *Anger Kills* by Redford B. Williams, M.D., and Virginia Williams, Ph.D. Copyright © 1993 by Redford B. Williams, M.D. and Virginia Williams, Ph.D. Reprinted by permission of Random House, Inc.

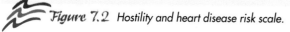

Figure 7.2 Hostility and heart disease risk scale.

Stress Vulnerability Questionnaire

Item	Strongly Agree	Mildly Agree	Mildly Disagree	Strongly Disagree
1. I try to incorporate as much physical activity* as possible in my daily schedule.	1	2	3	4
2. I exercise aerobically 20 minutes or more at least three times per week.	1	2	3	4
3. I regularly sleep 7 to 8 hours per night.	1	2	3	4
4. I take my time eating at least one hot, balanced meal a day.	1	2	3	4
5. I drink fewer than two cups of coffee (or equivalent) per day.	1	2	3	4
6. I am at recommended body weight.	1	2	3	4
7. I enjoy good health.	1	2	3	4
8 I do not use tobacco in any form.	1	2	3	4
9. I limit my alcohol intake to no more than one drink per day.	1	2	3	4
10. I do not use hard drugs (chemical dependency).	1	2	3	4
11. I have someone I love, trust, and can rely on for help if I have a problem or need to make an essential decision.	1	2	3	4
12. There is love in my family.	1	2	3	4
13. I routinely give and receive affection.	1	2	3	4
14. I have close personal relationships with other people who provide me with a sense of emotional security.	1	2	3	4
15. There are people close by whom I can turn to for guidance in time of stress.	1	2	3	4
16. I can speak openly about feelings, emotions, and problems with people I trust.	1	2	3	4
17. Other people rely on me for help.	1	2	3	4
18. I am able to keep my feelings of anger and hostility under control.	1	2	3	4
19. I have a network of friends who enjoy the same social activities I do.	1	2	3	4
20. I take time to do something fun at least once a week.	1	2	3	4
21. My religious beliefs provide guidance and strength to my life.	1	2	3	4
22. I often provide service to others.	1	2	3	4
23. I enjoy my job (major or school).	1	2	3	4
24. I am a competent worker.	1	2	3	4
25. I get along well with co-workers (or students).	1	2	3	4
26. My income is sufficient for my needs.	1	2	3	4
27. I manage time adequately.	1	2	3	4
28. I have learned to say "no" to additional commitments when I am already pressed for time.	1	2	3	4
29. I take daily quiet time for myself.	1	2	3	4
30. I practice stress management as needed.	1	2	3	4

Total Points: ☐

Scoring:

0–30 points	Excellent (great resistance to stress)
31–40 points	Good (little vulnerability to stress)
41–50 points	Average (somewhat vulnerable to stress)
51–60 points	Fair (vulnerable to stress)
≥61 points	Poor (highly vulnerable to stress)

*Walk instead of driving, avoid escalators and elevators, or walk to neighboring offices, homes, and stores.

From *Lifetime Physical Fitness & Wellness,* by W. W. K. Hoeger and S. A. Hoeger (Englewood, CO: Morton Publishing, 1998), p. 273.

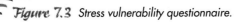 **Figure 7.3** *Stress vulnerability questionnaire.*

Changing a Type A Personality

🏃 Make a contract with yourself to slow down and take it easy. Put it in writing. Post it in a conspicuous spot, then stick to the terms you set up. Be specific. Abstracts ("I'm going to be less uptight") don't work.

🏃 Work on only one or two things at a time. Wait until you change one habit before you tackle the next one.

🏃 Eat more slowly, and eat only when you are relaxed and sitting down.

🏃 If you smoke, quit.

🏃 Cut down on your caffeine intake, as it increases the tendency to become irritated and agitated.

🏃 Take regular breaks throughout the day, even as brief as 5 or 10 minutes, when you totally change what you're doing. Get up, stretch, get a drink of cool water, walk around for a few minutes.

🏃 Work on fighting your impatience. If you're standing in line at the grocery store, study the interesting things people have in their carts instead of getting upset.

🏃 Work on controlling hostility. Keep a written log. When do you flare up? What causes it? How do you feel at the time? What preceded it? Look for patterns, and figure out what sets you off. Then do something about it. Either avoid the situations that cause you hostility or practice reacting to them in different ways.

🏃 Plan some activities just for the fun of it. Load a picnic basket in the car and drive to the country with a friend. After a stressful physics class, stop at a theater and see a good comedy.

🏃 Choose a role model, someone you know and admire who does not have a Type A personality. Observe the person carefully, then try out some techniques the person demonstrates.

🏃 Simplify your life so you can learn to relax a little bit. Figure out which activities or commitments you can eliminate right now, then get rid of them.

🏃 If morning is a problem time for you and you get too hurried, set your alarm clock half an hour earlier.

🏃 Take time out during even the most hectic day to do something truly relaxing. Because you won't be used to it, you may have to work at it at first. Begin by listing things you'd really enjoy that would calm you. Include some things that take only a few minutes: Watch a sunset, lie out on the lawn at night and look at the stars, call an old friend and catch up on news, take a nap, sauté a pan of mushrooms and savor them slowly.

🏃 If you're under a deadline, take short breaks. Stop and talk to someone for 5 minutes, take a short walk, or lie down with a cool cloth over your eyes for 10 minutes.

🏃 Pay attention to what your own body clock is saying. You've probably noticed that every 90 minutes or so, you lose the ability to concentrate, get a little sleepy, and have a tendency to daydream. Instead of fighting the urge, put down your work and let your mind wander for a few minutes. Use the time to imagine and let your creativity run wild.

🏃 Learn to treasure unplanned surprises: a friend dropping by unannounced, a hummingbird outside your window, a child's tightly clutched bouquet of wildflowers.

🏃 Savor your relationships. Think about the people in your life. Relax with them and give yourself to them. Give up trying to control others, and resist the urge to end relationships that don't always go as you'd like them to.

From *Wellness: Guidelines for a Healthy Lifestyle* by B. Q. Hafen and W. W. K. Hoeger (2d ed.) (Englewood, CO: Morton Publishing, 1998), p. 30.

questionnaire are related to health, social support, self-worth, and nurturance (sense of being needed). All of the factors are crucial for a person's physical, social, mental, and emotional well-being. The questionnaire will help you identify specific areas in which you can make improvements to help you cope more efficiently.

The benefits of physical fitness are discussed extensively in this book. Further, social support, self-worth, and nurturance are essential to cope effectively with stressful life events. These factors render a supportive and protective role in people's lives. The more integrated people are in society, the less vulnerable they are to stress and illness.

Positive correlations have been found between social support and health outcomes. People can draw upon social support to weather crises. Knowing that someone else cares, that people are there to lean on, that support is out there, is valuable for survival (or growth) in times of need.[4]

As you take the test, you will notice that many of the items describe situations and behaviors that are within your own control. To make yourself less vulnerable to stress, you will want to improve the behaviors that make you more vulnerable to stress. You should start by modifying the behaviors that are easiest to change before undertaking some of the most difficult ones.

Sources of Stress

Before addressing techniques that you can use to cope more effectively with stress, attempt to identify your current life stressors. To conduct this exercise, use the stress test provided in Figure 7.4. This test will help you determine stressors that you have encountered recently in your life. Think back over this past year and circle the "stress points" listed for each event that you experienced during this time. Then total the points and determine the amount of stress in your life during the past year according to the scale provided at the bottom of the scale.

Next, to help you cope more effectively, use the stress analysis form provided in Figure 7.5.

In this form, list the stressors that affect you the most in daily life. For each stressor, explain in the box provided the situation(s) under which it occurs, your response to it, the impact it is having in your life, and how you are presently

Common Symptoms of Stress

- headaches
- muscular aches (mainly in neck, shoulders, and back)
- grinding teeth
- nervous tick, finger tapping, toe tapping
- increased sweating
- increase in or loss of appetite
- insomnia
- nightmares
- fatigue
- dry mouth
- stuttering
- high blood pressure
- tightness or pain in the chest
- impotence
- hives
- dizziness
- depression
- irritation
- anger
- hostility
- fear, panic, anxiety
- stomach pain, flutters
- nausea
- cold, clammy hands
- poor concentration
- pacing
- restlessness
- rapid heart rate
- low-grade infection
- loss of sex drive
- rash or acne

Take the Stress Test

To get a feel for the possible health impact of the various recent changes in your life, think back over the past year and circle the "stress points" listed for each of the events that you experienced during that time. Then add up your points. A total score of anywhere from about 250 to 500 or so would be considered a moderate amount of stress. If you score higher than that, you may face an increased risk of illness; if you score lower than that, consider yourself fortunate.

Health

An injury or illness which:

kept you in bed a week or more, or sent you to the hospital	74
was less serious than that	44
Major dental work	26
Major change in eating habits	27
Major change in sleeping habits	26
Major change in your usual type or amount of recreation	28

Work

Change to a new type of work	51
Change in your work hours or conditions	35

Change in your responsibilities at work:

more responsibilities	29
fewer responsibilities	21
promotion	31
demotion	42
transfer	32

Troubles at work:

with your boss	29
with co-workers	35
with persons under your supervision	35
other work troubles	28
Major business adjustment	60
Retirement	52

Loss of job:

laid off from work	68
fired from work	79
Correspondence course to help you in your work	18

Home and family

Major change in living conditions	42

Change in residence:

move within the same town or city	25
move to a different town, city, or state	47
Change in family get-togethers	25
Major change in health or behavior of family member	55
Marriage	50
Pregnancy	67
Miscarriage or abortion	85

Gain of a new family member:

birth of a child	66
adoption of a child	65
a relative moving in with you	59
Spouse beginning or ending work	46

Child leaving home:

to attend college	41
due to marriage	41
for other reasons	45
Change in arguments with spouse	50
In-law problems	38

Change in the marital status of your parents:

divorce	59
remarriage	50

Separation from spouse:

due to work	53
due to marital problems	76
Divorce	96
Birth of grandchild	43
Death of spouse	119

Death of other family member:

child	123
brother or sister	102
parent	100

Personal and social

Change in personal habits	26
Beginning or ending school or college	38
Change of school or college	35
Change in political beliefs	24
Change in religious beliefs	29
Change in social activities	27
Vacation trip	24
New, close, personal relationship	37
Engagement to marry	45
Girlfriend or boyfriend problems	39
Sexual difficulties	44
"Falling out" of a close personal relationship	47
An accident	48
Minor violation of the law	20
Being held in jail	75
Death of a close friend	70
Major decision about your immediate future	51
Major personal achievement	36

Financial

Major change in finances:

increased income	38
decreased income	60
investment or credit difficulties	56
Loss or damage of personal property	43
Moderate purchase	20
Major purchase	37
Foreclosure on a mortgage or loan	58

Total score: [ ]

Source: Reprinted from the *Journal of Psychosomatic Research*, Vol. 43, Miller and Rahe, "Life Changes Scaling for the 1990's." 1997, with permission from Elsevier Science.

Figure 7.4 Stress test.

In the boxes provided below, list common stressors you encounter in daily life. For each stressor, explain the situation(s) under which it occurs, your response to it, the impact it is having in your life, and how you presently are handling the stressor. Also indicate what you can do to either avoid the stressor or cope with it more effectively in the future.

Stressor:

Stressor:

Stressor:

Figure 7.5   Stress analysis.

Stressor:

Stressor:

Stressor:

Figure 7.5 Stress analysis (continued).

handling the stressor. Based on what you have already learned, also indicate what you can do to either avoid the stressor or more effectively cope with it in the future. Upon completion of this exercise, proceed to the Relaxation Techniques section on page 146. Once you have learned and mastered some of these techniques, return to your stress analysis and reevaluate your approach to cope with each stressor.

Coping With Stress

The ways in which people perceive and cope with stress seems to be more important in the development of disease than the amount and type of stress itself. If individuals perceive stress as a definite problem in their lives, when it interferes with optimal level of health and performance, several techniques can help them cope more effectively.

First, of course, the person must recognize the existence of a problem. Many people either do not want to believe they are under too much stress or they fail to recognize some of the typical symptoms of distress. Noting some of the stress-related symptoms will help a person respond more objectively and initiate an adequate coping response.

When people have stress-related symptoms, they first should try to identify and remove the stressor or stress-causing agent. This is not as

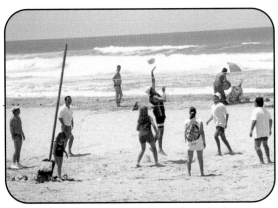

To prevent psychological burnout, add regular leisure-time physical activity to your schedule.

Releasing Anger the Healthy Way

🖎 Recognize the anger for what it is. Don't be afraid of it or try to suppress it.

🖎 Figure out what made you so angry, then decide whether it's worth being so upset. Chances are that it's really a minor irritation or hassle.

🖎 Stop before you act. Calm down first. Count to 10, take a deep breath, mentally recite the words to a favorite verse, or initiate some other distracting and relaxing activity. Then get ready to deal with the anger.

🖎 If you're ticked off at somebody else, use calm tact to say why, without ripping into the other person. Tell him or her how you're feeling, and try to negotiate some things.

🖎 Be generous with the other person. Maybe he just failed an exam. Maybe she just heard bad news from home. Maybe he's having a rotten day. Listen carefully to her side of things, and try as much as you can to understand.

🖎 When all else fails, forgive the other person. Everyone makes mistakes. Carrying a grudge will hurt you worse than it hurts the other person.

From *Wellness: Guidelines for a Healthy Lifestyle,* by B. Q. Hafen and W. W. K. Hoeger (2d ed,) (Englewood, CO: Morton Publishing, 1998), p. 34.

simple as it may seem, because in some situations eliminating the stressor is not possible, or a person may not even know the exact causing agent. If the cause is unknown, keeping a log of the time and days when the symptoms occur, as well as the events preceding and following the onset of symptoms, may be helpful.

For instance, a couple noted that every afternoon around 6 o'clock, the wife became nauseated and had abdominal pain. After seeking professional help, both were instructed to keep a log of daily events. It soon became clear that the symptoms did not occur on weekends but always started just before the husband came home from work during the week. Following some personal interviews with the couple, it was determined that the wife felt a lack of attention from her husband and responded subconsciously by becoming ill to the point at which she required personal care and affection from her husband. Once the stressor was identified, appropriate behavior changes were initiated to correct the situation.

In many instances, however, the stressor cannot be removed. Examples of situations in which little or nothing can be done to eliminate the stress-causing agent are the death of a close family member, first year on the job, an intolerable boss, a change in work responsibility. Nevertheless, stress can be managed through time management and relaxation techniques.

Time Management

According to Benjamin Franklin, "Time is the stuff life is made of." The current "hurry-up" style of life is not conducive to wellness. The hassles involved in getting through a typical day often lead to stress-related illnesses. People who do not manage their time properly will experience chronic stress, fatigue, despair, discouragement, and illness.

Based on a 1990 Gallup Poll, almost 80% of Americans reported that time moves too fast for them, and 54% felt they had to get everything done. The younger the respondents, the more they struggled with lack of time. Almost half wished they had more time for exercise and recreation, hobbies, and family.

Healthy and successful people are good time managers, able to maintain a pace of life within their comfort zone. In a survey of 1954 Harvard graduates from the school of business, only 27% had reached the goals they established in college. Every one had rated himself as a superior time manager, and only 8% of the remaining graduates perceived themselves as superior time managers. The successful graduates attributed their success to "smart work," not necessarily "hard work."

Trying to achieve one or more goals in a limited time can create a tremendous amount of stress. Many people just don't seem to have enough hours in the day to accomplish their tasks. The greatest demands on our time, nonetheless, frequently are self-imposed: trying to do too much, too fast, too soon.

Although some time killers, such as eating, sleeping, and recreation, are necessary for health and wellness, in excess they will cause stress. To make better use of your time:

1. Find the time killers. Many people do not know how they spend each part of the day. Keep a 4- to 7-day log, and record your activities at half-hour intervals. As you go through your typical day, record the activities so you will remember all of them. At the end of each day, decide when you wasted time. You may be shocked by the amount of time you spent on the phone, sleeping (more than 8 hours per night), or watching television.

2. Set long-range and short-range goals. Setting goals requires some in-depth thinking

Common Time killers

- watching television
- listening to radio/music
- sleeping
- eating
- daydreaming
- shopping
- socializing/parties
- recreation
- talking on the telephone
- worrying
- procrastination
- drop-in visitors
- confusion (unclear goals)
- indecision (what to do next)
- interruptions
- perfectionism (every detail must be done)

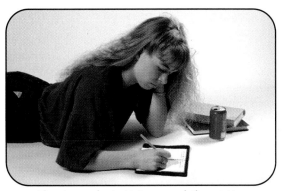

Planning and prioritizing your daily activities simplifies your days.

and helps put your life and daily tasks in perspective. Write down three goals that you want to accomplish: (a) in life, (b) 10 years from now, (c) this year, (d) this month, and (e) this week. You may want to file this form and review it in years to come.

3. Identify your immediate goals, and prioritize them for today and this week. Each day sit down and determine what you need to accomplish that day and that week. Rank your "today" and "this week" tasks in three categories: (a) top-priority, (b) medium-priority, and (c) "trash."

   Top-priority tasks are the most important ones. If you were to reap most of your productivity from 30% of your activities, which would they be? Medium-priority activities must be done but can wait a day or two. Trash activities are those that are not worth your time (for example, cruising the hallways).

4. Use a daily planner to help you organize and simplify your day. In this way you can access your priority list, appointments, notes, references, names, places, phone numbers, and addresses conveniently from your coat pocket or purse. Many individuals think that planning daily and weekly activities is a waste of time. A few minutes to schedule your time each day, however, will pay off in hours saved.

As you plan your day, be realistic and find your comfort zone. Determine what is the best way to organize your day. Which is the most productive time for work, study, errands? Are you a morning person, or are you getting most of your work done when other people are quitting for the day? Pick your best hours for top-priority activities. Be sure to schedule enough time for exercise and relaxation. Recreation is not necessarily wasted time. You need to take care of your physical and emotional well-being. Otherwise your life will be seriously imbalanced.

5. Take 10 minutes each night to figure out how well you accomplished your goals that day. Successful time managers evaluate themselves daily. This simple task will help you see the entire picture. Cross off the goals you accomplished, and carry over to the next day those you did not get done. You also may realize that some goals can be moved down to low-priority or be trashed.

In addition to the above steps, the following general suggestions can help you make better use of your time:

✍ *Delegate.* When possible, delegate activities that someone else can do for you. Having another person type your paper while you prepare for an exam might be well worth the expense and your time.

✍ *Say "no."* Learn to say no to activities that keep you from getting your top priorities done. You can do only so much in a single day. Nobody has enough time to do everything he or she would like to get done. Don't overload either. Many people are afraid to say no because they feel guilty if they do. Think ahead, and think of the consequences. Are you doing it to please others? What will it do to your well-being? Can you handle one more task? At some point you have to balance your activities and look at life and time realistically.

🏋️ *Protect against boredom.* Doing nothing can be a source of stress. People need to feel that they are contributing and that they are productive members of society. It also is good for self-esteem and self-worth. Set realistic goals, and work toward them each day.

🏋️ *Plan ahead for disruptions.* Even a careful plan of action can be disrupted. An unexpected phone call or visitor can ruin your schedule. Planning your response ahead of time will help you deal with these saboteurs.

🏋️ *Get it done.* Select only one task at a time, concentrate on it, and see it through. Many people do a little here, do a little there, then do something else. In the end nothing gets done. An exception to working on just one task at a time is when you are doing a difficult task. Rather than "killing yourself," interchange with another activity that is not as hard.

🏋️ *Eliminate distractions.* If you have trouble adhering to a set plan, remove distractions and trash activities from your eyesight. Television, radio, magazines, open doors, or studying in a park might distract you and become time killers.

🏋️ *Set aside "overtimes."* Regularly schedule time you did not think you would need as overtime to complete unfinished projects. Most people underschedule rather than overschedule time. The result is usually late-night burnout! If you schedule overtimes and get your tasks done, enjoy some leisure time, get ahead on another project, or work on some of your trash priorities.

🏋️ *Plan time for you.* Set aside special time for yourself daily. Life is not meant to be all work. Use your time to walk, read, or listen to your favorite music.

🏋️ *Reward yourself.* As with any other healthy behavior, positive change or a job well done deserves a reward. We often overlook the value of rewards, even if they are self-given. People practice behaviors that are rewarded and discontinue those that are not.

Relaxation Techniques

Stress management skills are essential to cope effectively and move forward in today's fast-paced world. Although benefits are reaped immediately after engaging in any of the several relaxation techniques described in this chapter, several months of regular practice may be necessary for total mastery. The relaxation exercises that follow should not be considered cure-alls or panaceas. If they do not prove to be effective, more specialized resources and professional help are indicated. In some instances a person's symptoms may not be caused by stress but, rather, may be related to a different medical disorder.

Physical Activity

Physical exercise is one of the simplest tools to control stress. Exercise and fitness are thought to reduce the intensity of stress and recovery from a stressful event. The value of exercise in reducing stress is related to several factors, the main one being less muscular tension.

For example, a person may be distressed because he or she has a miserable day at work and the job requires 8 hours of work in a smoke-filled room with an intolerable boss. To make matters worse, it is late and on the way home the car in front is going much slower than the speed limit. The body's fight or flight mechanism is activated. Heart rate and blood pressure shoot up, breathing quickens and deepens, muscles tense up, and all systems say "go." No action can be initiated, however, and the stress cannot be dissipated because you just cannot hit your boss or the car in front of you. A person surely could take action, though, by "hitting" the tennis ball, the weights, the swimming pool, or the jogging trail. By engaging in physical activity, a person is able to reduce the muscular tension and eliminate the physiological changes that triggered the fight-or-flight mechanism.

Physical exercise gives people an overall boost because it:

🏋️ Lessens feelings of anxiety, depression, frustration, aggression, anger, and hostility.

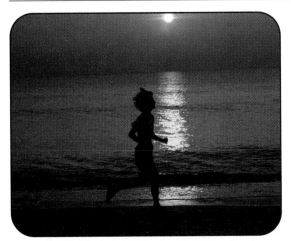

Physical activity is an excellent tool to control stress.

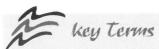 Alleviates insomnia.

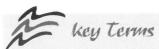 Provides an opportunity to meet social needs and develop new friendships.

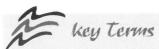 Allows people to share common interests and problems.

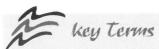 Develops self-discipline.

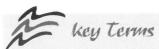 Provides the opportunity to do something enjoyable and constructive that will lead to better health and total well-being.

Although exercise has enhanced the health and quality of life of millions of people, for a small group of individuals, exercise can become an obsessive behavior with potentially addictive qualities. Compulsive exercisers often express feelings of guilt and discomfort when they miss a day's workout. These individuals sometimes continue to exercise even when they are injured or ill and should get proper rest for adequate recovery. Under these circumstances exercise becomes a biological stressor that will compromise performance and health.

As a biological stressor, compulsive exercise or overtraining produces both physiological and psychological symptoms. Many physical activities (for example, jogging, basketball, aerobics) performed at high intensity levels or for unusually long periods (overtraining) can be detrimental to a person's physical and emotional well-being.

Psychological symptoms of overtraining include lower motivation, depression, sleep disturbances, increased irritability, and lack of confidence. Physiological symptoms include musculoskeletal injuries, lower performance, slower recovery time, chronic fatigue, decreased appetite, loss of weight and lean tissue, fat gain, increased muscle tension, higher resting heart rate and blood pressure, and even ECG abnormalities. If you experience any of these symptoms, you need to reevaluate your exercise program and make adjustments accordingly. People who exceed the recommended guidelines for fitness development and maintenance (see Chapters 3 and 4) are exercising for reasons other than health, and some actually may be aggravating an already stressful situation.

Progressive Muscle Relaxation

One of the most popular methods used to dissipate stress is **progressive muscle relaxation,** which enables individuals to relearn the sensation of deep relaxation. Acute awareness of how it feels to progressively tighten and relax the muscles releases muscle tension and teaches the body to relax at will. Feeling the tension during the exercises also helps the person to be more alert to signs of distress because this tension is similar to that experienced in stressful situations. In everyday life these feelings then can cue the person to do relaxation exercises.

Relaxation exercises should be done in a quiet, warm, well-ventilated room. The exercises should encompass all muscle groups of the body. Most important is that the individual pay attention to the sensation he or she feels each time the muscles are tensed and relaxed. The instructions can be read to the person or memorized or tape-recorded. At least 20 minutes should be set aside to complete the entire sequence. Doing the

key Terms

Progressive muscle relaxation A relaxation technique that involves contracting, then relaxing muscle groups in the body in succession.

exercises any faster will defeat their purpose. Ideally, the sequence should be done twice a day.

First, the individual performing the exercises stretches out comfortably on the floor, face up, with a pillow under the knees, and assumes a passive attitude, allowing the body to relax as much as possible. Each muscle group is to be contracted in sequence, taking care to avoid any strain. Muscles should be tightened to only about 70% of the total possible tension to avoid cramping or some type of injury to the muscle itself.

To produce the relaxation effects, the person must pay attention to the sensation of tensing up and relaxing. The person holds each contraction about 5 seconds and then allows the muscles to go totally limp. The person should take enough time to contract and relax each muscle group before going on to the next. An example of a complete progressive muscle relaxation sequence is as follows:

1. Point your feet, curling the toes downward. Study the tension in the arches and the top of the feet. Hold, and continue to note the tension, then relax. Repeat once again.

2. Flex the feet upward toward the face, and note the tension in your feet and calves. Hold, and relax. Repeat once more.

3. Push your heels down against the floor as if burying them in the sand. Hold, and note the tension at the back of the thigh. Relax. Repeat once more.

4. Contract the right thigh by straightening the leg, gently raising the leg off the floor. Hold, and study the tension. Relax. Repeat with the left leg. Hold and relax. Repeat each leg again.

5. Tense the buttocks by raising your hips ever so slightly off the floor. Hold, and note the tension. Relax. Repeat once again.

6. Contract the abdominal muscles. Hold them tight and note the tension. Relax. Repeat one more time.

7. Suck in your stomach. Try to make it reach your spine. Flatten your lower back to the floor. Hold, and feel the tension in the stomach and lower back. Relax. Repeat once more.

8. Take a deep breath and hold it, then exhale. Repeat. Note your breathing becoming slower and more relaxed.

9. Place your arms at the side of your body and clench both fists. Hold, study the tension, and relax. Repeat a second time.

10. Flex the elbow by bringing both hands to the shoulders. Hold tight and study the tension in the biceps. Relax. Repeat one more time.

11. Place your arms flat on the floor, palms up, and push the forearms hard against the floor. Note the tension on the triceps. Hold, and relax. Repeat once more.

12. Shrug your shoulders, raising them as high as possible. Hold, and note the tension. Relax. Repeat once again.

13. Gently push your head backward. Note the tension in the back of the neck. Hold, relax. Repeat one more time.

14. Gently bring the head against the chest, push forward, hold, and note the tension in the neck. Relax. Repeat a second time.

15. Press your tongue toward the roof of your mouth. Hold, study the tension, and relax. Repeat once more.

16. Press your teeth together. Hold, and study the tension. Relax. Repeat one more time.

17. Close your eyes tightly. Hold them closed and note the tension. Relax, leaving your eyes closed. Do this one more time.

18. Wrinkle your forehead and note the tension. Hold, and relax. Repeat one more time.

When time is a factor during the daily routine and an individual is not able to go through the entire sequence, he or she may do only the exercises specific to the area that feels most tense. Performing a partial sequence is better than not doing the exercises at all. Completing the entire sequence, of course, yields the best results.

Breathing Techniques

Breathing exercises, too, also can be an antidote to stress. These exercises have been used for centuries in Asian countries to improve mental, physical, and emotional stamina. In breathing exercises the person concentrates on "breathing away" the tension and inhaling fresh air to the entire body. Breathing exercises can be learned in only a few minutes and require considerably less time than the progressive muscle relaxation exercises.

As with any other relaxation technique, these exercises should be done in a quiet, pleasant, well ventilated room. Any of the three examples of breathing exercises presented here will help relieve tension induced by stress.

1. *Deep breathing.* Lie with your back flat against the floor, and place a pillow under your knees, feet slightly separated, with toes pointing outward. (The exercise also may be done while sitting up in a chair or standing straight up). Place one hand on your abdomen and the other hand on your chest.

   Breathe in and out slowly so the hand on your abdomen rises when you inhale and falls as you exhale. The hand on the chest should not move much at all. Repeat the exercise about 10 times. Then scan your body for tension, and compare your present tension with the tension you felt at the beginning of the exercise. Repeat the entire process once or twice more.

2. *Sighing.* Using the abdominal breathing technique, breathe in through your nose to a specific count (e.g., 4, 5, or 6). Now exhale through pursed lips to double the intake count (e.g., 8, 10, or 12). Repeat the exercise eight to 10 times whenever you feel tense.

3. *Complete natural breathing.* Sit in an upright position or stand straight up. Breathing through your nose, fill your lungs gradually from the bottom up. Hold your breath for several seconds. Now exhale slowly by allowing your chest and abdomen

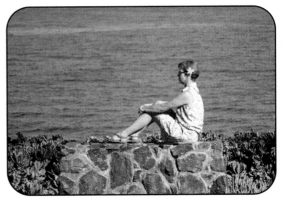

Meditation is an effective way to reduce stress.

to relax completely. Repeat the exercise eight to 10 times.

Meditation

More than 700 scientific studies have verified that **meditation** induces relaxation and alleviates the harmful physiological effects of stress. This technique can be learned rather quickly and can be used frequently during times of increased stress.

Initially the person who is learning to meditate should choose a room that is comfortable, quiet, and free of all disturbances (including telephones). After learning the technique, the person will be able to meditate just about anywhere. A time block of approximately 15 minutes, twice a day, is suggested for meditation.

1. Sit in a chair in an upright position with the hands resting either in your lap or on the arms of the chair. Close your eyes and focus on your breathing. Allow your body to relax as much as possible. Do not consciously try to relax, because trying means work. Rather, assume a passive attitude and concentrate on your breathing.

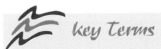

key Terms

Meditation A mental exercise in which the objective is to gain control over one's attention, clearing the mind and blocking out stressor(s).

2. Allow your body to breathe regularly, at its own rhythm, and repeat in your mind the word "one" every time you inhale, and the word "two" every time you exhale. Paying attention to these two words keeps distressing thoughts from entering into your mind.

3. Continue to breathe in this way about 15 minutes. Because the objective of meditation is to bring about a hypometabolic state leading to body relaxation, do not use an alarm clock to remind you that the 15 minutes have expired. The alarm will only trigger the stress response again, defeating the purpose of the exercise. Opening your eyes once in a while to keep track of the time is fine, but do not rush or anticipate the end of the 15 minutes. This time has been set aside for meditation, and you need to relax, take your time, and enjoy the exercise.

Which Technique Is Best?

Each person reacts to stress differently. Therefore, the best strategy to alleviate it depends mostly on the individual. Which technique is used does not matter as long as it works. You may want to experiment with all of them to find out which works best. A combination of two or more works best for many people.

All of the coping strategies discussed in this chapter help to block out stressors and promote mental and physical relaxation by diverting the attention to a different, nonthreatening action. Some of the techniques are easier to learn and take less time per session. Regardless of which technique you select, the time spent doing stress management exercises (several times a day, as needed) is well worth the effort when stress becomes a significant problem in life.

People need to learn to relax and take time out for themselves. Stress is not what makes people ill but, rather, the way they react to the stress-causing agent. Individuals who learn to be diligent and start taking control of themselves find that they can enjoy a better, happier, and healthier life.

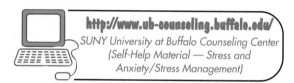

http://www.ub-counseling.buffalo.edu/
SUNY University at Buffalo Counseling Center
(Self-Help Material — Stress and
Anxiety/Stress Management)

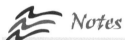 *Notes*

1. Hans Selye, *Stress Without Distress* (New York: Signet, 1974).

2. See Ray Rosenman, "Do You Have Type 'A' Behavior?" *Health and Fitness* (supplement), 1987; Redford Williams, *The Trusting Heart: Great News About Type A Behavior* (New York: Times Books, 1989), p. 120; Howard Friedman, *The Self-Healing Personality* (New York: Henry Holt & Co., 1991).

3. Redford Williams, *The Trusting Heart* (New York: Times Books, Division of Random House, 1989).

4. D. Girdano and G. Everly, *Controlling Stress and Tension: A Holistic Approach* (Englewood Cliffs, NJ: Prentice Hall, 1992); W. Schafer, *Stress Management for Wellness* (Ft. Worth: HBJ College Publishers, 1995).

A Healthy Lifestyle Approach

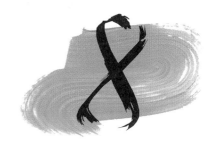

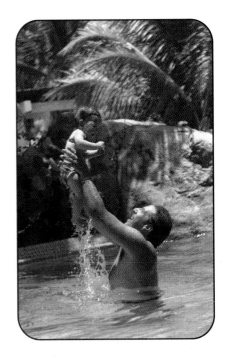

*T*he present lifestyle of many North Americans is such a serious threat to their health that it actually leads to premature illness and death. Improving the quality, and most likely the length, of our lives is a matter of personal choice. The combination of a fitness program and a healthy lifestyle program — the wellness approach — can lead to better health and quality of life.

As defined in Chapter 1, wellness is the constant and deliberate effort to stay healthy and achieve the highest potential for well-being. Wellness incorporates healthy lifestyle factors such as good fitness and nutrition, stress management, disease prevention, social support and self-worth, spirituality, substance abuse control, personal safety, and health education (see Figure 8.1). Ten simple lifestyle habits can increase longevity significantly:

1. Be physically active (including exercise).
2. Do not use tobacco.
3. Eat a healthy diet.
4. Maintain recommended body weight.
5. Sleep 7 to 8 hours each night.
6. Decrease stress levels.
7. Drink alcohol moderately or not at all.
8. Surround yourself with healthy relationships.
9. Be informed about the environment and avoid environmental risk factors.
10. Take personal safety measures.

Of all deaths in the United States, more than 64% are caused by cardiovascular disease and cancer.[1] Close to 80% of these deaths could be

Objectives

🏊 Understand the importance of implementing a healthy lifestyle program.

🏊 Identify the major risk factors for coronary heart disease.

🏊 Become acquainted with cancer-prevention guidelines.

🏊 Recognize the relationship between spirituality and wellness.

🏊 Learn the health consequences of chemical abuse and irresponsible sex.

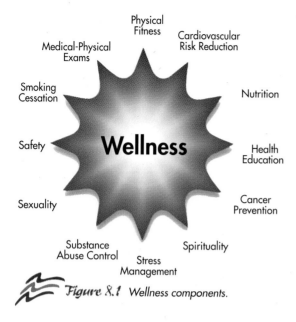

Figure 8.1 Wellness components.

prevented by following a healthy lifestyle. The third and fourth leading causes of death, chronic and obstructive pulmonary disease and accidents, also are preventable, primarily by abstaining from tobacco and other drugs, wearing seat belts, and using common sense. In looking at the underlying causes of death in the United States,[2] (see Figure 8.2) 9 of the 10 causes are related to lifestyle and lack of common sense. The "big three" — tobacco use, poor diet and inactivity, and alcohol abuse — are responsible for more than 800,000 annual deaths.

Diseases of the Cardiovascular System

The most prevalent degenerative conditions in the United States are **cardiovascular diseases**. One in six men and one in eight women age 45 and older have had a heart attack or stroke.[3] Based on 1995 vital statistics, 42% of all deaths in the United States were attributable to heart and blood vessel disease.[4] Some examples of cardiovascular diseases are coronary heart disease, peripheral vascular disease, congenital heart

disease, rheumatic heart disease, atherosclerosis, strokes, high blood pressure, and congestive heart failure. According to estimates, if all deaths from the major cardiovascular diseases were eliminated, life expectancy in the United States would increase by about 10 years.[5] Table 8.1 provides the estimated prevalence and annual number of deaths caused by the major types of cardiovascular disease.

According to the American Heart Association, the estimated cost of heart and blood vessel disease in the United States exceeded $274 billion in 1998. About 1.5 million people have heart attacks each year, and close to half a million of them die as a result. More than half of these deaths occur within 1 hour of the onset of symptoms, before the person reaches the hospital.[6]

Although heart and blood vessel disease is still the number-one health problem in the United States, the incidence declined by 36% in the two decades between 1970 and 1990 (see

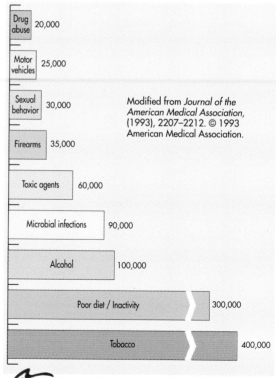

Modified from *Journal of the American Medical Association*, (1993), 2207–2212. © 1993 American Medical Association.

Figure 8.2 Underlying causes of death in the United States.

Table 8.1 *Estimated Prevalence and Yearly Number of Deaths from Cardiovascular Disease 1995*

	Prevalence	Deaths
Major forms of cardiovascular diseases[*]	58,200,000	960,592
Coronary heart disease	13,900,000[**]	
Heart attack	1,500,000	481,287
Stroke	4,080,000	157,991
High blood pressure	50,000,000	39,981[***]
Rheumatic fever/rheumatic heart disease	1,800,000	5,147

[*]Includes people with one or more forms of cardiovascular disease.
[**]Number of deaths included under heart attack.
[***]Mortality figures appear to be low because many heart attacks and stroke deaths are caused by high blood pressure.

Sources: American Heart Association, *Heart Stroke Facts* (Dallas: AHA, 1996); American Heart Association, *1995 Heart and Stroke Statistical Update* (Dallas: AHA, 1997).

Figure 8.3). The main reason for this dramatic decrease is health education. More people now are aware of the risk factors for cardiovascular disease and are changing their lifestyle to lower their potential risk for these diseases.

The heart and the coronary arteries are illustrated in Figure 8.4. The major form of cardiovascular disease is **coronary heart disease (CHD)**. In CHD the arteries that supply the heart muscle with oxygen and nutrients are narrowed by fatty deposits such as cholesterol and triglycerides. Narrowing of the coronary arteries diminishes the blood supply to the heart muscle, which can precipitate a heart attack. CHD is the single leading cause of death in the United States, accounting for approximately 21% of all deaths and about half of all cardiovascular

Warning Signals of a Heart Attack

The following symptoms may not all be present during a heart attack. If any start to occur, seek medical attention immediately. Failure to do so may result in death.

- Discomfort, pressure, fullness, squeezing, or pain in the middle of the chest that persists for several minutes. It may go away and return later.
- Pain that radiates to the shoulders, neck, or arms.
- Chest discomfort with lightheadedness, shortness of breath, nausea, sweating, or fainting.

Adapted from American Heart Association, *Heart Stroke Facts*, (Dallas: AHA, 1996).

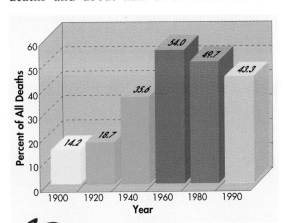

Figure 8.3 *Incidence of cardiovascular disease in the United States for selected years: 1900–1990.*

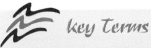

key Terms

Cardiovascular diseases Array of conditions that affect the heart and the blood vessels.

Coronary heart disease (CHD) Condition caused by obstruction of coronary arteries by plaque formation.

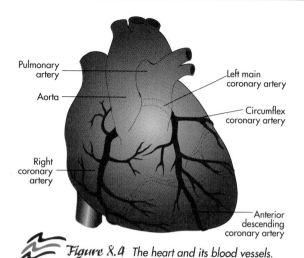

Figure 8.4 The heart and its blood vessels.

deaths.[7] More than half of the people who died suddenly from CHD had no previous symptoms of the disease. Further, the risk of death is greater in the least educated segment of the population.[8]

Risk Factors

The leading contributors to the development of CHD are:

- Physical inactivity
- High blood pressure
- Excessive body fat
- Low HDL-cholesterol
- Elevated LDL-cholesterol
- Elevated triglycerides
- Elevated homocysteine
- Diabetes
- Abnormal electrocardiograms (ECG)
- Tobacco use
- Stress
- Personal and family history of cardiovascular disease
- Gender
- Age

An important concept in CHD risk management is that — with the exception of age, gender, family history of heart disease, and certain electrocardiographic abnormalities — the risk factors are preventable and reversible. Approximately 90% of CHD can be prevented if people practice healthy lifestyle habits.[9] The above risk factors are discussed in the following pages.

Physical Inactivity

Improving cardiorespiratory endurance through aerobic exercise has perhaps the greatest impact in reducing the overall risk for cardiovascular disease. In this day and age of mechanized societies, we cannot afford *not* to exercise. Research data on the benefits of aerobic exercise in reducing cardiovascular disease are too impressive to be ignored.

Guidelines for implementing an aerobic exercise program are discussed thoroughly in Chapter 3. Following these guidelines will promote cardiorespiratory fitness, enhance health, and extend the lifespan. Even moderate amounts of aerobic exercise can reduce cardiovascular risk considerably. As shown in Figure 8.5, work conducted at the Aerobics Research Institute in

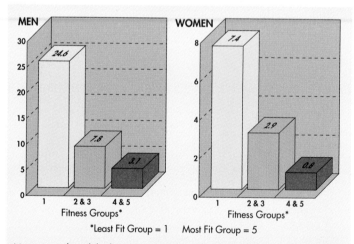

Note: Age-adjusted death rates per 10,000 person-years of follow-up, 1978–1985

From "Physical Fitness and All-Cause Mortality: A Prospective Study of Healthy Man and Woman" by S. N. Blair, H. W. Kohl, III, R. S. Paffenbarger, Jr., D. B. Clark, D. H. Cooper, and L. W. Gibbons, *Journal of the American Medical Association*, 262 (1985), 2395–2401.

Figure 8.5 The relationship between fitness levels and cardiovascular mortality.

Dallas showed a much higher incidence of cardiovascular deaths in unfit people (group 1) as compared to moderately fit people (groups 2 and 3).[10]

A regular aerobic exercise program helps to control most of the major risk factors that lead to heart and blood vessel disease. Aerobic exercise will:

- 🖋️ increase cardiorespiratory endurance.
- 🖋️ decrease and control blood pressure.
- 🖋️ reduce body fat.
- 🖋️ lower blood lipids (cholesterol and triglycerides).
- 🖋️ improve HDL-cholesterol (see later discussion).
- 🖋️ help control or decrease the risk for diabetes.
- 🖋️ increase and maintain good heart function, sometimes improving certain ECG abnormalities.
- 🖋️ motivate toward smoking cessation.
- 🖋️ alleviate stress.
- 🖋️ counteract a personal history of heart disease.

The significance of physical inactivity in contributing to cardiovascular risk was shown clearly in 1992 when the American Heart Association added physical inactivity as one of the five major risk factors for cardiovascular disease. (The other four are smoking, a poor cholesterol profile, high blood pressure, and obesity.)

High Blood Pressure (Hypertension)

Blood pressure should be checked regularly, regardless of whether it is or is not elevated. The pressure is measured in milliliters of mercury (mm Hg) and usually expressed in two numbers. The higher number reflects the *systolic pressure*, the pressure exerted during the forceful contraction of the heart. The lower value, *diastolic pressure*, is taken during the heart's relaxation phase, when no blood is being ejected.

Ideal blood pressure is 120/80 or below. The American Heart Association considers all blood pressures over 140/90 as **hypertension**. High blood pressure can be controlled with different types of medications, along with the lifestyle changes described below for people with mild hypertension. Because people respond differently to these medications, a physician may try out several to find out which produces the best results with the fewest side effects.

Recommended for people with mild hypertension are regular aerobic exercise, weight control, a low-salt/low-fat and high potassium/high calcium diet, lower alcohol and caffeine intake, smoking cessation, and stress management. People with high blood pressure should follow their physician's advice and stay on any prescribed medication.

Excessive Body Fat (Obesity)

As defined in Chapter 2, body composition is used in reference to the fat and nonfat components of the human body. If a person has too much fat weight, he or she is overweight or obese. Obesity long has been recognized as a risk factor for coronary heart disease, and in June 1998, the American Heart Association added it to its list of major risks for this disease. Maintaining recommended body weight (fat percent) is essential in any cardiovascular risk reduction program. For individuals with excessive body fat, even a modest weight reduction of 5% to 10% can reduce high blood pressure and total cholesterol levels. The causes of obesity are complex, including an individual's combination of genetics, behavior, and lifestyle factors. Guidelines for a comprehensive weight management program are given in Chapter 6.

Abnormal Cholesterol Profile

The term **blood lipids** is used mainly with reference to cholesterol and triglycerides. Because these substances cannot float around freely

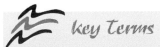

key Terms

Blood pressure The force of the blood exerted against artery walls.
Hypertension Blood pressure exceeding 140/90.
Blood Lipids Fat-soluble substances in the body.

in the water-based medium of the blood, they are packaged and transported in the blood by complex molecules called lipoproteins.

If you never have had a blood lipid test, it is highly recommended. The blood test includes total cholesterol, high-density lipoprotein cholesterol (HDL-cholesterol), low-density lipoprotein cholesterol (LDL-cholesterol), and triglycerides. A significant elevation in blood lipids has been linked to heart and blood vessel disease.

A poor blood lipid profile is thought to be the most important predisposing factor in the development of CHD, accounting for almost half of all cases. The general recommendation by the National Cholesterol Education Program (NCEP) is to keep total cholesterol levels below 200 mg/dl (see Table 8.2). The risk for heart attack risk increases 2% for every 1% increase in total cholesterol.[11]

Cholesterol levels between 200 and 239 mg/dl are borderline high, and levels of 240 mg/dl and above indicate high risk for disease. Approximately 51%, or 96.8 million American adults, have total cholesterol values of 200 mg/dl or higher, and 20% (37.7 million adults) have values at or above 240 mg/dl.[12]

Many preventive medicine practitioners recommend a lower total cholesterol level, ranging between 160 and 180 mg/dl. For children the level should be below 170 mg/dl. In the well known Framingham Heart Study, a 50-year ongoing project in the community of Framingham, Massachusetts, not a single individual with a total cholesterol level of 150 mg/dl or lower had a heart attack in the study period reported in 1986.[13]

Perhaps even more significant is the way cholesterol is carried in the bloodstream. **Cholesterol**, found only in animal fats and oil, is transported primarily by **high-density lipoproteins** (**HDL**) (a steroid alcohol) and **low-density lipoproteins** (**LDL**). HDL tends to attract cholesterol, which is carried to the liver to be metabolized and excreted. It acts as a scavenger, removing cholesterol from the body and preventing **atherosclerosis**.

Of the body's cholesterol, 60% to 80% is transported by LDL. If the blood has too much LDL cholesterol, it may adhere to the lining of the arteries and cause atherosclerosis. An LDL-cholesterol value below 130 mg/dl is desirable, between 130 and 159 mg/dl is borderline-high, and 160 mg/dl and above is high risk for cardiovascular disease. For people with cardiovascular problems, LDL should be 100 mg/dl or lower.[14]

The more HDL-cholesterol, the better. It is the "good cholesterol" and offers some protection against heart disease. Evidence suggests that low levels of HDL-cholesterol could be the best predictor of CHD and may be more significant than the total cholesterol value. Substantial research supports the evidence that a low level of HDL-cholesterol has the strongest relationship to CHD at all levels of total cholesterol, including levels below 200 mg/dl. The recommended HDL-cholesterol values to minimize the risk for CHD are 45 mg/dl or higher. A level below 35 mg/dl is viewed as having high risk for CHD. An HDL level above 60 mg/dl is believed to decrease the risk for coronary disease.

Increasing the HDL-cholesterol improves the cholesterol profile and reduces the risk for CHD. Habitual aerobic exercise (an intensity level above 6 METs), proper weight loss, and quitting smoking have all been shown to raise

Table 8.2 Standards for Blood Lipids

Total Cholesterol	≤200 mg/dl	Desirable
	201–239 mg/dl	Borderline high
	≥240 mg/dl	High risk
LDL-Cholesterol	≤130 mg/dl	Desirable
	131–159 mg/dl	Borderline high
	≥160 mg/dl	High risk
HDL-Cholesterol	≥45 mg/dl	Desirable
	36–44 mg/dl	Moderate risk
	≤35 mg/dl	High risk
Triglycerides	≤125 mg/dl	Desirable
	126–499 mg/dl	Borderline high
	≥500 mg/dl	High risk

Source: National Cholesterol Education Program

HDL-cholesterol. Getting enough beta-carotene, substituting monounsaturated oils for saturated fat in the diet (not to exceed 30% of all calories consumed during the day), and engaging in drug therapy also promote higher HDL-cholesterol levels.

If LDL-cholesterol is higher than ideal, it can be lowered by losing body fat, manipulating the diet, and taking medication. A diet low in fat, saturated fat, transfatty acids, and cholesterol and high in fiber is recommended to decrease LDL-cholesterol. The National Cholesterol Education Program (NCEP) recommends replacing saturated fat with monounsaturated fat (for example, olive, canola, peanut, and sesame oils), because the latter does not cause a reduction in HDL-cholesterol and actually may lower LDL-cholesterol.

Many experts believe that, to have a significant effect in lowering LDL-cholesterol, total fiber intake must be in the range of 25 to 30 grams per day (see the discussion on fiber in Chapter 5); total fat consumption must be significantly lower than the current 30% of total daily caloric intake guidelines; saturated fat consumption has to be under 10% of the total daily caloric intake; and the average cholesterol consumption should be much lower than 300 mg per day.

Most people in the United States have an average fiber intake of less than 12 grams per day. Fiber — in particular the soluble type — has been shown to lower cholesterol by helping bind and excrete fats from the body. The incidence of heart disease is low in populations where daily fiber intake exceeds 30 grams per day. Further, a 1996 Harvard University Medical School study on 43,000 middle-age men followed for more than 6 years showed that increasing fiber intake to 30 daily grams resulted in a 41% reduction in heart attacks.[15]

Saturated fats are found mostly in meats and dairy products but seldom in foods of plant origin. Poultry and fish contain less saturated fat than beef but should be eaten in moderation (about 3 to 6 ounces per day). Transfatty acids are partially saturated fats whose chemical structures have been changed during a fat-hardening

process called hydrogenation. This process is done to increase shelf life and to solidify these fats so they are more spreadable (for example, margarine). Unsaturated fats are mainly of plant origin and cannot be converted to cholesterol.

The antioxidant effect of Vitamins C and E and beta-carotene also can reduce the risk for CHD.[16] Scientific information suggests that a single unstable free radical (oxygen compound produced in normal metabolism) can damage LDL particles. Vitamin C seems to inactivate free radicals, and vitamin E protects LDL from oxidation. Beta-carotene not only absorbs free radicals, keeping them from causing damage, but it also may help increase HDL levels. One to two medium-size carrots (raw) per day provide the recommended daily amount of beta-carotene antioxidant nutrients.

Research on the effects of a 30%-fat diet has shown that it has little or no effect in lowering cholesterol and that CHD actually continues to progress in people who have the disease. The good news came in a 1991 study published in the *Archives of Internal Medicine*,[17] which reported that the men and women in the study lowered their cholesterol by an average of 23% in only 3 weeks following a 10% or less fat-calorie diet combined with a regular aerobic exercise program, primarily walking. In this diet, cholesterol intake was limited to less than 25 mg/day. The author of the study concluded that, although the exact percent fat guideline (10% or 15%) is unknown (it also varies from individual

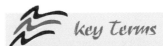

key terms

Cholesterol A waxy substance, technically a steroid alcohol, found only in animal fats and oil; used in making cell membranes, as a building block for some hormones, in the fatty sheath around nerve fibers, and in other necessary substances.

High-density lipoproteins (HDL) Substances in the blood that attract, transport, and remove cholesterol.

Low-density lipoproteins (LDL) Cholesterol-transporting molecules in the blood (bad cholesterol).

Atherosclerosis Harmful accumulation of plaque in the arteries.

to individual), 30% total fat calories is definitely too high a level when attempting to decrease cholesterol.

A daily 10% total-fat diet requires that the person limit fat intake to an absolute minimum. Some health-care professionals contend that a diet like this is difficult to follow indefinitely. People with high cholesterol levels, however, may not need to follow that diet indefinitely but should adopt the 10% fat diet while attempting to lower cholesterol. Thereafter, eating a 30%-fat diet may be adequate to maintain recommended cholesterol levels (national data indicate that current fat consumption in the United States averages 37% of total calories; see Figure 5.1 in Chapter 5).

A drawback of very low fat diets (less than 25% fat) is that they tend to lower HDL-cholesterol and increase triglycerides. If HDL-cholesterol is low already, monounsaturated fat should be added to the diet. Olive oil and nuts are sample food items that are high in monounsaturated fat. A specialized nutrition book should be consulted to determine food items that are high in monounsaturated fat.

The following dietary guidelines are recommended to lower LDL-cholesterol levels:

- Consume between 25 and 30 grams of fiber daily.
- Eat fewer than three eggs per week.
- Consume red meats (3 ounces per serving) fewer than three times per week, and no organ meats (such as liver and kidneys).
- Do not eat commercially baked foods.
- Drink low-fat milk (1% or less fat, preferably) and low-fat dairy products.
- Do not use coconut oil, palm oil, or cocoa butter.
- Eat fish instead of red meat.
- Bake, broil, grill, poach, or steam food instead of frying.
- Refrigerate cooked meat before adding to other dishes. Remove fat hardened in the refrigerator before mixing the meat with other foods.
- Avoid fatty sauces made with butter, cream, and cheese.
- Maintain recommended body weight.

Elevated Triglycerides

Triglycerides, also known as free fatty acids, in combination with cholesterol, speed up the formation of plaque. **Very low-density lipoproteins** (VLDLs) and chylomicrons carry triglycerides in the bloodstream. These fatty acids are found in poultry skin, lunch meats, and shellfish, but they are manufactured mainly in the liver, from refined sugars, starches, and alcohol. A high intake of alcohol and sugars (honey included) significantly raises triglyceride levels. The level can be lowered by cutting down on these foods along with reducing weight (if overweight) and doing aerobic exercise. A normal blood triglyceride level is less than 125 mg/dl (see Table 8.2). For people with cardiovascular problems, this level should be below 100 mg/dl.[18]

Elevated Homocysteine

Clinical data indicating that many heart attack victims have normal cholesterol levels have led researchers to look for other risk factors that may contribute to atherosclerosis. Although it is not a blood lipid, a high concentration of **homocysteine** in the blood is thought to enhance plaque formation and subsequent blockage of the arteries.[19] The body uses homocysteine to help build proteins and carry out cellular metabolism. It is an intermediate amino acid in the interconversion of two other amino acids: methionine and cysteine. This interconversion requires the B vitamin folate (folic acid) and vitamins B_6 and B_{12}.

Typically, homocysteine is metabolized rapidly, so it does not accumulate in the blood or damage the arteries. Many people, however, have high blood levels of homocysteine. This might be attributable to either a genetic inability to metabolize homocysteine or a deficiency in the vitamins required for its conversion. Homocysteine accumulation is theorized to be toxic because it may:

1. Cause damage to the inner lining of the arteries (the initial step in the process of atherosclerosis);
2. Stimulate the proliferation of cells that contribute to plaque formation; and
3. Encourage clotting that may completely obstruct an artery.

Keeping homocysteine from accumulating in the blood seems to be as simple as eating the recommended daily servings of vegetables, fruits, grains, and some meat and legumes. Increasing evidence that folate can prevent heart attacks has led to the recommendation that people consume 400 mcg per day of folate. Unfortunately, estimates indicate that less than 88% of Americans get 400 daily mcg of folate.[20] Five daily servings of fruits and vegetables can provide sufficient levels of folate and vitamin B_6 to remove and clear homocysteine from the blood. People who consume these five servings are unlikely to derive extra benefits from a vitamin B complex supplement.

Vitamin B_{12} is found primarily in animal flesh and animal products. Vitamin B_{12} deficiency is rarely a problem, as 1 cup of milk or an egg provides the daily requirement. The body also recycles most of this vitamin; therefore, it takes years to develop a deficiency.

Because of the mounting evidence of the benefits of nutrient supplementation, Dr. William Castelli, medical director of the Framingham Cardiovascular Institute, offers the following daily supplement recommendations to prevent heart disease:[21]

- 400 IU of vitamin E (d-alpha tocopherol)
- 500 to 1000 mg of vitamin C
- 200 mcg of selenium
- A vitamin B complex supplement

For people who have elevated cholesterol, 500 mg of daily niacin (also a B vitamin) can help lower cholesterol. Niacin supplementation, nonetheless, may produce side effects such as flushing, tingling, and itching. These symptoms usually disappear in a few days but may return if the dose is altered or the supplement is not taken at the same time each day. Dr. Castelli, nonetheless, points out that vitamin and mineral supplements do not replace a diet with ample amounts of daily fruits, vegetables, and whole grains.

Diabetes

In people who have **diabetes mellitus** the pancreas totally stops producing insulin, or does not produce enough to meet the body's needs, or the cells become resistant to the effects of insulin. The role of insulin is to "unlock" the cells and escort glucose into the cell.

The incidence of cardiovascular disease and death in the diabetic population is quite high. More than 80% of people with diabetes mellitus die from cardiovascular disease. People with chronically elevated blood glucose levels may have problems in metabolizing fats, which can make them more susceptible to atherosclerosis, coronary disease, heart attacks, high blood pressure, and strokes. Diabetics also have lower HDL-cholesterol and higher triglyceride levels.

Chronic high blood sugar also can lead to nerve damage, vision loss, kidney damage, and decreased immune function (making the individual more susceptible to infections). Diabetics are four times as likely to become blind and 20 times more likely than nondiabetics to develop kidney failure. Nerve damage in the lower extremities decreases the person's awareness to injury and infection. A small untreated sore can cause severe infection, gangrene, and even lead to an amputation.[22]

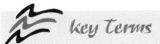

Key Terms

Triglycerides Fats formed by glycerol and three fatty acids.

Very low density lipoprotein (VLDL) Proteins that transport cholesterol and triglycerides in the bloodstream.

Homocysteine An amino acid used to build proteins and carry out cell metabolism.

Diabetes mellitus A disease in which the body doesn't produce or properly utilize insulin.

An 8-hour fasting blood glucose level above 126 mg/dl on two separate tests confirms a diagnosis of diabetes. A level of 126 or higher should be brought to the attention of a physician. This guideline has changed from previous years, in which a level above 140 had been used to diagnose diabetes. The guideline was revised in 1997.

Diabetes is of two types:

1. Type I, or insulin-dependent diabetes (IDDM). Also called juvenile diabetes because it is found mainly in young people.
2. Type II, or non-insulin-dependent diabetes (NIDDM).

In Type I the pancreas produces little or no insulin. With type II, the pancreas either does not produce sufficient insulin or it produces adequate amounts but the cells become insulin-resistant, keeping glucose from entering the cell.

Although diabetes has a genetic predisposition, adult-onset (Type II) diabetes is related closely to overeating, obesity, and lack of physical activity. More than 80% of Type II diabetics are overweight or have a history of excessive weight. In most cases this condition can be corrected through a special diet, a weight-loss program, and a regular exercise program.

A diet high in complex carbohydrates and water-soluble fibers (found in fruits, vegetables, oats, and beans), low in saturated fat, and low in sugar is helpful in treating diabetes. Several research reports have shown that a habitual aerobic exercise program (walking, cycling, or swimming four to five times per week) increases the body's receptivity to insulin. More recently, both moderate-intensity and vigorous physical activity have been associated with increased insulin sensitivity and decreased risk for diabetes.[23] The key to increase and maintain proper insulin sensitivity is *regularity* of the exercise program. Failure to maintain habitual physical activity voids the benefits.

Aggressive weight loss, especially if combined with increased activity, often allows diabetic patients to normalize their blood sugar level without the use of medication. Individuals who have high blood glucose levels should consult a physician to decide on the best treatment.

Abnormal Electrocardiograms (ECGs)

Electrocardiograms (ECGs) are taken at rest, during the stress of exercise, and during recovery. An **exercise ECG** also is known as a graded exercise stress test or a maximal exercise tolerance test. Similar to a high-speed road test on a car, a **stress ECG** reveals the heart's tolerance to high-intensity exercise. Based on the findings, ECGs may be interpreted as normal, equivocal, or abnormal.

A stress ECG frequently is used to diagnose coronary heart disease. It also is administered to determine cardiorespiratory fitness levels, to screen individuals for preventive and cardiac rehabilitation programs, to detect abnormal blood pressure response during exercise, and to establish actual or functional maximal heart rate for purposes of exercise prescription.

Not every adult who wishes to start or continue in an exercise program needs a stress ECG. The following guidelines can help you determine when this type of test should be conducted:

1. Men over age 40 and women over age 50.
2. A total cholesterol level above 200 mg/dl, or an HDL-cholesterol level below 35 mg/dl.
3. Hypertensive and diabetic patients.
4. Cigarette smokers.
5. Individuals with a family history of CHD, syncope, or sudden death before age 60.
6. People with an abnormal resting ECG.
7. All individuals with symptoms of chest discomfort, dysrhythmias, syncope, or chronotropic incompetence (a heart rate that increases slowly during exercise and never reaches maximum).

Tobacco Use

Cigarette smoking is the single largest preventable cause of illness and premature death in the United States. When considering all related deaths, tobacco is responsible for 400,000 unnecessary deaths per year.[24] Smoking has been

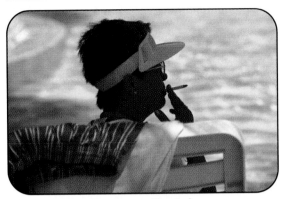

Cigarette smoking is the single largest preventable cause of illness and premature death in the United States.

linked to cardiovascular disease, cancer, bronchitis, emphysema, and peptic ulcers.

About 53,000 of those yearly deaths are nonsmokers who were exposed to secondhand smoke in daily life. Both fatal and nonfatal cardiac events are increased greatly in people exposed to passive smoking. Some 37,000 yearly deaths from heart disease are attributed to secondhand smoke. Because of the slight adaptation to the harmful effects of smoking in regular smokers, adverse effects of passive smoking are much greater to the nonsmoker. Secondhand smoke is ranked behind active smoking and alcohol as the third leading preventable cause of death in the United States.[25] Passive smoking is a significant risk factor for heart disease in children and adults alike.

In relation to coronary disease, not only does smoking speed up the process of atherosclerosis, but it also produces a threefold increase in the risk of sudden death following a myocardial infarction. Smoking increases heart rate and blood pressure and irritates the heart, which can trigger fatal cardiac arrhythmias (irregular heart rhythms). As far as the extra load on the heart is concerned, giving up one pack of cigarettes per day is the equivalent of losing between 50 and 75 pounds of excess body fat! Another harmful effect is a decrease in HDL-cholesterol, the "good" type that helps control blood lipids.

Cigarette smoking, a poor cholesterol profile, low fitness, and high blood pressure are the four major risk factors for coronary heart disease. The risk for cardiovascular disease starts to decrease the moment you quit smoking. The risk approaches that of a lifetime nonsmoker after cessation.

Pipe and cigar smoking and chewing tobacco also increase the risk for heart disease. Even if no smoke is inhaled, toxic substances are absorbed through the membranes of the mouth and end up in the bloodstream.

Quitting tobacco use is not easy. The addictive properties of nicotine make quitting difficult, and physical and psychological withdrawal symptoms set in.

A six-step plan to help people stop smoking is contained in Figure 8.6. The most important factor in quitting cigarette smoking is a sincere desire to do so. More than 95% of successful ex-smokers have been able to quit on their own, either by quitting cold turkey or by using self-help kits available from organizations such as the American Cancer Society, the American Heart Association, and the American Lung Association. Only 3% of ex-smokers quit as a result of formal cessation programs.

Stress

Stress has become a part of life. People have to deal daily with goals, deadlines, responsibilities, pressures. The stressor itself is not what creates the health hazard but, rather, the individual's response to it.

The human body responds to stress by producing more catecholamines to prepare the body for "fight or flight." If the person fights or flees, the higher levels of catecholamines are

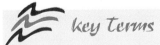

key terms

Electrocardiogram (ECG or EKG) A recording of the electrical impulses that stimulate the heart to contract.

Exercise ECG A recording of heart activity during high-intensity activity.

Stress ECG See Exercise ECG.

SIX-STEPS TO QUIT SMOKING

The following six-step plan has been developed as a guide to help you quit smoking. The total program should be completed in 4 weeks or less. Steps one through four should take no longer than 2 weeks. A maximum of 2 additional weeks are allowed for the rest of the program.

Step One   Decide positively that you want to quit. Now prepare a list of the reasons why you smoke and why you want to quit.

Step Two   Initiate a personal diet and exercise program. Exercise and decreased body weight cause a greater awareness of healthy living and increase motivation for giving up cigarettes.

Step Three   Decide on the approach you will use to stop smoking. You may quit cold turkey or gradually decrease the number of cigarettes smoked daily. Many people have found that quitting cold turkey is the easiest way to do it. Although it may not work the first time, after several attempts, all of a sudden smokers are able to overcome the habit without too much difficulty. Tapering off cigarettes can be done in several ways. You may start by eliminating cigarettes that you do not necessarily need, you can switch to a brand lower in nicotine or tar every couple of days, you can smoke less of each cigarette, or you can simply decrease the total number of cigarettes smoked each day.

Step Four   Set the target date for quitting. In setting the target date, choosing a special date may add a little extra incentive. An upcoming birthday, anniversary, vacation, graduation, family reunion — all are examples of good dates to free yourself from smoking.

Step Five   Stock up on low-calorie foods — carrots, broccoli, cauliflower, celery, popcorn (butter- and salt-free), fruits, sunflower seeds (in the shell), sugarless gum, and plenty of water. Keep such food handy on the day you stop and the first few days following cessation. Replace it for cigarettes when you want one.

Step Six   This is the day that you will quit smoking. On this day and the first few days thereafter, do not keep cigarettes handy. Stay away from friends and events that trigger your desire to smoke. Drink large amounts of water and fruit juices, and eat low-calorie foods. Replace the old behavior with new behavior. You will need to replace smoking time with new positive substitutes that will make smoking difficult or impossible. When you desire a cigarette, take a few deep breaths and then occupy yourself by doing a number of things such as talking to someone else, washing your hands, brushing your teeth, eating a healthy snack, chewing on a straw, doing dishes, playing sports, going for a walk or bike ride, going swimming, and so on.

If you have been successful and stopped smoking, a lot of events still can trigger your urge to smoke. When confronted with such events, people rationalize and think, "One won't hurt." It will not work! Before you know it, you will be back to the regular nasty habit. Be prepared to take action in those situations. Find adequate substitutes for smoking. Remind yourself of how difficult it has been and how long it has taken you to get to this point. As time goes on, it will only get easier rather than worse.

Figure 8.6 Six-step smoking cessation approach.

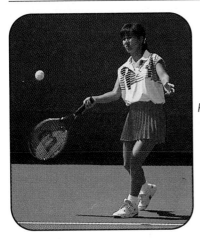

*Physical activity is
an excellent way
to relieve stress.*

metabolized and the body is able to return to a normal state. If, however, a person is under constant stress and unable to take action (as in the death of a close relative or friend, loss of a job, trouble at work, financial insecurity), the catecholamines remain elevated in the bloodstream.

People who are not able to relax have a constant low-level strain on the cardiovascular system that could manifest itself in heart disease. In addition, when a person is in a stressful situation, the coronary arteries that feed the heart muscle constrict, reducing the oxygen supply to the heart. If the blood vessels are largely blocked by atherosclerosis, abnormal heart rhythms or even a heart attack may follow.

Individuals who are under a lot of stress and do not cope well with it need to take measures to counteract the effects of stress in their lives. They must identify the sources of stress and learn how to cope with them. People need to take control of themselves, examine and act upon the things that are most important in their lives, and ignore less meaningful details.

Physical activity is one of the best ways to relieve stress. When a person takes part in physical activity, the body metabolizes excess catecholamines and is able to return to a normal state. Exercise also steps up muscular activity, which contributes to muscular relaxation.

Many executives in large cities are choosing the evening hours for their physical activity programs, stopping after work at the health or fitness club. In doing this, they are able to "burn up" the excess tension accumulated during the day and enjoy the evening hours. This has proven to be one of the best stress management techniques.

Personal and Family History

Individuals who have a family history of, or already have experienced cardiovascular problems, are at higher risk than those who never have had a problem. People with this sort of history should be encouraged strongly to keep the other risk factors as low as possible. Because most risk factors are reversible, the risk for future problems will decrease significantly.

Age and Gender

Age becomes a risk factor for men over age 45 and women over age 55. The greater incidence of heart disease may stem in part from lifestyle changes as we get older (less physical activity, poor nutrition, obesity, and so on). Men are at greater risk for cardiovascular disease than women earlier in life. Following menopause, women's risk increases. Based on final mortality statistics for 1995, more women (505,440) than men (455,152) died from cardiovascular disease.[26]

Young people should not think that heart disease will not affect them. The process begins early in life, as shown in American soldiers who died during the Korean and Vietnam conflicts. Autopsies conducted on soldiers killed at 22 years of age and younger revealed that approximately 70% had early stages of atherosclerosis. Other studies found elevated blood cholesterol levels in children as young as 10 years old.

Even though the aging process cannot be stopped, it certainly can be slowed. Chronological age versus physiological age is an important concept in longevity. Some individuals in their 60s or older have the body of a 20-year-old. And 20-year-olds often are in such poor condition and health that they almost seem to have the body of a 60-year-old. Risk factor management and positive lifestyle habits are the best ways to slow natural aging.

Cancer

Cell growth is controlled by **deoxyribonucleic acid (DNA)** and ribonucleic acid (RNA). When nuclei lose their ability to regulate and control cell growth, cell division is disrupted and mutant cells may develop. Some of these cells may grow uncontrollably and abnormally, forming a mass of tissue called a tumor, which can be either **benign** or **malignant**. Benign tumors can interfere with normal bodily functions, but they rarely cause death. More than 23% of all deaths in the United States come from cancer. Over 1.2 million new cases are reported, and more than half a million people die each year from cancer.[27]

More than 100 types of **cancer** can develop in the body. Cancer cells grow for no reason and multiply, destroying normal tissue. If the spread of cells is not controlled, death ensues. A cell may duplicate as many as 100 times. Normally, the DNA molecule is duplicated perfectly during cell division. In a few cases the DNA molecule is not replicated exactly, but specialized enzymes make repairs quickly. Occasionally cells with defective DNA keep dividing and ultimately form a small tumor. As more mutations occur, the altered cells continue to divide and can become malignant. A decade or more can pass between carcinogenic exposure or mutations and the time cancer is diagnosed.

A critical turning point in the development of cancer is when a tumor reaches about one million cells. At this stage it is referred to as **carcinoma in situ**. It is at an early stage and has not spread. If undetected, the tumor may go for months and years without any significant growth.

While encapsulated, a tumor does not pose a serious threat to human health. To grow, the tumor requires more oxygen and nutrients. In time, a few of the cancer cells start producing chemicals that enhance **angiogenesis**. Through the new blood vessels cells break away from a malignant tumor and migrate to other parts of the body, in a process called **metastasis**, where they can cause new cancer.

Although the immune system and the blood turbulence destroy most cancer cells, only one abnormal cell lodging elsewhere can start a new cancer. These cells also will grow and multiply uncontrollably, destroying normal tissue.

Once cancer cells metastasize, treatment becomes more difficult. Therapy can kill most cancer cells, but a few cells may become resistant to treatment. These cells then can grow into a new tumor that will not respond to the same treatment.

As with cardiovascular disease, cancer is largely preventable. As much as 80% of all human cancer is related to lifestyle or environmental factors (including diet, tobacco use, excessive use of alcohol, sexual and reproductive activity, and exposure to environmental hazards). Equally important is that more than 8 million Americans with a history of cancer were alive in 1998. Currently, 4 of 10 people diagnosed with cancer are expected to be alive 5 years from the initial diagnosis.

Guidelines for Cancer Prevention

The biggest factor in fighting cancer today is health education. People need to be informed about the risk factors for cancer and the guidelines for early detection. The most effective way to protect against cancer is to change negative lifestyle habits and behaviors. Figure 8.7 presents a questionnaire regarding the risk factors and preventive measures, which are also discussed below.

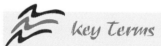 *key terms*

Deoxyribonucleic acid (DNA) Genetic material in the nucleus of each body cell.

Benign Noncancerous.

Malignant Cancerous.

Cancer A group of diseases characterized by uncontrolled growth and spread of abnormal cells into malignant tumors.

Carcinoma in situ An encapsulated malignant tumor.

Angiogenesis Formation of blood vessels.

Metastasis Movement of bacteria or body cells from one part of the body to another; usually refers to the spread of cancer.

ARE YOU TAKING CONTROL?

Today, scientists think most cancers may be related to lifestyle and environment — what you eat, drink, if you smoke, and where you work and play. So the good news is that you can help reduce your own cancer risk by taking control of things in your daily life.

10 Steps to a Healthier Life and Reduced Cancer Risk

		Yes	No
1.	**Are you eating more cabbage-family vegetables?** They include broccoli, cauliflower, brussels sprouts, all cabbages, and kale.	☐	☐
2.	**Are high-fiber foods included in your diet?** Fiber occurs in whole grains, fruits, and vegetables including peaches, strawberries, potatoes, spinach, tomatoes, wheat and bran cereals, rice, popcorn, and whole-wheat bread.	☐	☐
3.	**Do you choose foods with vitamin A?** Fresh foods with beta-carotene such as carrots, peaches, apricots, squash and broccoli are the best source, not vitamin pills.	☐	☐
4.	**Is vitamin C included in your diet?** You'll find vitamin C naturally in lots of fresh fruits and vegetables such as grapefruit, cantaloupe, oranges, strawberries, red and green peppers, broccoli and tomatoes.	☐	☐
5.	**Do you exercise and monitor calorie intake to avoid weight gain?** Walking is ideal exercise for many people.	☐	☐
6.	**Are you cutting overall fat intake?** This is done by eating lean meat, fish, skinned poultry, and low-fat dairy products.	☐	☐
7.	**Do you limit salt-cured, smoked, nitrite-cured foods?** Choose bacon, ham, hotdogs, or salt-cured fish only occasionally if you like it a lot.	☐	☐
8.	**If you smoke, have you tried quitting?**	☐	☐
9.	**If you drink alcohol, are you moderate in your intake?**	☐	☐
10.	**Do you respect the sun's rays?** Protect yourself with sunscreen — at least #15 — wear long sleeves and a hat, especially during midday hours — 11 a.m. to 3 p.m.	☐	☐

If you answer yes to most of these questions, congratulations. You are taking control of simple lifestyle factors that will help you feel better and reduce your risk for cancer.

Source: Texas Division of American Cancer Society.

Figure 8.7 *Cancer prevention questionnaire.*

Dietary Changes

The American Cancer Society estimates that one-third of all cancers in the United States are related to nutrition. A healthy diet, therefore, is critical to decrease the risk for cancer. The diet should be low in fat and high in fiber, and contain vitamins A and C from natural sources. Protein intake should be within the RDA guidelines. Cruciferous vegetables and green tea are encouraged. Alcohol should be consumed in moderation, and obesity should be avoided.

High fat intake has been linked primarily to breast, colon, and prostate cancers. Total fat intake should be limited to less than 20% of total daily calories.[28] Low intake of fiber seems to increase the risk for colon cancer. Also recommended is the consumption of at least 25 grams of fiber daily.[29] Foods high in vitamins A and C may deter cancers of the larynx, esophagus, and lung. Salt-cured, smoked, and nitrite-cured foods have been associated with cancer of the esophagus and stomach. Vitamin C seems to discourage the formation of nitrosamines. These potentially cancer-causing compounds are formed when nitrites and nitrates, which are used to prevent the growth of harmful bacteria in processed meats, combine with other chemicals in the stomach.

Carrots, squash, sweet potatoes, and cruciferous vegetables (cauliflower, broccoli, cabbage, Brussels sprouts, and kohlrabi) seem to protect against cancer. These vegetables contain a lot of beta-carotene (a precursor to vitamin A) and vitamin C. Researchers believe the antioxidant effect of these vitamins protects the body from oxygen-free radicals. As discussed in Chapter 5, during normal metabolism most of the oxygen in the human body is converted into stable forms of carbon dioxide and water. A small amount, however, ends up in an unstable form known as oxygen-free radicals, which are thought to attack and damage the cell membrane and DNA, leading to the formation of cancers. Antioxidants absorb free radicals before they can cause damage, and they also interrupt the sequence of reactions once damage has begun.

Green tea contains many nutrients, but in particular polyphenols, potent cancer-fighting antioxidants found in fresh fruits and vegetables and many grains. The antioxidant effect of one of the polyphenols in green tea, epigallocatechin gallate, or EGCG, is at least 25 times more effective than vitamin E and 100 times more effective than vitamin C at protecting cells and the DNA from damage believed to cause cancer, heart disease, and other diseases associated with free radicals.[30]

Polyphenols are thought to fight cancer by shutting off the formation of cancer cells, turning up the body's natural detoxification defenses, and suppressing the progression of the disease. EGCG is also twice as strong as the red wine antioxidant resveratrol, which helps prevent heart disease.

Green tea seems to be especially helpful in preventing gastrointestinal cancers, including those of the stomach, small intestines, pancreas, and colon. Polyphenols are known to block the formation of nitrosamines and quell the activation of carcinogens. Green tea consumption also has been linked to a lower incidence of lung, esophageal, and estrogen-related cancers, including most breast cancers. In Japan, where people drink green tea regularly but smoke twice as much as people in the United States, the incidence of lung cancer is about half that of the United States. Drinking two or more cups of green tea daily is recommended in a cancer-prevention diet.

A promising new horizon in cancer prevention is the discovery of phytochemicals. These compounds, found in abundance in fruits and vegetables, seem to exert a powerful effect in cancer prevention by blocking the formation of cancerous tumors and disrupting the process at almost every step of the way.[31] Phytochemicals exert their protective action by:[32,33]

- Removing carcinogens from cells before they cause damage.
- Activating enzymes that detoxify cancer-causing agents.
- Keeping carcinogens from locking onto cells.
- Preventing carcinogens from binding to DNA.

🍃 Breaking up cancer-causing precursors to benign forms.

🍃 Disrupting the chemical combination of cell molecules that can produce carcinogens.

🍃 Keeping small tumors from accessing capillaries (small blood vessels) to get oxygen and nutrients.

Nutritional guidelines also discourage excessive intake of protein. Daily protein intake for some Americans is almost twice the amount the human body needs. Too much animal protein seems to decrease blood enzymes that prevent precancerous cells from developing into tumors.

Some research suggests that grilling protein (fat or lean) at high temperatures for a long time increases the formation of carcinogenic substances on the skin or surface of the meat. Microwaving the meat for a couple of minutes before barbecuing decreases the risk, as long as the fluid released by the meat is discarded. Most of the potential carcinogens collect in this solution. Removing the skin of poultry before serving, and longer cooking at lower temperatures also seems to lower the risk.[34] Soy and soy products may help because they contain chemicals that prevent cancer. Soy protein seems to decrease the formation of carcinogens during cooking of meats.[35]

Alcohol should be consumed in moderation, as too much alcohol raises the risk for developing certain cancers, especially when it is combined with tobacco smoking or smokeless tobacco. In combination, these substances significantly increase the risk for mouth, larynx, throat, esophagus, and liver cancers. Approximately 17,000 cancer deaths yearly are attributed to excessive use of alcohol, often in combination with smoking. The combined action of heavy use of alcohol and tobacco can increase cancer of the oral cavity fifteenfold.

Maintaining recommended body weight also is encouraged. Obesity may be associated with cancers of the colon, rectum, breast, prostate, gallbladder, ovary, and uterus.

Abstaining From Tobacco

Current estimates indicate that 25.9 million men (27.8%) and 23.5 million women (23.3%) in the United States are cigarette smokers. Another 4.4 million young people between the ages of 12 and 17 years are smokers.[36] Cigarette smoking by itself is a major health hazard. When considering all related deaths, smoking is responsible for about 400,000 yearly unnecessary deaths in the United States. The World Health Organization estimates that smoking causes 3 million deaths worldwide each year. The average life expectancy for a chronic smoker is about 15 years less than for a nonsmoker.[37]

The biggest carcinogenic exposure in the workplace is cigarette smoke. The American Cancer Society reports that 87% of lung cancers and at least 29% of all cancers are linked to smoking. The use of smokeless tobacco also can lead to nicotine addiction and dependence and carries an increased risk for mouth, larynx, throat, and esophageal cancers.[38]

Avoiding Excessive Sun Exposure

Too much exposure to ultraviolet radiation (both UVB and UVA rays) is a major contributor to skin cancer. The most common sites of skin cancer are those exposed to the sun most often (face, neck, and back of the hands). The three types of skin cancer are:

1. Basal cell carcinoma
2. Squamous cell carcinoma
3. Malignant melanoma.

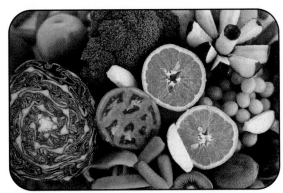

Phytochemicals, found in abundance in fruits and vegetables, seem to have a powerful effect in decreasing the risk for cancer.

Nearly 90% of the almost 1 million cases of basal cell or squamous cell skin cancers reported yearly in the United States could have been prevented by protecting the skin from the sun's rays. Melanoma is the most deadly, causing approximately 7,300 deaths in 1998. One in every six Americans will develop some type of skin cancer eventually.

Nothing is healthy about a "healthy tan." Tanning of the skin is the body's natural reaction to permanent and irreversible damage from too much exposure to the sun. Even small doses of sunlight add up to a greater risk for skin cancer and premature aging. Whereas tan fades at the end of the summer season, the underlying skin damage does not disappear. People with sensitive skin in particular should avoid sun exposure between 10:00 a.m. and 4:00 p.m.

The stinging sunburn comes from ultraviolet B rays (UVB), which also are thought to be the main cause of premature wrinkling and skin aging, roughened/leathery/sagging skin, and skin cancer. Unfortunately, the damage may not become evident until up to 20 years later. In comparison, skin that has not been overexposed to the sun remains smooth and unblemished and, over time, shows less evidence of aging.

Sunlamps and tanning parlors provide mainly ultraviolet A rays (UVA). Once thought to be safe, we now know that they also are damaging and have been linked to melanoma, the most serious form of skin cancer. As few as 15 to 30 minutes of exposure to UVA can be as dangerous as a day spent in the sun.[39]

Sunscreen lotion should be applied about 30 minutes before lengthy exposure to the sun

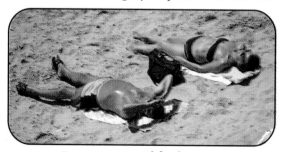

Tanning poses a risk for skin cancer from overexposure to the sun's ultraviolet rays.

because the skin takes that long to absorb the protective ingredients. A sun protection factor (SPF) of at least 15 is recommended. SPF 15 means that the skin takes 15 times longer to burn than with no lotion. If you ordinarily get a mild sunburn after 20 minutes of noonday sun, an SPF 15 allows you to remain in the sun about 300 minutes before burning. The higher the number, the more the protection. When swimming or sweating, waterproof sunscreens should be reapplied more often because all sunscreens lose strength when they are diluted.

Monitoring Estrogen, Radiation Exposure, and Potential Occupational Hazards

Estrogen intake has been linked to endometrial cancer but can be taken safely under careful supervision by a physician. Although radiation exposure increases the risk for cancer, the benefits of x-rays may outweigh the risk involved, and most medical facilities use the lowest dose possible to keep the risk to a minimum. Occupational hazards, such as asbestos fibers, nickel and uranium dusts, chromium compounds, vinyl chloride, and bischlormethyl ether, increase the risk for cancer. Cigarette smoking magnifies the risk from occupational hazards.

Physical Activity

A more active lifestyle seems to offer a protective effect against cancer. Although the mechanism is not clear, physical fitness and cancer mortality in men and women may have a graded and consistent inverse relationship.[40] A daily 30-minute, moderate-intensity exercise program lowers the risk for colon cancer and may lower the risk for cancers of the breast and reproductive system. In addition, growing evidence suggests that the body's autoimmune system may play a role in preventing cancer. Studies have indicated that moderate exercise improves the autoimmune system.[41]

Early Detection

Fortunately, many cancers can be controlled or cured through early detection. The real problem comes when cancerous cells spread, because they are difficult to wipe out then. Therefore, effective prevention, or at least early detection, is crucial. Herein lies the importance of periodic screening. Table 8.3 summarizes the American Cancer Society recommendations for early detection of cancer.

Other Factors

The contribution of many of the other much publicized factors is not as significant as those just pointed out. Intentional food additives, saccharin, processing agents, pesticides, and packaging materials currently used in the United States and other developed countries seem to have minimal consequences. High levels of stress and poor coping may affect the autoimmune system negatively and render the body less effective in dealing with the various cancers.

Genetics plays a role in susceptibility in about 10% of all cancers. Most of the effect is seen in the early childhood years. Some cancers are a combination of genetic and environmental liability. Genetics may add to the environmental

Table 8.3 Summary of Recommendations for Early Detection of Cancer in Asymptomatic People

Site	Recommendation
Cancer-related Checkup	A cancer-related checkup is recommended every 3 years for people aged 20–40 and every year for people age 40 and older. This exam should include health counseling and, depending on a person's age, might include examinations for cancers of the thyroid, oral cavity, skin, lymph nodes, testes, and ovaries, as well as for some nonmalignant diseases.
Breast	Women 40 and older should have an annual mammogram, an annual clinical breast exam (CBE) performed by a health-care professional, and should perform monthly breast self-examination. The CBE should be conducted close to the scheduled mammogram.
	Women ages 20–39 should have a clinical breast exam performed by a health care professional every 3 years and should perform monthly breast self-examination.
Colon & Rectum	Men and women aged 50 or older should follow *one* of the examination schedules below: • A fecal occult blood test every year and a flexible sigmoidoscopy every five years.* • A colonoscopy every 10 years.* • A double-contrast barium enema every 5 to 10 years.* • A digital rectal exam should be done at the same time as sigmoidoscopy, colonoscopy, or double-contrast barium enema. People who are at moderate or high risk for colorectal cancer should talk with a doctor about a different testing schedule.
Prostate	The ACS recommends that both the prostate-specific antigen (PSA) blood test and the digital rectal examination be offered annually, beginning at age 50, to men who have a life expectancy of at least 10 years and to younger men who are at high risk. Men in high-risk groups, such as those with a strong familial predisposition (e.g., two or more affected first-degree relatives) or African Americans, may begin at a younger age (e.g., 45 years.)
Uterus	**Cervix:** All women who are or have been sexually active or who are 18 and older should have an annual Pap test and pelvic examination. After three or more consecutive satisfactory examinations with normal findings, the Pap test may be performed less frequently. Discuss the matter with your physician.
	Endometrium: Women at high risk for cancer of the uterus should have a sample of endometrial tissue examined when menopause begins.

© 1998, American Cancer Society, Inc. Used by permission.

risk of certain types of cancers. The biggest carcinogenic exposure in the workplace is cigarette smoke. Environment, however, means more than pollution and smoke. It incorporates diet, lifestyle-related events, viruses, and physical agents such as x-rays and exposure to the sun.

Warning Signals

Everyone should become familiar with the following seven warning signals for cancer and bring them to a physician's attention if any are present:

1. Change in bowel or bladder habits.
2. Sore that does not heal.
3. Unusual bleeding or discharge.
4. Thickening or lump in breast or elsewhere.
5. Indigestion or difficulty in swallowing.
6. Obvious change in wart or mole.
7. Nagging cough or hoarseness.

Scientific evidence and testing procedures for prevention and early detection of cancer do change. Studies continue to provide new information. The intent of cancer prevention programs is to educate and guide individuals toward a lifestyle that will help prevent cancer and enable early detection of malignancy. The Recommendations for Early Detection of Cancer in Asymptomatic People by the American Cancer Society, outlined in Table 8.3, should be heeded in regular physical examinations as part of a cancer-prevention program.

Treatment of cancer always should be left to specialized physicians and cancer clinics. Current treatment modalities include surgery, radiation, radioactive substances, chemotherapy, hormones, and immunotherapy.

Chronic Obstructive Pulmonary Disease

Chronic obstructive pulmonary disease (COPD) encompasses diseases that limit air flow, such as chronic bronchitis, emphysema, and a reactive airway component similar to that of asthma.

The incidence of COPD increases proportionately with cigarette smoking (and other forms of smoked tobacco) and exposure to certain types of industrial pollution. In the case of emphysema, genetic factors also may play a role.

Accidents

Even though most people do not consider accidents a health problem, accidents are the fourth leading cause of death in the United States, affecting the total well-being of millions of Americans each year. Accident prevention and personal safety also are part of a health enhancement program aimed at achieving a higher quality of life. Proper nutrition, exercise, abstinence from cigarette smoking, and stress management are of little help if the person is involved in a disabling or fatal accident caused by distraction, a single reckless decision, or not wearing safety seat belts properly.

Accidents do not always just happen. We sometimes cause accidents. Other times we are victims of accidents. Although some factors in life — earthquakes, tornadoes, and airplane crashes, for example — are completely beyond our control, more often than not personal safety and accident prevention are a matter of common sense. Most accidents result from poor judgment and a confused mental state. Frequently accidents happen when we are upset, not paying attention to the task with which we are involved, or abusing alcohol and other drugs.

Alcohol abuse is the number-one cause of all accidents. Alcohol intoxication is the leading cause of fatal automobile accidents. Other drugs commonly abused in society alter feelings and perceptions, cause mental confusion, and impair judgment and coordination, greatly increasing the risk for accidental morbidity and mortality.

Spiritual Well-Being

The definition of **spirituality** by the National Interfaith Coalition on Aging encompasses Christians and non-Christians alike. It assumes that all people are spiritual in nature. Spiritual health provides a unifying power that integrates the other dimensions of wellness (see Figure 8.8). Basic characteristics of spiritual people include a sense of meaning and direction in life, a relationship to a higher being, freedom, prayer, faith, love, closeness to others, peace, joy, fulfillment, and altruism.

Religion has been a major part of cultures since the beginning of time. Although not everyone claims an affiliation with a certain religion or denomination, various surveys indicate that more than 90% of the U.S. population believes in God or a universal spirit functioning as God.

People, furthermore, believe to a varying extent that (a) a relationship with God is meaningful; (b) God can grant help, guidance, and assistance in daily living; and (c) mortal existence has a purpose. If we accept any or all of these statements, attaining spirituality will have a definite effect on our happiness and well-being. Although the reasons why religious affiliation enhances wellness are difficult to determine, possible reasons include the promotion of healthy lifestyle behaviors, social support, assistance in times of crisis and need, and counseling to overcome one's weaknesses.

Altruism, a key attribute of spiritual people, seems to enhance health and longevity. Altruism has been the focus of several studies in recent years. Researchers believe that doing good for others is good for oneself, especially for the immune system.

In a study of more than 2,700 people in Michigan,[42] the investigators found that people who did regular volunteer work lived longer. People who did not perform regular volunteer work (at least once a week) had a 250% greater mortality risk during the course of the study. In this same study the authors found that the health benefits of altruism could be so powerful that even just watching films of altruistic endeavors enhances the formation of an immune system chemical that helps fight disease.

Wellness requires a balance between physical, mental, spiritual, emotional, and social well-being. The relationship between spirituality and wellness, therefore, is meaningful in our quest for a better quality of life. As with other parameters of wellness, optimum spirituality requires development of the spiritual nature to its fullest potential.

Substance Abuse

Chemical dependencies presently encompasses some of the most serious self-destructive forms of addiction in society. Abused substances include alcohol, hard drugs, and cigarettes (the latter has been discussed already in this chapter). Problems associated with substance abuse are drunken or impaired driving, mixing drug prescriptions, family difficulties, and drugs to improve athletic performance (anabolic steroids).

Recognizing that all forms of substance abuse are unhealthy, the following information focuses on three of the most self-destructive addictive substances: alcohol, marijuana, and cocaine.

Spiritual

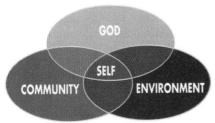

Well-being

 Figure 8.8 Components of spiritual well-being.

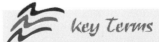 **key Terms**

Spirituality An affirmation of life in a relationship with God, self, community, and environment that nurtures and celebrates wholeness (National Interfaith Coalition on Aging).

Altruism True concern for and action on behalf of others (opposite of egoism) or a sincere desire to serve others above one's personal needs.

Alcohol

Alcohol represents one of the most significant health-related drug problems in the United States today. Estimates indicate that seven in 10 adults, or more than 100 million Americans 18 years and older, are drinkers. Approximately 10 million of them will have a drinking problem, including alcoholism, during their lifetime. Another 3 million teenagers are thought to have a drinking problem.

Alcohol intake cuts down on peripheral vision, impairs the ability to see and hear, causes slower reactions, reduces concentration and motor performance (including swaying and poor judgment of distance and speed of moving objects), lessens fear, increases risk-taking behaviors, causes more frequent urination, and induces sleep. A single large dose of alcohol also may lower sexual function. One of the most unpleasant, dangerous, and life-threatening consequences of drinking is the synergistic action of alcohol when combined with other drugs, particularly central nervous system depressants.

Long-term manifestations of alcohol abuse can be serious and life-threatening. These conditions include cirrhosis of the liver (scarring of the liver, often fatal); greater risk for oral, esophageal, and liver cancer; cardiomyopathy (a disease that affects the heart muscle); high blood pressure; greater risk for strokes; inflammation of the esophagus, stomach, small intestine, and pancreas; stomach ulcers; sexual impotence; malnutrition; brain cell damage and consequent loss of memory; depression, psychosis, and hallucinations.

Illegal Drugs

Approximately 60% of the world's production of illegal drugs is consumed in the United States. Each year we spend more than $100 billion on illegal drugs, surpassing the total dollars taken in from all crops produced by U.S. farmers. According to the U.S. Department of Education, today's drugs are stronger and more addictive, posing a greater risk than ever before. Drugs lead to physical and psychological dependence. If used regularly, they integrate into the body's chemistry, raising drug tolerance and forcing the person to increase the dosage constantly for similar results. In addition to the serious health problems caused by drug abuse, more than half of all adolescent suicides are drug-related.

Marijuana

Marijuana (pot or grass) is the most widely used illegal drug in the United States. Approximately 20 million people in the country use marijuana regularly. Earlier studies in the 1960s indicated that the potential effects of marijuana were exaggerated and that the drug was relatively harmless. The drug as it is used today, however, is as much as 10 times stronger than it was when the initial studies were conducted. Long-term harmful effects of marijuana use include atrophy of the brain leading to irreversible brain damage, as well as decreased resistance to infectious diseases, chronic bronchitis, lung cancer, and possible sterility and impotence.

Cocaine

Similar to marijuana, for many years cocaine was thought to be a relatively harmless drug. This misconception came to an abrupt halt in 1980s when two well known athletes, Len Bias (basketball) and Don Rogers (football), died suddenly following cocaine overdose. An estimated 4 to 8 million people in the United States use cocaine, 96% of whom had used marijuana previously.

Sustained cocaine snorting can lead to a constant runny nose, nasal congestion and inflammation, and perforation of the nasal septum. Long-term consequences of cocaine use in general include loss of appetite, digestive disorders, weight loss, malnutrition, insomnia, confusion, anxiety, and cocaine psychosis (characterized by paranoia and hallucinations). Large overdoses of cocaine can end in sudden death from respiratory paralysis, cardiac arrhythmias, and severe convulsions. For individuals who lack an enzyme used in metabolizing cocaine, as few as two to three lines of cocaine may be fatal.

Recognizing the hazards of chemical use, families, teams, and communities can assist each other in preventing problems, as well as help those who have problems with chemical use. Moreover, treating chemical dependency (including alcohol) seldom is accomplished without professional guidance and support. To secure the best available assistance, people in need should contact a physician or obtain a referral from a local mental health clinic (see Yellow Pages in the phone book.)

Sexually Transmitted Diseases

As the name implies, sexually transmitted diseases (STDs) are diseases spread through sexual contact. STDs have reached epidemic proportions in the United States. Of the more than 25 known STDs, some are still incurable. The American Social Health Association projected that 25% of all Americans will acquire at least one STD in their lifetime. Each year more than 12 million people are newly infected with STDs, including more than 4 million cases of chlamydia, 800,000 cases of gonorrhea, between a half a million and one million cases of genital warts, half a million of herpes, and nearly 100,000 cases of syphilis. Attracting most of the attention because of its life-threatening potential were more than 65 thousand new cases of AIDS in the United States in 1996.

HIV/AIDS

AIDS, acquired immunodeficiency virus is the most frightening of all STDs because it has no known cure and none is predicted for the near future. It is the end result of **human immunodeficiency virus (HIV)** that spreads among individuals who engage in risky behavior such as unprotected sex or the sharing of hypodermic needles. When a person becomes infected with HIV, the virus multiplies and attacks and destroys white blood cells. These cells are part of the immune system, whose function is to fight off infections and diseases in the body.

As the number of white blood cells killed increases, the body's immune system breaks down

gradually or may be destroyed totally. Without the immune system a person becomes susceptible to opportunistic infections or cancers not ordinarily seen in healthy people.

HIV is a progressive disease. At first people who contract the virus may not know they are infected. An incubation period of weeks, months, or years may go by during which time no symptoms appear. The virus may live in the body 10 years or longer before any symptoms emerge. As of 1994, almost 44% of the people infected with HIV in the United States did not know they were infected until they began developing AIDS-related symptoms.[43]

As the infection progresses to the point at which certain diseases develop, the person is said to have AIDS. HIV itself doesn't kill. Nor do people die from AIDS. AIDS is the term used to define the final stage of HIV infection. Death is caused by a weakened immune system that is unable to fight off opportunistic diseases.

On the average, 7 to 8 years elapse after infection before the individual develops the symptoms that fit the case definition of AIDS. From that point on, the person may live another 2 to 3 or more years. In essence, from the point of infection, the individual may endure a chronic disease for 8 to 10 years.

No one has to become infected with HIV. Once infected with the virus, a person will never become uninfected. The only answer is to protect oneself against this disease. No one should be so ignorant as to believe that it can never happen to him or her!

HIV is transmitted by the exchange of cellular body fluids — blood, semen, vaginal secretions, and maternal milk. These fluids may be exchanged during sexual intercourse, by using

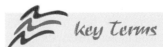

key terms

Acquired immunodeficiency syndrome (AIDS) End stage of infection by the human immunodeficiency virus (HIV).

Human immunodeficiency virus (HIV) A chronic infectious disease, the end result of which is AIDS, spread by exchange of bodily fluids through sexual contact and shared needles in drug use.

hypodermic needles used previously by infected individuals, between a pregnant woman and her developing fetus, babies from an infected mother during childbirth, less frequently during breast feeding, and rarely from a blood transfusion or organ transplant.

AIDS is an "equal opportunity epidemic." People do not get HIV because of who they are but, rather, because of what they do. HIV and AIDS threaten anyone, anywhere: men, women, children, teenagers, young people, older adults, Whites, Blacks, Hispanics, homosexuals, heterosexuals, bisexuals, druggies, Americans, Africans, Asians, Europeans. Nobody is immune to HIV.

You cannot tell if people are infected with HIV or have AIDS simply by looking at them or taking their word. Not you, not a nurse, not even a doctor can tell, unless an HIV antibody test is done. Therefore, every time you engage in risky behavior, you run the risk of contracting HIV. The two most basic risky behaviors are: (a) having unprotected vaginal, anal, or oral sex with an HIV-infected person, and (b) sharing hypodermic needles or other drug paraphernalia with someone who is infected.

Based on estimates by the U.S. Surgeon General, one in every 250 Americans is infected with HIV. Around the world an estimated 17 million people are infected, more than 4 million of whom have developed AIDS. Because of the lengthy incubation period, about 20% of the AIDS patients in the United States today are believed to have been infected as teenagers. By the end of 1966, a total of 575,850 AIDS cases had been diagnosed in the United States and over 350,000 had died from the diseases caused by HIV. Most of the people who die are in the 20- to 45-year-old age group.

Although more than half of all AIDS cases in the United States initially occurred in homosexual or bisexual men, HIV infection now is spreading at a faster rate in heterosexuals. Many heterosexuals practice unprotected sex because they don't believe it can happen to their segment of the population. HIV is an epidemic that does not discriminate by sexual orientation. Worldwide about 75% of the AIDS cases have been reported in heterosexuals.

As with any other serious illness, AIDS patients deserve respect, understanding, and support. Rejection and discrimination are traits of immature, hateful, and ignorant people. Education, knowledge, and responsible behaviors are the best ways to minimize fear and discrimination.

Guidelines for Preventing STDs

With all the grim news about STDs, the good news is that you can do things to prevent their spread, and take precautions to keep yourself from becoming a victim. The facts are in: The best prevention technique is a mutually monogamous sexual relationship, sex with only one person who has sexual relations only with you. That one behavior will remove you almost completely from any risk for developing an STD.

Unfortunately, in today's society, trust is an elusive concept. You may be led to believe you are in a monogamous relationship when your partner actually: (a) may be cheating on you and gets infected, (b) ends up having a one-night stand with someone who is infected, (c) got the virus several years ago before the present relationship and still doesn't know of the infection, (d) may not be honest with you and chooses not to tell you about the infection, or (e) is shooting up drugs and becomes infected. In any of these cases, HIV can be passed on to you.

Because your future and your life are at stake, and because you may never know if your partner is infected, you should give serious and careful consideration to postponing sex until you believe you have found a lifetime monogamous relationship. In doing so, you will not have to live with the fear of catching HIV or other STDs or deal with an unplanned pregnancy.

As strange as this may seem to some, many people postpone sexual activity until they are married. This is the best guarantee against HIV. Young people should understand that married life will provide plenty of time for fulfilling and rewarding sex.

If you choose to delay sex, do not let peers pressure you into having sex. Some people would have you believe you are not a real man or woman if you don't have sex. Manhood and womanhood are not proven during sexual intercourse but, instead, through mature, responsible, and healthy choices.

Other people lead you to believe that love doesn't exist without sex. Sex in the early stages of a relationship is not the product of love but is simply the fulfillment of a physical, and often selfish, drive. A loving relationship develops over a long time with mutual respect for each other.

Teenagers are especially susceptible to peer pressure leading to premature sexual intercourse. As a result, more than a million teens become pregnant each year, with a 43% pregnancy rate for all girls at least once as a teenager. Too many young people wish they had postponed sex and silently admire those who do. Sex lasts only a few minutes. The consequences of irresponsible sex may last a lifetime. In some cases they are fatal.

Then there are those who enjoy bragging about their sexual conquests and mock people who choose to wait. In essence, many of these conquests are only fantasies expounded in an attempt to gain popularity with peers.

Sexual promiscuity never leads to a trusting, loving, and lasting relationship. Mature people respect others' choices. If someone does not respect your choice to wait, he or she certainly does not deserve your friendship or, for that matter, anything else.

There is no greater sex than that between two loving and responsible individuals who mutually trust and admire each other. Contrary to many beliefs, these relationships are possible. They are built upon unselfish attitudes and behaviors.

As you look around, you will find people who have these values. Seek them out and build your friendships and future around people who respect you for who you are and what you believe. You don't have to compromise your choices or values. In the end you will reap the greater rewards of a fulfilling and lasting relationship, free of AIDS and other STDs.

Also, be prepared so that you will know your course of action before you get into an intimate situation. Look for common interests, and work together toward them. Express your feelings openly: "I'm not ready for sex; I just want to have fun and kissing is fine with me." If your friend does not accept your answer and is not willing to stop the advances, be prepared with a strong response. Statements like "Please stop" or "Don't!" are for the most part ineffective. Use a firm statement such as: "No, I'm not willing to do it" or "I've already thought about this, and I'm not going to have sex." If this still doesn't work, label the behavior as rape: "This is rape, and I'm going to call the police."

What about those who do not have — or do not desire — a monogamous relationship? Risky behaviors that significantly increase the chances of contracting an STD, including HIV infection, are:

1. Multiple or anonymous sexual partners such as a pickup or prostitute.

2. Anal sex with or without a condom.

3. Vaginal or oral sex with someone who shoots drugs or engages in anal sex.

4. Sex with someone you know who has several sex partners.

5. Unprotected sex (without a condom) with an infected person.

6. Sexual contact of any kind with anyone who has symptoms of AIDS or who is a member of a group at high risk for AIDS.

7. Sharing toothbrushes, razors, or other implements that could become contaminated with blood with anyone who is, or might be, infected with the HIV virus.

Avoiding risky behaviors that destroy quality of life and life itself is a critical component of a healthy lifestyle. Learning the facts so you can make responsible choices can protect you and those around you from startling and unexpected conditions. Using alcohol moderately (or not at all), refraining from substance abuse, and preventing sexually transmitted diseases are keys to averting both physical and psychological damage.

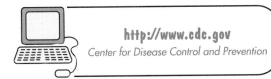

http://www.cdc.gov
Center for Disease Control and Prevention

Notes

1. U. S. Department of Health and Human Services, National Center for Health Statistics, *Monthly Vital Statistics Report: Advance Report of Final Mortality Statistics*, 45:11, Supplement 2, June 12, 1997.

2. J. M. McGinnis and W. H. Foege, "Actual Causes of Death in the United States," *Journal of the American Medical Association,* 270(1993), 2207–2212.

3. American Heart Association, *Heart and Stroke Facts: 1995* (Statistical Supplement) (Dallas: AHA, 1994).

4. U. S. Department of Health and Human Services.

5. American Heart Association, *Heart and Stroke Facts* (Statistical Supplement) (Dallas: AHA, 1997).

6. American Heart Association, 1997.

7. U. S. Department of Health and Human Services.

8. American Heart Association, 1997.

9. P. N. Hopkins and R. R. Williams, "Identification and Relative Weight of Cardiovascular Risk Factors," *Cardiology Clinics*, 4(1986), 3–32.

10. S. N. Blair, H. W. Kohl III, R. S. Paffenbarger, Jr., D. G. Clark, K. H. Cooper, and L. W. Gibbons, "Physical Fitness and All-Cause Mortality: A Prospective Study of Healthy Men and Women," *Journal of the American Medical Association*, 262(1989), 2395–2401.

11. "Lipid Research Clinics Program: The Lipid Research Clinic Coronary Primary Prevention Trial Results," *Journal of the American Medical Association*, 251(1984), 351–364.

12. American Heart Association, *Fact Sheet on Heart Attack, Stroke and Risk Factors* (Dallas: AHA, 1997).

13. W. P. Castelli and K. Anderson, "A Population at Risk: Prevalence of High Cholesterol Levels in Hypertensive Patients in the Framingham Study," *American Journal of Medicine*, 80, Supplement 2A(1986), 23–32.

14. W. Castelli, "Smart Heart Strategies: Best Ways to Beat Heart Disease," *Bottom Line/Personal*, 19:4(1998), 1–3.

15. E. B. Rimm, A. Ascherio, E. Giovannucci, D. Spiegelman, M. J. Stampfer, and W. C. Willett, "Vegetable, Fruit, and Cereal Fiber Intake and Risk of Coronary heart Disease Among Men," *Journal of the American Medical Association*, 275(1996), 447–451.

16. J. M. Gaziano and C. H. Hennekens, "A New Look at What Can Unclog Your Arteries," *Executive Health Report*, 27:8(1991), 16.

17. R. J. Barnard, "Effects of Lifestyle Modification on Serum Lipids," *Archives of Internal Medicine*, 151(1991), 1389–1394.

18. Castelli.

19. O. Nygard, J. E. Nordreahaug, H. Refsum, P. M. Ueland, M. Farstad, and S. E. Vollset, "Plasma Homocysteine Levels and Mortality in Patients with Coronary heart Disease," *New England Journal of Medicine*, 337(1997), 230–236.

20. C. J. Boushey, S. A. A. Beresford, G. S. Omenn, and A. G. Motulsky, "A Quantitative Assessment of Plasma Homocysteine as a Risk Factor for Vascular Disease," *Journal of the American Medical Association*, 274(1995), 1049–1057.

21. Castelli.

22. "Diabetes: Weight Control and Exercise May Keep You Off the Road to High Blood Sugar," Medical Essay, supplement to *Mayo Clinic Health Letter*, February 1998.

23. E. J. Mayer et al., "Intensity and Amount of Physical Activity in Relation to Insulin Sensitivity," *Journal of the American Medical Association*, 279(1998), 669–674.

24. McGinnis and Foege.

25. S. A. Glantz and W. W. Parmley. "Passive Smoking and Heart Disease," *Journal of the American Medical Association*, 273(1995), 1047–1053.

26. American Heart Association, 1997.

27. American Cancer Society, 1998 *Cancer Facts and Figures* (New York: ACS, 1998).

28. J. H. Weisburger and G. M. Williams, "Causes of Cancer," *American Cancer Society Textbook of Clinical Oncology* (Atlanta: ACS, 1995), 10–39.

29. Weisburger and Williams.

30. L. Mitscher and V. Dolby, *The Green Tea Book — China's Fountain of Youth.* (New York: Avery Press, 1997; L. Mitscher, "Strongest Known Disease-fighting Antioxidant," Bottom Line/Personal, 18:4(1997), 3.

31. S. Begley, "Beyond Vitamins," *Newsweek*, April 25, 1994, pp. 45–49.

32. Begley.

33. "Antioxidant Vitamins: Are They the Only Cancer-Phyters?" *Cancer Smart*, 1:3(1995),4–5.

34. "Your Barbecue Grill: A Smoking Gun?" *Cancer Smart*, 1:2(1995), 4–5.

35. Weisburger and Williams.

36. American Heart Association, *Fact Sheet on Heart Attack, Stroke and Risk Factors* (Dallas: AHA, 1997).

37. American Cancer Society, 1995 *Cancer Facts and Figures* (New York: ACS, 1995).

38. American Cancer Society, 1998.

39. "Questions & Answers," *Cancer Smart*, 4(1998), 12.

40. Blair et al.

41. I-Min Lee, "Exercise and Physical Health: Cancer and Immune Function," *Research Quarterly for Exercise and Sport*, 66(1995), 286–291.

42. E. R. Growald and A. Lusks, "Beyond Self," *American Health*, March 1988, pp. 51–53.

43. E. Pennisi, "AIDS Becomes More of an Equal Opportunity Epidemic," *American Society for Microbiology News* 61:5(1995), 236-240.

Relevant Questions and Answers about Fitness and Wellness

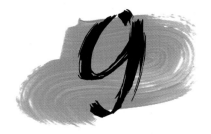

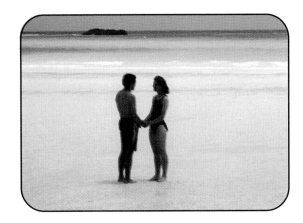

Some of the most frequently asked questions about various aspects of physical fitness and wellness are addressed in this chapter. The answers will further clarify concepts discussed throughout the book, as well as put to rest several myths that misinform fitness and wellness participants.

Safety of Exercise Participation and Injury Prevention

Q. Can aerobic exercise make a person immune to heart and blood vessel disease?

A. Scientific evidence clearly indicates that aerobically fit individuals have a much lower incidence of cardiovascular disease. A regular aerobic exercise program by itself, however, is not an absolute guarantee against diseases of the heart and blood vessels. Several factors increase a person's risk for cardiovascular disease.

Though physical inactivity is one of the most significant risk factors, studies have documented that multiple interrelations usually exist between these risk factors. Physical inactivity, for instance, often contributes to an increase in (a) body fat, (b) LDL-cholesterol, (c) triglycerides, (d) stress, (e) blood pressure, and (f) risk for diabetes (see Figure 9.1). As discussed in Chapter 8, most risk factors are preventable and reversible. Overall risk factor management is the best advice to minimize the risk for cardiovascular disease. Research also indicates that the odds of surviving a heart attack are much higher for people who engage in a regular aerobic exercise program.

Objectives

- Dispel common misconceptions related to physical fitness and wellness.
- Give practical advice and tips regarding safety.
- Address some concerns specific to women.
- Clarify additional concepts regarding nutrition and weight control.
- Answer some questions regarding wellness and aging.
- Provide guidelines related to fitness/wellness consumer issues.

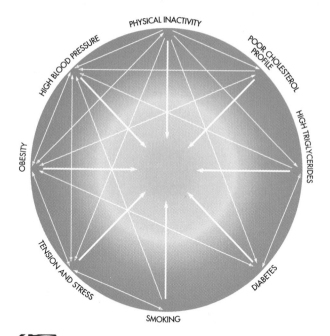

PHYSICAL INACTIVITY
HIGH BLOOD PRESSURE
POOR CHOLESTEROL PROFILE
OBESITY
HIGH TRIGLYCERIDES
TENSION AND STRESS
DIABETES
SMOKING

Figure 9.1 Interrelationships among leading cardiovascular risk factors.

Q What amount of aerobic exercise is optimal for decreasing the risk for cardiovascular disease significantly?

A The amount of exercise required to maintain cardiorespiratory fitness is a training session approximately every 48 hours for 20 to 30 minutes in the appropriate target training zone (see Chapter 3). People who accumulate 30 minutes of moderate-intensity physical activity on most days of the week can expect to reap many of the health benefits provided by a regular exercise program.[1]

The amount of exercise required to offset the risk cannot be pinpointed specifically because of the many individual differences (genetic and lifestyle) between people. Research, however, is beginning to shed some light on this subject. One of the earlier studies indicated that about 300 calories should be expended daily through aerobic exercise to obtain a certain degree of protection against cardiovascular disease.[2] A study by Dr. Ralph Paffenbarger and his

co-researchers on Harvard alumni (see Figure 1.6 in Chapter 1) found that expending 2,000 calories per week as a result of physical activity yielded the lowest risk for cardiovascular disease in this group of almost 17,000 alumni. The 2,000 calories per week represents about 300 calories per daily exercise session.

The work alluded to in Chapter 8 (see Figure 8.5), conducted at the Aerobics Research Institute in Dallas, indicated that even moderate fitness levels can reduce the incidence of cardiovascular problems substantially.[3] The minimum dose for moderate fitness requires an expenditure of about 200 calories five to seven times per week.[4] Slightly greater protection is achieved at higher fitness levels.

Clinical data on individuals with or at risk for coronary heart disease suggest that more than 1,400 calories per week may have to be expended to improve cardiorespiratory fitness, more than 1,500 weekly calories to stop the progression of atherosclerotic lesions, and over 2,200 calories per week or the equivalent of 5 to 6 hours of weekly exercise, for regression of lesions.[5] As noted in the previous question, physical activity or exercise by themselves do not provide an absolutely risk-free guarantee against cardiovascular disease.

Q At what age should I start concerning myself with cardiovascular disease?

A The disease process, not only for cardiovascular disease but also cancer, starts early in life as a result of poor lifestyle habits. Studies have shown beginning stages of atherosclerosis and elevated blood lipids in children as young as 10 years old.

Many positive habits can be established early in life within the walls of one's own home. If people are taught at a young age that they should avoid excessive calories, sweets, salt and

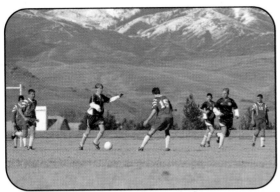

Regular physical activity during youth enhances the likelihood of lifetime participation in an exercise program.

alcohol, not to use tobacco, and to participate in physical activity, their chances of leading a healthier life are much greater than is true with the present generation. When it comes to teaching, some of the best advice to humanity is: "Come and follow me." If you cultivate positive health habits in your own life, your children will be more likely to follow.

Q Can I exercise after donating blood?

A The average amount of blood taken in a donation is about 500 ml (half liter), compared to a total body volume of 5 liters. This volume is replenished immediately by reserve blood components stored in the body. Unless you are given special instructions not to exercise, you should continue with your regular program.

Q Will exercise offset the detrimental effects of cigarette smoking?

A Physical exercise often motivates toward smoking cessation but does not offset any ill effects of smoking. Smoking greatly decreases the ability of the blood to transport oxygen to working muscles. Oxygen is carried in the circulatory system by hemoglobin, the iron-containing pigment of the red blood cells. Carbon monoxide, a byproduct of cigarette smoke, has 210 to 250 times greater affinity for hemoglobin than oxygen does. Consequently, carbon monoxide combines much faster with hemoglobin,

decreasing the oxygen-carrying capacity of the blood.

Chronic smoking also increases airway resistance, requiring the respiratory muscles to work much harder and consume more oxygen to ventilate a given amount of air. If you quit smoking, exercise does help increase the functional capacity of the pulmonary system.

Q Will exercise help me feel better?

A Yes. Many studies have found that exercise helps people feel better, improve self-esteem and self-confidence, relieve stress, and even alleviate depression. As with the physiological benefits of exercise, psychological benefits are enjoyed through regular participation. Hence, a lifetime of physical activity is just as important for mental wellness.

Q How can I tell if I'm exceeding the safe limits for exercising?

A The best method to determine whether you are exercising too strenuously is to check your heart rate and make sure it does not exceed the limits of your target zone. Exercising above this target zone may not be safe for unconditioned or high-risk individuals. You do not need to exercise beyond your target zone to gain the desired benefits for the cardiorespiratory system.

In addition, several physical signs will tell you when you are exceeding functional limitations: rapid or irregular heart rate, difficult breathing, nausea, vomiting, lightheadedness, headaches, dizziness, pale skin, flushness, extreme weakness, lack of energy, shakiness, sore muscles, cramps, and tightness in the chest. These are all signs of exercise intolerance, the physical aversion to exercise conducted at intensity levels beyond a person's functional capacity. Learn to listen to your body. If you notice any of these symptoms, seek medical attention before continuing your exercise program.

Q Can I exercise when I have a cold or the flu?

A The most important consideration is to use common sense and pay attention to your symptoms. Typically, you may continue exercise if your symptoms include a runny nose, sneezing, or a scratchy throat. If you are running a fever or your muscles ache, you are vomiting, have diarrhea, or have a hacking cough, you should avoid exercise. Following an illness, be sure to ease back gradually into your program. Do not attempt to return at the same intensity and duration that you were used to prior to your illness.

Q How fast should heart rate decrease following aerobic exercise?

A To a certain extent, recovery heart rate is related to fitness level. The better your cardiorespiratory fitness level, the faster your heart rate will decrease following exercise. As a rule of thumb, heart rate should be below 120 beats per minute 5 minutes into recovery. If your heart rate is above 120, you most likely have overexerted yourself or possibly could have some other cardiac abnormality. If you decrease the intensity or duration of exercise, or both, and you still have a fast heart rate 5 minutes into recovery, consult your physician.

Q How fast does a person lose the benefits of exercise after stopping an exercise program?

A How quickly the benefits of exercise are lost differs among the various components of physical fitness and also depends on the condition the person achieves before discontinuing the exercise. Specifically with regard to cardiorespiratory endurance, it has been estimated that 4 weeks of aerobic training are completely reversed in 2 consecutive weeks of physical inactivity.

On the other hand, if you have been exercising regularly for months or years, 2 weeks of inactivity will not hurt you as much as it will someone who has exercised only a few weeks. Generally speaking, within 2 to 3 days of aerobic inactivity, the cardiorespiratory system starts to lose some of its capacity. Flexibility can be maintained with two or three stretching sessions per week, and strength is maintained with just one maximal training session per week. If you have to interrupt the program for reasons beyond your control, do not attempt to resume your training at the same level you left off but, instead, build up gradually again.

A regular fitness program should be maintained even during traveling and vacation periods. When traveling, plan ahead and examine your options before you leave home. Many hotels provide in-house fitness facilities. Although the equipment often is limited, it's generally sufficient for an adequate cardiorespiratory and strength workout. Frequent travelers would benefit from joining a nationally franchised health club, a YMCA, or a YWCA. In this manner you can continue the same exercise program while visiting different cities.

Activities that require a minimum of equipment and no facilities, such as jogging or rope jumping, are excellent alternatives for the road. If you are going to venture out in a new city, always ask for safe places to jog. Nearby parks or a high school track usually are safe and help you stay away from traffic and stoplights. The strength-training (without equipment) and flexibility exercises provided in Appendices B and C can be used to maintain your strength and flexibility. If visiting a resort area, fitness rental equipment, such as bikes and roller blades, is often available.

Q What type of clothing should I wear when I exercise?

A The type of clothing you wear during exercise is important. In general, clothing should fit comfortably and allow free movement of the various body parts. Select clothing according to air temperature, humidity, and exercise intensity. Avoid nylon and rubberized materials and tight clothes that interfere with the cooling mechanism of the human body or obstruct normal blood flow. Fabrics made from polypropylene, Capilene, Thermax, and synthetics are best. These types of fabrics draw moisture away from the skin, enhancing evaporation and cooling the body. Exercise intensity also is important because the harder you exercise, the more heat the body produces.

When exercising in the heat, avoid the hottest time of the day, between 11:00 a.m. and 5:00 p.m. Avoid surfaces such as asphalt, concrete, and artificial turfs, as they absorb heat, which then radiates to the body. (Also see the discussion on exercise in hot and humid conditions in this chapter).

Only a minimal amount of clothing is necessary during exercise in the heat, to allow for maximal evaporation. Clothing should be lightweight, light-colored, loose-fitting, airy, and absorbent. Examples of commercially available products that can be used during exercise in the heat include Asci's Perma Plus, Cool-max, and Nike's Dri-F.I.T. Double-layer acrylic socks are more absorbent than cotton and help to prevent blistering and chafing of the feet. A straw-type hat can be worn to protect the eyes and head from the sun. Clothing for exercise in the cold is discussed later in this chapter.

A good pair of shoes is vital to prevent lower-limb injuries. Shoes manufactured specifically for your choice of activity are a must. When selecting proper footwear, body type, tendency toward pronation or supination, and exercise surfaces must be considered. Shoes should have good stability, motion control, and comfortable fit. Purchase shoes in the middle of the day when feet have expanded and might be one-half size larger. For increased breathability, choose shoes with nylon or mesh uppers. Generally, salespeople at reputable athletic shoe stores are knowledgeable and can help you select a good shoe that fits your needs. Examine your

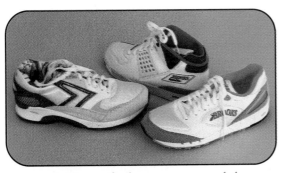

Activity-specific shoes are recommended to prevent injuries.

shoes after 500 miles or 6 months, and obtain a new pair if they are worn out. Old shoes frequently are responsible for lower-limb injuries.

Q What time of the day is best for exercise?

A A person can exercise at almost any time of the day except about 2 hours following a regular meal, or the noon and early afternoon hours on hot and humid days. Many people enjoy exercising early in the morning because it gives them a good boost to start the day. Others prefer the lunch hour for weight-control reasons. By exercising at noon, they do not eat as big a lunch, which helps keep down daily caloric intake. Highly stressed people seem to like the evening hours because of the relaxing effects of exercise.

Q How long should a person wait after a meal before engaging in strenuous physical exercise?

A The length of time to wait before exercising after a meal depends on the amount of food eaten. On the average, after a regular meal a person should wait about 2 hours before participating in strenuous physical activity. Light physical activity, such as a walk, is fine. If anything, it helps burn extra calories and may help the body metabolize fats more efficiently.

Q How should acute sports injuries be treated?

A The best treatment always has been prevention. If an activity causes unusual discomfort or chronic irritation, you need to treat the cause by decreasing the intensity, switching activities, substituting equipment, or upgrading clothing, such as proper-fitting shoes.

In cases of acute injury, the standard treatment is rest, cold application, compression or splinting (or both), and elevation of the affected body part. The acronym is RICE: R = rest, I = ice application, C = compression, and E = elevation. Cold should be applied three to five times a day for 15 to 20 minutes at a time during the first 24 to 36 hours, by submerging the injured area in cold water, using an icebag, or applying ice massage to the affected part. An elastic bandage or wrap can be used for compression. Elevating the body part decreases blood flow to it. The purpose of these treatment modalities is to minimize swelling in the area, which hastens recovery time.

After the first 36 to 48 hours, heat can be used if the injury shows no further swelling or inflammation. If you have doubts regarding the nature or seriousness of the injury (such as suspected fracture), you should seek a medical evaluation.

Obvious deformities (such as in fractures, dislocations, or partial dislocations) call for splinting, cold application with an icebag, and medical attention. Never try to reset any of these conditions by yourself, as muscles, ligaments, and nerves could be damaged further. These injuries should be treated by specialized medical personnel. A quick reference guide for the signs or symptoms and treatment of exercise-related problems is provided in Table 9.1.

Table 9.1 *Reference Guide for Exercise-Related Problems*

Injury	Signs/Symptoms	Treatment*
Bruise (contusion)	Pain, swelling, discoloration	Cold application, compression, rest
Dislocations/Fractures	Pain, swelling, deformity	Splinting, cold application, seek medical attention
Heat cramps	Cramps, spasms and muscle twitching in the legs, arms, and abdomen	Stop activity, get out of the heat, stretch, massage the painful area, drink plenty of fluids
Heat exhaustion	Fainting, profuse sweating, cold/clammy skin, weak/rapid pulse, weakness, headache	Stop activity, rest in a cool place, loosen clothing, rub body with cool/wet towel, drink plenty of fluids, stay out of heat for 2–3 days
Heat stroke	Hot/dry skin, no sweating, serious disorientation, rapid/full pulse, vomiting, diarrhea, unconsciousness, high body temperature	Seek immediate medical attention, request help and get out of the sun, bathe in cold water/spray with cold water/rub body with cold towels, drink plenty of cold fluids
Joint sprains	Pain, tenderness, swelling, loss of use, discoloration	Cold application, compression, elevation, rest, heat after 36 to 48 hours (if no further swelling)
Muscle cramps	Pain, spasm	Stretch muscle(s), use mild exercises for involved area
Muscle soreness and stiffness	Tenderness, pain	Mild stretching, low-intensity exercise, warm bath
Muscle strains	Pain, tenderness, swelling, loss of use	Cold application, compression, elevation, rest, heat after 36 to 48 hours (if no further swelling)
Shin splints	Pain, tenderness	Cold application prior to and following any physical activity, rest, heat (if no activity is carried out)
Side stitch	Pain on the side of the abdomen below the rib cage	Decrease level of physical activity or stop altogether, gradually increase level of fitness
Tendinitis	Pain, tenderness, loss of use	Rest, cold application, heat after 48 hours

* Cold should be applied 3 to 4 times a day for 15 minutes
  Heat can be applied 3 times a day for 15 to 20 minutes.

Q. What causes muscle soreness and stiffness?

A. Muscle soreness and stiffness are common in individuals who (a) begin an exercise program or participate after a long layoff from exercise, (b) exercise beyond their customary intensity and duration, and (c) perform eccentric training. The acute soreness that sets in during the first few hours after exercise is thought to be related to a lack of blood (oxygen) flow and general fatigue of the exercised muscles. The delayed soreness that appears several hours after exercise (usually 12 hours or so later) and lasts 2 to 4 days may be related to tiny tears in muscle tissue, muscle spasms that increase fluid retention and thereby stimulate the pain nerve endings, and overstretching or tearing of connective tissue in and around muscles and joints.

Two types of contraction accompany muscular activity with movement (see Chapter 3 discussion on dynamic contractions) — concentric muscle contraction and eccentric muscle contraction. **Concentric muscle contraction** is *a dynamic contraction in which the muscle shortens as it develops tension.* **Eccentric muscle contraction** is *a dynamic contraction in which the muscle fibers lengthen while developing tension.*

For example, during the arm-curl exercise the elbow flexor muscles (biceps, brachioradialis, and brachialis) shorten as the weight is brought toward the shoulder (concentric contraction). On the way down the muscles contract eccentrically as they lengthen while the person lowers the weight slowly to the starting position.

When running, as you place your foot on the ground, the muscles contract eccentrically to absorb the weight of the body as you strike the ground. This eccentric contraction is followed by a concentric contraction of the leg as you push off the ground to propel the body forward. Unlike running, cycling requires only concentric contractions of the leg muscles as you pedal the bicycle. A concentric contraction of the quadriceps muscles is produced as you push down on the pedal. If you use toe clips, a concentric contraction of the hamstring muscles occurs as you pull the pedal back up to the top of the circle. Eccentric training has been shown to produce more muscle soreness than concentric training. A hard running workout, therefore, produces greater muscle soreness than a hard cycling workout of similar intensity and duration.

To prevent soreness and stiffness, the recommended approach is to warm up gradually before physical activity and stretch adequately after exercise. Do not attempt to do too much too quickly. If you become sore and stiff, you have overdone your workout. In these cases, mild stretching, low-intensity exercise to stimulate blood flow, and a warm bath can bring relief.

Stretching may be of greatest significance following exercise. Tired muscles tend to contract to a shorter than normal length. Byproducts of exercise metabolism also may cause muscle spasms. Post-exercise stretching thus can help return a muscle to its normal length.

Q. How should I care for shin splints?

A. The **shin splint,** one of the most common injuries to the lower limbs, usually results from one or more of the following: (a) lack of proper and gradual conditioning, (b) doing physical activities on hard surfaces (wooden floors, hard tracks, cement, and asphalt), (c) fallen arches in the feet, (d) chronic overuse, (e) muscle fatigue, (f) faulty posture, (g) improper shoes, and (h) participating in weight-bearing activities when excessively overweight.

To manage shin splints:

1. Remove or reduce the cause (exercise on softer surfaces, wear better shoes or arch supports, or completely stop exercise until the shin splints heal).

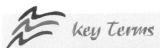

key Terms

Concentric muscle contraction A dynamic contraction in which the muscle shortens as it develops tension.

Eccentric muscle contraction A dynamic contraction in which the muscle fibers lengthen while developing tension.

Shin splint Injury to the lower leg characterized by pain and irritation at the front of the leg.

2. Do stretching exercises before and after physical activity.

3. Use ice massage for 10 to 20 minutes before and after physical exercise.

4. Apply active heat (whirlpool and hot baths) for 15 minutes, two to three times a day.

5. Use supportive taping during physical activity (the proper taping technique can be learned readily from a qualified athletic trainer).

Q What causes side stitch?

A Side stitch happens primarily in the early stages of exercise participation. The exact cause of this sharp pain in the side that occurs sometimes during exercise is unknown. Some experts suggest that it could relate to a lack of blood flow to the respiratory muscles during strenuous physical exertion. Side stitch occurs primarily in unconditioned beginners and in trained individuals when they exercise at higher intensities than usual. As one's physical condition improves, this problem disappears unless training is intensified. Some people, however, encounter side stitch during downhill running. If side stitch is a problem for you, slow down, and if it persists, stop altogether. Lying down on your back and gently bringing both knees to the chest and holding that position for 30 to 60 seconds also helps.

Some people also get side stitch if they eat or drink juice shortly before exercise. Drinking only water an hour to two prior to exercise can prevent side stitch. Other individuals have problems with commercially available carbohydrate solutions during high-intensity exercise. Unless carbohydrate replacement is crucial to complete an event (marathon, triathlon), drink cool water for fluid replacement, or try a different carbohydrate solution. Fluid and carbohydrate replacement during prolonged exercise or exercise in the heat are discussed later in this chapter.

Q What causes muscle cramps, and what should be done when they occur?

A Muscle cramps are caused by the body's depletion of essential electrolytes or a breakdown in coordination between opposing muscle groups. If you have a muscle cramp, first attempt to stretch the muscle(s) involved. In the case of the calf muscle, for example, pull your toes up toward the knees. After stretching the affected muscles, rub them down gently, and finally do some mild exercises requiring the use of those particular muscles.

In pregnant and lactating women muscle cramps often are related to a lack of calcium. If women get cramps during these times, calcium supplements usually relieve the problem. Tight clothing also can cause cramps because it restricts blood flow to active muscle tissue.

Q Why is exercising in hot and humid conditions unsafe?

A When a person exercises, only 30%–40% of the energy the body produces is used for mechanical work or movement. The rest of the energy (60%–70%) is converted into heat. If this heat cannot be dissipated properly because the weather is too hot or the relative humidity is too high, body temperature increases and in extreme cases can result in death.

The specific heat of body tissue (the heat required to raise the temperature of the body by 1°C) is .38 calories per pound of body weight per 1°C (.38 cal/lb/°C). This indicates that if no body heat is dissipated, a 150-pound person has to burn only 57 calories (150 × .38) to increase total body temperature by 1°C. If this person were to engage in an exercise session requiring 300 calories (about 3 miles running) without dissipating any heat, the inner body temperature would increase by 5.3°C, the equivalent of going from 98.6 to 108.1°F.

This example clearly illustrates the need for caution when exercising in hot or humid weather. If the relative humidity is too high, body heat cannot be lost through evaporation because the atmosphere already is saturated with water vapor. In one instance, a football casualty occurred at a temperature of only 64°F but at a relative humidity of 100%. As a general rule, care must be taken when air temperature is above 90°F and relative humidity is above 60%.

The American College of Sports Medicine has recommended that individuals should not engage in strenuous physical activity when the readings of a wet bulb globe thermometer exceed 82.4°F. With this type of thermometer, the wet bulb is cooled by evaporation, and on dry days it shows a lower temperature than the regular (dry) thermometer. On humid days the cooling effect is less because of less evaporation; hence, the difference between the wet and dry readings is not as great.

Following are descriptions of and first-aid measures for the three major signs of trouble when exercising in the heat:

1. *Heat cramps*. Symptoms include cramps and spasms and muscle twitching in the legs, arms, and abdomen. To relieve heat cramps, stop exercising, get out of the heat, massage the painful area, stretch slowly, and drink plenty of fluids (water, fruit drinks, or electrolyte beverages).

2. *Heat exhaustion*. Symptoms include fainting, dizziness, profuse sweating, cold, clammy skin, weakness, headache, and a rapid, weak pulse. If you incur any of these symptoms, stop and find a cool place to rest. Drink cool water only if conscious. Loosen or remove clothing, and rub your body with a cool/wet towel or ice packs. Place yourself in a supine position with legs elevated 8 to 12 inches. If you are not fully recovered in 30 minutes, seek immediate medical attention.

3. *Heat stroke*. Symptoms include serious disorientation; warm, dry skin; no sweating; rapid, full pulse; vomiting; diarrhea; unconsciousness; and high body temperature. As the body temperature climbs, unexplained anxiety sets in. When the body temperature reaches 104°F to 105°F, the individual may feel a cold sensation in the trunk of the body, goose bumps, nausea, throbbing in the temples, and numbness in the extremities. Most people become incoherent after this stage. When body temperature reaches 105°F to 106°F, disorientation, loss of fine-motor control, and muscular weakness set in. If the temperature exceeds 106°F, serious neurologic injury and death may be imminent.

Heat stroke requires immediate emergency medical attention. Request help and get out of the sun and into a cool, humidity-controlled environment. While you're waiting to be taken to the hospital's emergency room, you should be placed in a semi-seated position, and your body should be sprayed with cool water and rubbed with cool towels. If possible, cold packs should be placed in areas with abundant blood supply such as the head, neck, armpits, and groin. Fluids should not be given if you are unconscious. In any case of heat-related illness, if the person refuses water, vomits, or starts to lose consciousness, call for an ambulance immediately. Proper initial treatment of heat stroke is critical.

Q What are the recommended guidelines for fluid replacement during prolonged aerobic exercise?

A The main objective of fluid replacement during prolonged aerobic exercise is to maintain the blood volume so circulation and sweating can continue at normal levels. Adequate water replacement is the most important factor in preventing heat disorders. Drinking about 6 to 8 ounces of cool water every 15 to 20 minutes during exercise seems to be ideal to prevent

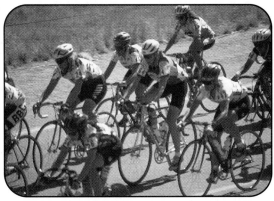

Fluid and carbohydrate replacement are essential during exercise of long duration.

dehydration. Cold fluids are absorbed more rapidly from the stomach.

Commercial fluid-replacement solutions (e.g., Exceed, All-Sport, Gatorade) contain about 6% to 8% glucose, which seems to be optimal for fluid absorption and performance in most cases. Sugar does not become available to the muscles until about 30 minutes after drinking a glucose solution.

Drinks high in fructose or with a glucose concentration above 8% will slow water absorption when exercising in the heat. Most soft drinks (cola, noncola) contain between 10% and 12% glucose, an amount that is too high for proper rehydration during exercise in the heat.

Commercially prepared sports drinks are recommended especially when exercise will be strenuous and carried out for more than an hour. For exercise lasting less than an hour, water is sufficient to replace fluid loss. The sports drinks you select should be based on your personal preference. Try different drinks at 6% to 8% glucose concentration to see which drink you tolerate best and suits your taste as well.

For long-distance events researchers recommend that 30 to 60 grams of carbohydrate (120 to 240 calories) be consumed every hour. This is best accomplished by drinking 8 ounces of a 6% to 8% carbohydrate sports drink every 15 minutes. The percentage of the carbohydrate drink is determined by dividing the amount of carbohydrate (in grams) by the amount of fluid (in ml) and multiplying by 100. For example, 18 grams of carbohydrate in 240 ml (8 oz) of fluid yields a drink at 7.5% (18 ÷ 240 × 100).

Q What precautions must a person take when exercising in the cold?

A When exercising in the cold, the two factors to consider are frostbite and **hypothermia**. In contrast to hot and humid conditions, exercising in the cold usually is not health-threatening because clothing for heat conservation can be selected and exercise itself increases the production of body heat.

Most people actually overdress for exercise in the cold. Because exercise increases body temperature, a moderate workout on a cold day makes you feel that it is 20°–30° warmer than the actual temperature. Overdressing for exercise can make the clothes damp from excessive perspiration. The risk for hypothermia increases when a person is wet or not moving around sufficiently to increase body heat. Initial warning signs of hypothermia include shivering, loss of coordination, and difficulty in speaking. With a continued drop in body temperature, shivering stops, the muscles weaken and stiffen, and the person feels elated or intoxicated and eventually loses consciousness. To prevent hypothermia, use common sense, dress properly, and be aware of environmental conditions.

The popular belief that exercising in cold temperatures (32°F and lower) freezes the lungs is false because the air is warmed properly in the air passages before it reaches the lungs. Cold is not what poses a threat. Rather, wind velocity is what affects the chill factor greatly.

For example, exercising at a temperature of 25°F with adequate clothing is not too cold, but if the wind is blowing at 25 miles per hour, the chill factor lowers the actual temperature to −5°F. This effect is even worse if a person is wet and exhausted. When windy, exercise (jog, cycle) against the wind on the way out and with the wind when you return.

Even though the lungs are under no risk when exercising in the cold, the face, head, hands, and feet should be protected, as they are subject to frostbite. Watch for numbness and discoloration — signs of frostbite. In cold temperatures as much as 50% of the body's heat can be lost through an unprotected head and neck. A wool or synthetic cap, hood, or hat will help to hold in body heat. Mittens are better than gloves because they keep the fingers together so the surface area from which to lose heat is less. Inner linings of synthetic material are recommended because they wick (draw) moisture away from the skin. Avoid cotton next to the skin because once it gets wet, whether from perspiration, rain, or snow, cotton loses its insulating properties.

Wearing several layers of lightweight clothing is preferable to wearing one single, thick layer because warm air is trapped between layers of clothes, enabling greater heat conservation. As body temperature increases, you can remove layers as necessary. For lengthy or long-distance workouts (cross-country skiing or long runs) take a small backpack to carry any clothing you remove. You also can carry extra warm and dry clothes in case you stop exercising away from shelter. If you remain outdoors following exercise, added clothing and continuous body movement are essential.

The first layer of clothes should wick moisture away from the skin. Polypropylene, Capilene, and Thermax are recommended. Next, a layer of wool, dacron, or polyester fleece insulates well even when wet. Lycra tights or sweatpants help to protect the legs. The outer layer should be waterproof, wind-resistant, and breathable. A synthetic material such as Gortex is best so moisture still can escape from the body. A ski or face mask helps protect the face. In extremely cold conditions petroleum jelly can be used to protect exposed skin such as the nose, cheeks, or around the eyes.

Special Considerations For Women

Q What are the physiological differences between men and women as related to exercise?

A Men and women have several basic differences that affect their physical performance. On the average, men are about 3 to 4 inches taller and 25 to 30 pounds heavier than women. The average body fat in college males is about 12% to 16%, whereas in college females it is 22% to 26%.

Maximal oxygen uptake (aerobic capacity) is about 15% to 30% greater in men, related primarily to a higher hemoglobin concentration and lower body fat content in men. The higher hemoglobin concentration allows men to carry a greater amount of oxygen during exercise, which is advantageous during aerobic events.

The quality of muscle in men and women is the same. Men, however, are stronger because they have a greater amount of muscle mass and a greater capacity for muscle hypertrophy, the muscle's ability to increase in size. The larger capacity for muscle hypertrophy is related to sex-specific hormones. Strength differences are significantly less, though, when taking into consideration body size and composition.

Men also have wider shoulders, longer extremities, and a 10% greater bone width, except for pelvic width. Notwithstanding all these gender differences in physiological characteristics, the two sexes respond to training in a similar way.

Q If the potential for muscle hypertrophy in women is not as great, why do so many women body builders develop such heavy musculature?

A The idea that strength training allows women to develop muscle hypertrophy to the same extent as men do is as false as the notion that playing basketball will turn women into giants. Masculinity and femininity are established by genetic inheritance, not by the amount of physical activity. Variations in the extent of masculinity and femininity are determined by individual differences in hormonal secretions of androgen, testosterone, estrogen, and progesterone. Women with a bigger-than-average build often are inclined to participate in sports because of their natural physical advantage. As a result, many women have associated participation in sports and strength training with large muscle size.

As the number of women who participate in sports has increased steadily during the last few years, the misconception that strength training in women leads to large increases in muscle size has abated somewhat. For example, per pound of body weight, women gymnasts are considered

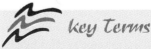

key Terms

Hypothermia A breakdown in the body's ability to generate heat and a drop in body temperature below 95°F.

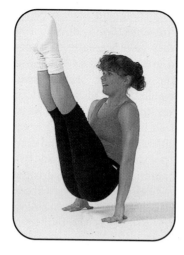

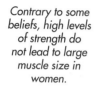

Contrary to some beliefs, high levels of strength do not lead to large muscle size in women.

to be among the strongest athletes in the world. These athletes engage regularly in serious strength-training programs. Yet, female gymnasts have some of the most well-toned and graceful figures of all women. In recent years improved body appearance has become the rule rather than the exception for women who participate in strength-training programs. Some of the most attractive female movie stars and beauty pageant participants also train with weights to improve their personal image.

At the same time, you may ask, "If weight training doesn't masculinize women, why do so many women body builders develop such heavy musculature?" In the sport of body building, the athletes follow intense training routines consisting of two or more hours of constant weight lifting with short rest intervals between sets. Many times body-building training routines call for back-to-back exercises using the same muscle groups. The objective of this type of training is to pump extra blood into the muscles, which makes the muscles appear much bigger than they really are in a resting condition. Based on the intensity and the length of the training session, the muscles can remain filled with blood and appear measurably larger for several hours after completing the training session. Therefore, in real life, these women are not as muscular as they seem when they are "pumped up" for a contest.

In the sport of body building, a big point of controversy is the use of **anabolic steroids** and human growth hormones, by women as well as men. These hormones produce detrimental and undesirable side effects, which some women deem tolerable (for example, hypertension, fluid retention, smaller breasts, deepening of the voice, facial whiskers, and growth of body hair). Anabolic steroid use in general, except for medical reasons and when monitored carefully by a physician, can have serious health consequences.

Use of anabolic steroids by women body builders is widespread. According to several sportsmedicine physicians and women body builders, about 80% of women body builders have used steroids. Furthermore, according to several women's track-and-field coaches, as many as 95% of women athletes in this sport around the world used anabolic steroids to remain competitive at the international level.

Undoubtedly, women who take steroids will build heavy musculature and, if they take the steroids long enough, will show masculinizing effects. As a result, the International Federation of Body Building instituted a mandatory steroid-testing program for women participating in the Miss Olympia contest. When drugs are not used to promote development, improved body image is the rule rather than the exception in women who participate in body building, strength training, and sports in general.

Q Does participation in exercise hinder menstruation?

A In some instances highly trained athletes develop amenorrhea during training and competition. This condition is seen most often in extremely lean women who also engage in sports that require strenuous physical effort over a sustained time. It is by no means irreversible. At present we do not know whether the condition is caused by physical stress or emotional stress related to high-intensity training, excessively low body fat, or other factors.

Although women on the average have a lower physical capacity during menstruation, women have broken Olympic and world records at all stages of the menstrual cycle. Menstruation should not keep a woman from participating in athletics, and it will not necessarily have a negative impact on performance.

Q Does exercise help relieve dysmenorrhea?

A Although exercise has not been shown to either cure or aggravate **dysmenorrhea,** it has been shown to help relieve menstrual cramps because it improves circulation to the uterus. Particularly, stretching exercises of the muscles in the pelvic region seem to reduce and prevent painful menstruation that is not the result of a disease.

Q Is exercising safe during pregnancy?

A Women should not forsake exercise during pregnancy. If anything, they should exercise to strengthen the body and prepare for delivery. Moderate exercise during pregnancy helps to prevent excessive weight gain and speed recovery following birth. Pregnant women in American Indian tribes continue to do all of their difficult work chores up to the very day of delivery, and a few hours after the baby's birth they resume their normal activities. Women athletes have competed in sports during the early stages of pregnancy. The woman and her personal physician should make the final decision regarding her exercise program.

Stretching exercises are to be performed gently because hormonal changes during pregnancy increase the laxity of muscles and connective tissue. These changes facilitate delivery, but they also make women more susceptible to injuries during exercise. In 1994 the American College of Obstetricians and Gynecologists released the latest set of its guidelines for exercise during pregnancy.[6] Among the recommendations for pregnant women with no additional risk factors are:

1. Continue to exercise at a mild-to-moderate pace throughout the pregnancy, but decrease exercise intensity by about 25% from the prepregnancy program.

2. Exercise regularly a minimum of three times a week instead of doing occasional exercise bouts.

3. Pay attention to the body's signals of discomfort and distress. Stop exercise when tired. Never exercise to exhaustion. Stop if unusual symptoms arise, such as pain of any kind, cramping, nausea, bleeding, leaking of amniotic fluid, faintness, dizziness, palpitations, numbness in any part of the body, or decreased fetal activity.

4. After the first trimester avoid exercises that require you to lie on your back. This position can block blood flow to the uterus and the baby.

5. Do nonweight-bearing activities such as cycling, swimming, or water aerobics, which minimize the risk of injury and may allow continuation of exercise throughout pregnancy.

6. Avoid activities that could precipitate a loss of balance or cause even mild trauma to the abdomen.

7. Get proper nourishment. (Pregnancy requires approximately 300 extra calories per day.)

8. During the first 3 months in particular, avoid exercising in the heat. Wear clothing that allows for proper dissipation of heat and drink plenty of water.

Q What is osteoporosis, and how can it be prevented?

A Osteoporosis is the softening, deterioration, or loss of total body bone. Bones become so weak and brittle that the person is vulnerable to fractures, primarily of the hip, wrist, and spine. Osteoporosis is preventable. It begins slowly in the third and fourth decades of life.

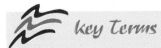 *key Terms*

Anabolic steroids A synthetic version of the male sex hormone testosterone, which promotes muscle development and hypertrophy.

Dysmenorrhea Painful menstruation.

The importance of normal estrogen levels, adequate calcium intake, and physical activity cannot be overemphasized in maximizing bone density in young women and lowering the rate of bone loss later in life. All three factors are crucial in preventing osteoporosis. The absence of any one of these three factors leads to bone loss, for which the other two never compensate completely.

Prevention of osteoporosis should begin early in life by having enough calcium in the diet (RDA of 800 to 1,200 mg per day) and by participating in a lifetime exercise program. Also, vitamin D, which is necessary for optimal calcium absorption, may have to be taken in supplements. To further enhance calcium absorption and decrease calcium loss, alcohol, caffeine, and protein intake should be controlled; cigarettes should be eliminated; and an extremely high-fiber diet should be avoided. A list of selected foods and their respective calcium content is provided in Table 9.2. Weight-bearing exercises such as walking, jogging, and weight training are especially helpful. Not only do they tone muscles, but they also produce stronger and thicker bones.

Prevailing research tells us that estrogen is the most important factor in preventing bone loss. Lumbar bone density in women with regular menstrual cycles exceeds that of women with a history of **oligomenorrhea**, and amenorrhea interspaced with regular cycles. Furthermore, the lumbar density of these two groups of women is higher than that of women who never had regular cycles.

Women are especially susceptible to osteoporosis after menopause because the accompanying estrogen loss hastens the rate at which bone mass is broken down. Following menopause, every woman should consider hormone replacement therapy and discuss it with her physician. Women who have estrogen therapy do not lose bone mineral density at the rate that nontherapy women do. Neither exercise nor calcium supplementation will offset the damaging effects of lower estrogen levels.

Although osteoporosis is viewed primarily as a women's disease, more than 30% of all men will be affected by age 75. It therefore is recommended that all adults over age 50 consume 1200 mg of calcium and 400 to 800 IU of vitamin D daily.

Table 9.2 Low-Fat Calcium-Rich Foods

Food	Amount	Calcium (mg)	Calories	Calories from Fat
Beans, red kidney, cooked	1 cup	70	218	4%
Beet, greens, cooked	1/2 cup	72	13	—
Broccoli, cooked, drained	1 small stalk	123	36	—
Burrito, bean	1	173	307	28%
Cottage cheese, 2% low-fat	1/2 cup	78	103	18%
Milk, nonfat, powdered	1 tbsp	52	27	1%
Milk, skim	1 cup	296	88	3%
Ice milk (vanilla)	1/2 cup	102	100	27%
Instant breakfast, whole milk	1 cup	301	280	26%
Kale, cooked, drained	1/2 cup	103	22	—
Okra, cooked, drained	1/2 cup	74	23	—
Shrimp, boiled	3 oz.	99	99	9%
Spinach, raw	1 cup	51	14	—
Yogurt, fruit	1 cup	345	231	8%
Yogurt, low-fat, plain	1 cup	271	160	20%

Q Do women have special needs for iron?

A Iron is a key element of hemoglobin in the blood, which carries oxygen from the lungs to all tissues of the body. The RDA of iron for adult women is 15 mg per day (10 mg for men). According to a survey by the U.S. Department of Agriculture, 19- to 50-year-old women in the United States consumed only 60% of the RDA for iron. People who do not have enough iron in the body can develop iron-deficiency anemia, in which the concentration of hemoglobin in the red blood cells is less than it should be.

Physically active women also may have a greater than average need for iron. Heavy training creates a demand for iron that is higher than the recommended intake because small amounts of iron are lost through sweat, urine, and stools. Mechanical trauma, caused by pounding of the feet on the pavement during extensive jogging, also may lead to the destruction of iron-containing red blood cells.

Among female endurance athletes, a large percentage is reported to have iron deficiency. Blood ferritin level, a measure of stored iron in the human body, should be checked frequently in women who participate in intense physical training.

The rates of iron absorption and iron loss vary from person to person. In most cases, though, people can get enough iron by eating more iron-rich foods such as beans, peas, green leafy vegetables, enriched grain products, egg yolk, fish, and lean meats. Although organ meats such as liver are especially good sources, they also are high in cholesterol. A list of foods high in iron content is given in Table 9.3.

Nutrition and Weight Control

Q What is the difference between a calorie and a kilocalorie (kcal)?

A Calorie is the unit of measure indicating the energy value of food and cost of physical activity. Technically, a kilocalorie (kcal), or large

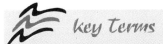

key Terms

Oligomenorrhea Irregular menstrual cycles.

Table 9.3 Iron-Rich Foods

Food	Amount	Iron (mg)	Calories	Cholesterol	Calories from Fat
Beans, red kidney, cooked	1 cup	4.4	218	0	4%
Beef, ground lean	3 oz.	3.0	186	81	48%
Beef, sirloin	3 oz.	2.5	329	77	74%
Beef, liver, fried	3 oz.	7.5	195	345	42%
Beet greens, cooked	1/2 cup	1.4	13	0	—
Broccoli, cooked, drained	1 sm stalk	1.1	36	0	—
Burrito, bean	1	2.4	307	14	28%
Egg, hard cooked	1	1.0	72	250	63%
Farina (Cream of Wheat), cooked	1/2 cup	6.0	51	0	—
Instant breakfast, whole milk	1 cup	8.0	280	33	26%
Peas, frozen, cooked, drained	1/2 cup	1.5	55	0	—
Shrimp, boiled	3 oz.	2.7	99	128	9%
Spinach, raw	1 cup	1.7	14	0	—
Vegetables, mixed, cooked	1 cup	2.4	116	0	—

calorie, is the amount of heat necessary to raise the temperature of 1 kilogram of water 1°C. For simplification, people call it a calorie rather than kcal. For example, if the caloric value of a food is 100 calories (kcal), the energy in this food could raise the temperature of 100 kilograms of water by 1°C.

Q Does cooking affect the caloric content of food?

A Cooking does not alter the caloric content of food significantly. The only exception is meat, in which broiling and barbecuing drain off some of the fat and decrease the caloric content. Frying, on the other hand, increases the caloric content of food significantly because of the large number of calories in the oil in which the food is fried.

Q In many instances, why don't the different fats listed on food labels add up to the total amount of fat listed on the labels?

A If present, transfatty acids and glycerol are included in the total fat figure of the food label. They constitute only a small part of the total fat in most foods. Transfatty acids are partially saturated fats and are not included on the label because they do not fit into any of the classifications of saturated, monounsaturated, and polyunsaturated fat. Glycerol also is included in the total amount of fat because it is used as a building block for fatty acids (triglycerides).

Q Is it true that calories don't count if I'm on a low-fat diet?

A Some self-proclaimed nutrition experts would have you believe that the answer to the previous question is yes. A "nonfat" label doesn't mean 0 calories or nonfattening when a person is overindulging. Calories do count. And though most low-fat diets are also low in calories, you can't assume that all are. Eating too many calories, regardless of the source, results in weight gain. In addition, what you eat along with your carbohydrates make a difference. Salads and

pasta are carbohydrate-rich, but many dressings and sauces that go along with them are not.

Q Does heavy perspiration during exercise help a person lose weight?

A Intense exercise, especially in warm or hot conditions, greatly enhances water loss (perspiration) from the body. You sweat off water, not fat. Without fluid replacement, a person can lose between 3 and 8 pounds of weight (water) per hour, depending on body size and ambient temperature. Once fluid is replaced after exercise, the weight is regained quickly. Fluids, however, should be replaced regularly *during* exercise. As pointed out earlier, fluid replacement is crucial for optimal performance and proper heat balance.

Q Are rubberized sweatsuits and steam baths effective in losing weight?

A The answer to this question is simply no! When a person wears a sweatsuit or steps into a sauna, the weight lost is not fat but is merely a significant amount of water. Sure, it looks nice when you step on the scale immediately afterward, but this represents a false loss of weight. As soon as you replace body fluids, you gain back the weight quickly.

Wearing rubberized sweatsuits not only hastens the rate of body fluid loss — fluid that is vital during prolonged exercise — but at the same time raises the body's core temperature. This combination puts a person in danger of dehydration, which impairs cellular function and in extreme cases even can cause death.

Q Are mechanical vibrators useful in losing weight?

A Some people will try almost anything to lose weight as long as they can still overindulge. In an attempt to solve their weight problem, these people can be deceived easily and often resort to quick fixes. Mechanical vibrators are worthless in a weight-control program. Vibrating belts and turning rollers may feel good, but they require no effort whatsoever. A person would have to vibrate continuously for 76 hours to lose the energy equivalent to 1 pound of fat! Fat cannot be "shaken off"; the body uses it as an energy substrate, and it is lost most efficiently by burning it in muscle tissue.

Q Is coffee detrimental to good health?

A Caffeine is a drug and, as such, can produce several undesirable side effects. Caffeine doses of more than 200 to 500 mg can cause an inordinately rapid heart rate, abnormal heart rhythms, a rise in blood pressure, higher body temperature, and oversecretion of gastric acids, leading to stomach problems. It also may have some link to birth defects in unborn children. It, too, may induce symptoms of anxiety, depression, nervousness, and dizziness. The caffeine content of various types of coffee ranges from 65 mg per 6 ounces for instant coffee to as high as 180 mg for drip coffee. Soft drinks, mainly colas, range in caffeine content from 30 mg to 80 mg per 12-ounce can.

Q Do athletes or individuals who train for long periods need a special diet?

A In general, athletes do not require special supplementation or any other special type of diet. Unless the diet is deficient in basic nutrients, no special, secret, or magic diet will help people perform better or develop faster as a result of what they eat. As long as the diet is balanced, based on a large variety of nutrients from the basic food groups, athletes do not require additional supplements other than the antioxidant recommendations made in Chapter 5. Even in strength training and body building, protein in excess of 20% of total daily caloric intake is not necessary.

The main difference between a sedentary person and a highly active individual is in the total number of calories required daily and the amount of carbohydrate intake during bouts of prolonged physical activity. During training, people consume more calories because of the greater energy expenditure required as a result of intense physical training.

A regular diet should be altered to include about 70% carbohydrates (carbohydrate loading) during several days of heavy aerobic training or when a person is going to participate in a long-distance event of more than 90 minutes (marathons, triathlons, road cycling races). For events shorter than 90 minutes, carbohydrate loading does not seem to enhance performance.

Exercise and Aging

Q What about exercise programs for older adults?

A Unlike any prior time in U.S. history, the elderly population constitutes the fastest growing segment. In 1880 less than 3% of the total population, fewer than 2 million people, was older than 65. By 1980 the elderly population had reached approximately 25 million, more than 11.3% of the population. According to estimates,[7] the elderly will make up more than 20% of the total U.S. population by the year 2035.

Even though fitness is just as important for older people as it is for young people, developers of fitness programs have neglected older adults. Much research remains to be done in this area, but studies thus far indicate that older individuals who are physically fit enjoy better health and quality of life.

The main objective of fitness programs for older adults should be to help them improve their functional health status. This implies the ability to maintain independent living and avoid disability. A committee of the American Alliance of Health, Physical Education, Recreation and Dance (AAHPERD) has defined *functional fitness* for older adults as "the physical capacity of the individual to meet ordinary and unexpected demands of daily life safely and effectively."[8] This definition clearly indicates the need for fitness programs that relate closely to activities this population normally encounters. The AAHPERD committee encourages participation in programs that will help develop cardiorespiratory endurance, localized muscular endurance, muscular flexibility, agility and balance, and

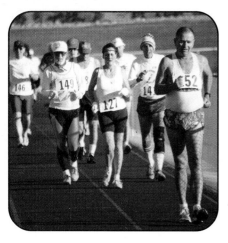

Exercise enhances quality of life and longevity.

motor coordination. A copy of the battery of fitness tests for older adults can be obtained from AAHPERD, Reston, Virginia.

Q What is the relationship between aging and physical work capacity?

A Although previous research studies have documented declines in physiological functioning and motor capacity as a result of aging, no hard evidence at present proves that declines in physical work capacity are related primarily to the aging process. Lack of physical activity — a common phenomenon as people age — may be accompanied by decreases in physical work capacity that are greater by far than the effects of aging itself.

Data on individuals who have taken part in systematic physical activity throughout life indicate that these groups of people maintain a higher level of functional capacity and do not experience the typical declines in later years. From a functional point of view, the typical sedentary American is about 25 years older than his or her chronological age indicates. Thus, an active 60-year-old person can have a work capacity similar to that of a sedentary 35-year-old.

Unhealthy behaviors precipitate premature aging. For sedentary people, productive life ends at about age 60. Most of

these people hope to live to be 65 or 70 and often must cope with serious physical ailments. These people stop living at age 60 but choose to be buried at age 70 (see Figure 9.2)!

Scientists believe a healthy lifestyle allows people to live a vibrant life — a physically, intellectually, emotionally, socially active, and functionally independent existence — to age 95. When death comes to active people, it usually is quick and not as a result of prolonged illness (see Figure 9.2). Such are the rewards of a wellness way of life.

Q Do older adults respond to physical training?

A The trainability of elderly men and women alike and the effectiveness of physical activity for enhancing health have been demonstrated in prior research.[9] Older adults who increase their level of physical activity go through significant changes in cardiorespiratory endurance, strength, and flexibility. The extent of the changes depends on their initial fitness level and the types of activities selected for their training (walking, cycling, strength training, and so on).

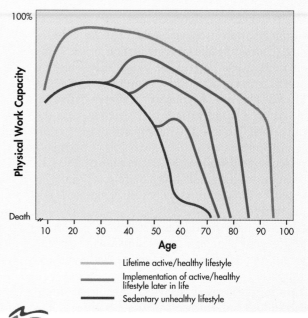

Figure 9.2 Relationship between physical work capacity, aging, and lifestyle habits.

Improvements in maximal oxygen uptake in older adults are similar to those of younger people, although older people seem to require a longer training period to achieve these changes. Declines in cardiorespiratory endurance (maximal oxygen uptake) per decade of life after age 25 seem to be about 9% for sedentary adults and 5% or less in active people.

Results of a study on the effects of aging on the cardiorespiratory system of male exercisers versus nonexercisers showed that the maximal oxygen uptake of regular exercisers was almost twice that of the nonexercisers.[10] The study revealed a decline in maximal oxygen uptake between the ages 50 and 68 of only 13% in the active group, compared to 41% in the inactive group. These changes indicate that about one-third of the loss in maximal oxygen uptake results from aging and two-thirds from inactivity. Blood pressure, heart rate, and body weight also were remarkably better in the exercising group.

Muscle strength declines by 10% to 20% between the ages of 20 and 50, and between ages 50 and 70 it drops by another 25% to 30%. Through strength training, frail adults in their 80s or 90s can double or triple their strength in just a few months. The amount of muscle hypertrophy achieved, however, decreases with age. Muscle flexibility drops by about 5% per decade of life. Stretching 10 minutes every other day can prevent most of this drop from developing with age.[11] In terms of body composition, inactive adults continue to gain body fat after age 60 despite the tendency toward lower body weight.

Older adults who wish to initiate or continue an exercise program are encouraged strongly to have a complete medical exam, including a stress electrocardiogram first (see Chapter 8). Recommended activities for older adults include calisthenics, walking, jogging, swimming, cycling, and water aerobics.

Older people should avoid isometric and other intense weight-training exercises. Activities that require all-out effort or require participants to hold their breath (valsalva maneuver) tend to lessen blood flow to the heart and cause a significant increase in blood pressure and load on the heart. Older adults should participate in activities that require continuous and rhythmic muscular activity (about 50% to 70% of functional capacity) and strength training with light weights. These activities do not cause large increases in blood pressure or place an intense overload on the heart.

As illustrated in Figure 9.2, physical fitness or physical work capacity can be increased at any age. Complete benefits of a healthy lifestyle, nonetheless, are best attained by starting early in life.

Fitness/Wellness Consumer Issues

Q How can I protect myself from fitness/wellness quackery and fraud?

A The rapid growth in fitness and wellness programs during the last three decades has spurred **quackery** and **fraud**. The promotion of fraudulent products that deceive consumers into adopting "miraculous," quick, and easy ways toward total well-being.

Today's market is saturated with "special" foods, diets, supplements, pills, cures, equipment, books, and videos that promise quick, dramatic results. Advertisements for these products often are based on testimonials, unproven claims, secret research, half-truths, and quick-fix statements that the uneducated consumer wants to hear. In the meantime, the organization or enterprise making the claims stands to reap a large profit from consumers' willingness to pay for astonishing and spectacular solutions to problems related to their unhealthy lifestyle.

Television, magazine, and newspaper advertisements are not necessarily reliable. For

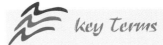

key Terms

Quackery/fraud The conscious promotion of unproven claims for profit.

instance, one piece of equipment sold through television and newspaper advertisements promised to "bust the gut" through 5 minutes of daily exercise that appeared to target the abdominal muscle group. This piece of equipment consisted of a metal spring attached to the feet on one end and held in the hands on the other end. According to handling and shipping distributors, the equipment was "selling like hotcakes," and companies could barely keep up with consumers' demands.

Three problems became apparent to the educated consumer. First, there is no such thing as spot-reducing; therefore, the claims could not be true. Second, 5 minutes of daily exercise burn hardly any calories and, therefore, have no effect on weight loss. Third, the intended abdominal (gut) muscles were not really involved during the exercise. The exercise engaged mostly the gluteal and lower-back muscles. This piece of equipment now can be found at garage sales for about a tenth of its original cost!

Many uneducated consumers are targets of deception by organizations making fraudulent claims for their products. Even though deceit is all around us, we can protect ourselves from consumer fraud. The first step is education. You have to be informed about the product you intend to purchase. If you do not have or cannot find the answers, seek the advice of a reputable professional. Ask someone who understands the product but does not stand to profit from the transaction. As examples, a physical educator or an exercise physiologist can advise you regarding exercise equipment; a registered dietitian can provide information on nutrition and weight-control programs; a physician can offer advice on treatment modalities. Also, be alert to those who bill themselves as "experts." Look for qualifications, degrees, professional experience, certifications, reputation.

Another clue to possible fraud is that if it sounds too good to be true, it probably is. Quick-fix, miraculous, special, secret, mail orders only, money-back guarantee, and testimonials often are announced in advertisements of fraudulent promotions. When claims are made, ask where the claims are published. Newspapers, magazines, and trade books are apt to be unreliable sources of information. Refereed scientific journals are the most reliable sources of information. When a researcher submits information for publication in a refereed journal, at least two qualified and reputable professionals in the field conduct blind reviews of the manuscript. A blind review means the author does not know who will review the manuscript and the reviewers do not know who submitted the manuscript. Acceptance for publication is based on this input and relevant changes.

If you have questions or concerns about a health product, you may write to the National Council Against Health Fraud (NCAHF), P.O. Box 1276, Loma Linda, CA 92354. The purpose of this organization is to monitor deceitful advertising, investigate complaints, and offer the public information regarding fraudulent health claims.

Q What guidelines should I follow when looking for a reputable health-fitness facility?

A As you follow a lifetime wellness program, you may want to consider joining a health/fitness facility. Or, if you have mastered the contents of this book and your choice of fitness activity is one you can pursue on your own (walking, jogging, cycling), you may not need to join a health club. Barring injuries, you may continue your exercise program outside the walls of a health club for the rest of your life. You also can conduct strength-training and stretching programs within the walls of your

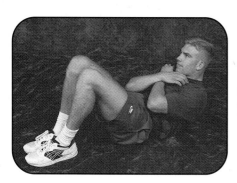

Spot-reducing does not work.

own home (see Chapters 3 and 4 and Appendices B, C, and D).

To stay up to date on fitness and wellness developments, you probably should buy a reputable and updated fitness/wellness book every 4 to 5 years. You also might subscribe to a credible health, fitness, nutrition, or wellness newsletter to stay current.

If you are contemplating membership in a fitness facility:

- Examine all exercise options in your community: health clubs/spas, YMCAs, gyms, colleges, schools, community centers, senior centers, and the like.

- Check to see if the facility's atmosphere is pleasurable and nonthreatening to you. Will you feel comfortable with the instructors and other people who go there? Is it clean and kept up well? If the answer is no, this may not be the right place for you.

Reliable Sources of Health, Fitness, Wellness, and Nutrition Information

Newsletter	Approx. Yearly Issues	Annual Cost
Consumer Reports Health Letter P.O. Box 56356 Boulder, CO 80323–2148	12	$24
Executive Health's Good Health Report P.O. Box 8880 Chapel Hill, NC 27515	12	$34
HealthNews P.O. Box 8963 Waltham, MA 02254-9959	12	$29
Tufts University Diet & Nutrition Letter P.O. Box 57857 Boulder, CO 80322–7857	12	$24
University of California Berkeley Wellness Letter P.O. Box 420148 Palm Coast, FL 32142	12	$24

- Analyze costs versus facilities, equipment, and programs. Take a look at your personal budget. Will you really use the facility? Will you exercise there regularly? Many people obtain memberships and allow dues to be withdrawn automatically from a local bank account, yet seldom attend the fitness center.

- Find out what types of facilities are available: running track, basketball/tennis/racquetball courts, aerobic exercise room, strength-training room, pool, locker rooms, saunas, hot tubs, handicapped access, and so on.

- Check the aerobic and strength-training equipment available. Does the facility have treadmills, bicycle ergometers, Stair Masters, cross-country skiing simulators, free weights, Universal Gym, Nautilus? Make sure the facilities and equipment meet your interests.

- Consider the location. Is the facility close, or do you have to travel several miles to get there? Distance often discourages participation.

- Check on times the facility is accessible. Is it open during your preferred exercise time (for example, early morning or late evening)?

- Work out at the facility several times before you become a member. Are people standing in line to use the equipment, or is it readily available during your exercise time?

- Inquire about instructors' qualifications. Do the fitness instructors have college degrees or professional certifications from organizations such as the American College of Sports Medicine (ACSM) or the International Dance Exercise Association (IDEA)? These organizations have rigorous standards to ensure professional preparation and quality of instruction.

- Consider the approach to fitness (including all health-related components of fitness). Is it well-rounded? Do the instructors spend time with members, or do members have to seek them out constantly for help and instruction?

✍ Ask about supplementary services. Does the facility provide or contract out for regular health and fitness assessments (cardiorespiratory endurance, body composition, blood pressure, blood chemistry analysis)? Are wellness seminars (nutrition, weight control, stress management) offered? Do these have hidden costs?

Q. What factors should I consider before purchasing exercise equipment?

A The first question you need to ask yourself is: Do I really need this piece of equipment? Most people buy on impulse because of television advertisements or because a salesperson convinces them that it is a great piece of equipment that will do wonders for their health and fitness. Again, if marketing claims seem too good to be true, they probably are. With some creativity, you can implement an excellent and comprehensive exercise program with little, if any, equipment (see Chapters 3 and 4).

Many people buy expensive equipment only to find they really do not enjoy that mode of activity. They do not remain regular users. Stationary bicycles (lower body only) and rowing ergometers were among the most popular pieces of equipment in the 1980s. Most of them are seldom used now and have become "fitness furniture" somewhere in the basement.

Exercise equipment does have its value for people who prefer to exercise indoors, especially during the winter months. It supports some people's motivation and adherence to exercise. The convenience of having equipment at home also allows for flexible scheduling. You can exercise before or after work or while you watch your favorite television show.

If you are going to purchase equipment, the best recommendation is to actually try it out several times before buying it. Ask yourself several questions: Did I enjoy the workout? Is the unit comfortable? Am I too short, tall, or heavy for it? Is it stable, sturdy, and strong? Do I have to assemble the machine? If so, how difficult is it to put together? How durable is it? Ask for references — people or clubs that have used the equipment extensively. Are they satisfied? Have they enjoyed the activity (the equipment)? Talk with professionals at colleges, sportsmedicine clinics, or health clubs.

Another consideration is to look at used units for signs of wear and tear. Quality is important. Cheaper brands may not be durable, wasting your investment.

Finally, watch out for expensive gadgets. Monitors that provide exercise heart rate, work output, caloric expenditure, speed, grade, and distance may help motivate you, but they are expensive, need repairs, and do not enhance the actual fitness benefits of the workout. Look at maintenance costs and check for service personnel in your community.

What's Next?

The objective of this book is to provide you with the basic information necessary to implement your personal healthy lifestyle program. Your activities over the last few weeks or months may have helped you develop positive habits that you should try to carry on throughout life.

Now that you are about to finish this course, the real challenge will be a lifetime commitment to fitness and wellness. Adhering to the program in a structured setting is a lot easier. Fitness and wellness is a continual process. As you proceed with the program, keep in mind that the greatest benefit is a higher quality of life.

Most people who adopt a wellness way of life recognize this new quality after only a few weeks into the program. In some instances — especially individuals who have led a poor lifestyle for a long time — establishing positive habits and gaining feelings of well-being might take a few months. In the end, however, everyone who applies the principles of fitness and wellness will reap the desired benefits.

Being diligent and taking control of yourself will provide you a better, happier, healthier, and more productive life. Be sure to maintain a program based on your needs and what you enjoy doing most. This will make the journey easier and more fun along the way. Once you reach the top, you will know there is no looking back. If you don't get there, you won't know what it's like. Improving the quality and longevity of your life now is in your hands. It will require persistence and commitment, but only you can take control of your lifestyle and thereby reap the benefits of wellness.

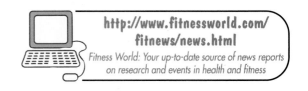

http://www.fitnessworld.com/
fitnews/news.html

Fitness World: Your up-to-date source of news reports on research and events in health and fitness

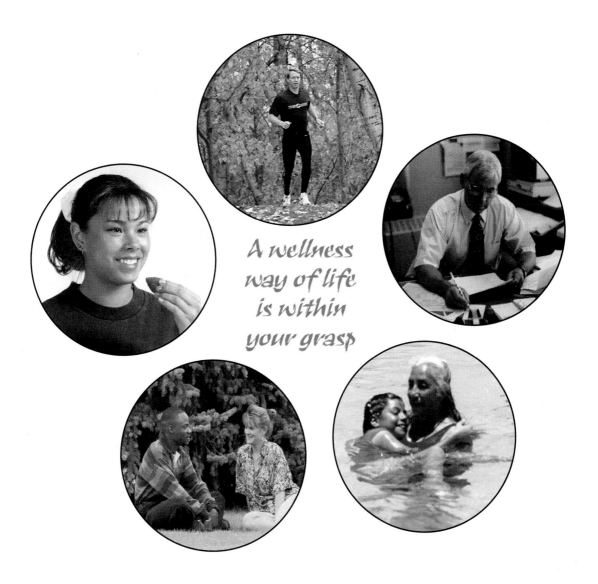

A wellness way of life is within your grasp

Notes

1. R. Pate et al., "Physical Activity and Public Health," *Journal of the American Medical Association*, 273(1995), 402–407.

2. R. S. Paffenbarger, Jr., R. T. Hyde, A. L. Wing, and C. H. Steinmetz. "A Natural History of Athleticism and Cardiovascular Health." *Journal of the American Medical Association*, 252(1984), 491–495.

3. S. N. Blair, H. W. Kohl III, R. S. Paffenbarger, Jr., D. G. Clark, K. H. Cooper, and L. W. Gibbons, "Physical Fitness and All-Cause Mortality: A Prospective Study of Healthy Men and Women," *Journal of the American Medical Association*, 262(1989), 2395–2401.

4. Pate.

5. R. Hambrecht et al., "Various Intensities of Leisure Time Physical Activity in Patients with Coronary Artery Disease: Effects on Cardiorespiratory Fitness and Progression of Coronary Atherosclerotic Lesions," *Journal of the American College of Cardiology*, 22(1993), 468–477.

6. American College of Obstetricians and Gynecologists, Guidelines for Exercise During Pregnancy, 1994.

7. L. DiPietro, "The Epidemiology of Physical Activity and Physical Function in Older People," *Medicine and Science in Sports and Exercise,* 28(1996), 596–600.

8. W. H. Osness, M. Adrian, B. Clark, W. Hoeger, D. Raab, and R. Wiswell, *Functional Fitness Assessment for Adults Over 60 Years* (Reston, VA: American Alliance for Health, Physical Education, Recreation, and Dance, 1990).

9. American College of Sports Medicine, Position Stand: "Exercise and Physical Activity for Older Adults," *Medicine and Science in Sports and Exercise,*" 30(1998), 992–1008.

10. F. W. Kash, J. L. Boyer, S. P. Van Camp, L. S. Verity, and J. P. Wallace. "The Effect of Physical Activity on Aerobic Power in Older Men (A Longitudinal Study)," *Physician and Sports Medicine*, 18:4(1990), 73–83.

11. "Exercise for the Ages," *Consumer Reports on Health* (Yonkers, NY: Editors, July, 1996).

Pre- and Post-Fitness Profiles

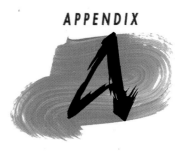

Personal Fitness Profile: Pre-Test

Date: _____ Course: _____ Section: _____

Name: _____ Age: _____ Male or Female: M / F

Body Weight: _____ . _____

Fitness Component	Test Data	Test Results	Fitness Classification	Fitness Goal
Cardiorespiratory Endurance	Time	$VO_{2max.}$		$VO_{2max.}$
1.5-Mile Run	_____ : _____	_____ . _____ _____		_____ . _____
	Time			
1.0-Mile Walk	_____ : _____			
	Heart Rate	$VO_{2max.}$		$VO_{2max.}$
	_____	_____ . _____ _____		_____ . _____
Muscular Strength / Endurance	Reps	Percentile		
Bench Jumps	_____	_____	_____	_____
Chair Dips / Mod. Push-Ups	_____	_____	_____	_____
Bent-Leg Curl-Ups/Abd. Crunches	_____	_____	_____	_____
Overall Fitness Category			_____	
Muscular Flexibility	Inches	Percentile		
Modified Sit-and-Reach	_____	_____	_____	_____
Body Rotation (R/L)	_____	_____	_____	_____
Overall Fitness Category			_____	
Body Composition	mm			
Chest / Triceps	_____			
Abdominal / Suprailium	_____			
Thigh	_____			
Sum of Skinfolds	_____			
Percent Body Fat		_____	_____	_____
Lean Body Mass (lbs.)		_____		_____

_____   _____   _____
Student Signature   Instructor Signature   Date

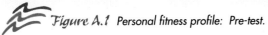

Figure A.1 Personal fitness profile: Pre-test.

Personal Fitness Profile: Post-Test

Date: _____ Course: _____ Section: _____

Name: _____ Age: _____ Male or Female: M / F

Body Weight: _____ . _____

Fitness Component	Test Data	Test Results	Fitness Classification
Cardiorespiratory Endurance	Time	$VO_{2\,max.}$	
1.5-Mile Run	_____ : _____	_____ . _____	_____
1.0-Mile Walk	Time _____ : _____		
	Heart Rate _____	$VO_{2\,max.}$ _____ . _____	_____
Muscular Strength / Endurance	Reps	Percentile	
Bench Jumps	_____	_____	_____
Chair Dips / Mod. Push-Ups	_____	_____	_____
Bent-Leg Curl-Ups/Abd. Crunches	_____	_____	_____
Overall Fitness Category			_____
Muscular Flexibility	Inches	Percentile	
Modified Sit-and-Reach	_____	_____	_____
Body Rotation (R/L)	_____	_____	_____
Overall Fitness Category			_____
Body Composition	mm		
Chest / Triceps	_____		
Abdominal / Suprailium	_____		
Thigh	_____		
Sum of Skinfolds	_____		
Percent Body Fat	_____	_____	_____
Lean Body Mass (lbs.)	_____	_____	_____

_____   _____   _____
Student Signature   IInstructor Signature   Date

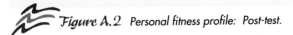

Figure A.2 *Personal fitness profile: Post-test.*

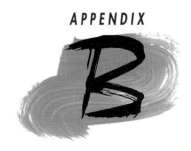
Strength-Training Exercises

Strength-Training Exercises Without Weights

1 Step-Up

Action: Step up and down using a box or chair approximately twelve to fifteen inches high. Conduct one set using the same leg each time you go up and then conduct a second set using the other leg. You could also alternate legs on each step-up cycle. You may increase the resistance by holding a child or some other object in your arms (hold the child or object close to the body to avoid increased strain in the lower back).

Muscles Developed: Gluteal muscles, quadriceps, gastrocnemius, and soleus.

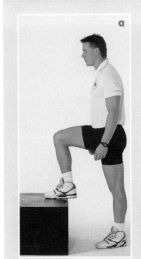
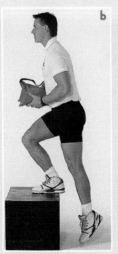

2 High-Jumper

Action: Start with the knees bent at approximately 150° and jump as high as you can, raising both arms simultaneously.

Muscles Developed: Gluteal muscles, quadriceps, gastrocnemius, and soleus.

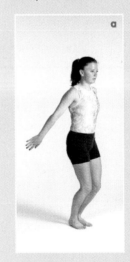
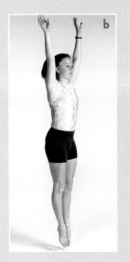

Photographs for Exercises 13, 14, 16, 17, 18, 19, 20, and 22 are courtesy of Universal Gym® Equipment, Inc., 930 27th Avenue, S.W., Cedar Rapids, IA 52406. Photographs for Exercises 15 and 21 are courtesy of Nautilus®, a registered trademark of Nautilus® Sports/Medical Industries, Inc., P.O. Box 809014, Dallas, TX 75380-9014.

3

Push-Up

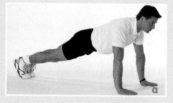
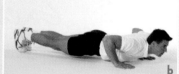

Action: Maintaining your body as straight as possible, flex the elbows, lowering the body until you almost touch the floor, then raise yourself back up to the starting position. If you are unable to perform the push-up as indicated, you can decrease the resistance by supporting the lower body with the knees rather than the feet (see illustration c) or using an incline plane and supporting your hands at a higher point than the floor (see illustration d). If you wish to increase the resistance, have someone else add resistance to your shoulders as you are coming back up (see illustrations e and f).

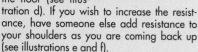
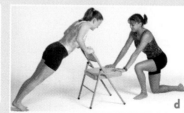
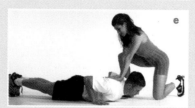
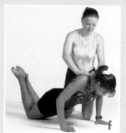

Muscles Developed: Triceps, deltoid, pectoralis major, erector spinae, and abdominals.

4

Abdominal Crunch and Bent-Leg Curl-Up

Action: Start with your head and shoulders off the floor, arms crossed on your chest, and knees slightly bent (the greater the flexion of the knee, the more difficult the curl-up). Now curl up to about 30° (abdominal crunch — see illustration b) or curl all the way up (bent-leg curl-up), then return to the starting position without letting the head or shoulders touch the floor, or allowing the hips to come off the floor. If you allow the hips to raise off the floor and the head and shoulders to touch the floor, you will most likely "swing up" on the next sit-up, which minimizes the work of the abdominal muscles. If you cannot curl up with the arms on the chest, place the hands by the side of the hips or even help yourself up by holding on to your thighs (illustrations d and e). Do not perform the curl-up exercise with your legs completely extended, as this will cause strain on the lower back.

Muscles Developed: Abdominal muscles (crunch) and hip flexors (complete curl-up).

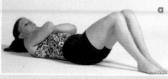
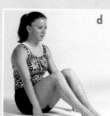
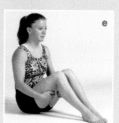
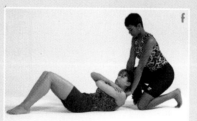

NOTE: The bent-leg curl-up exercise should be used only by individuals of at least average fitness without a history of lower back problems. New participants and those with a history of lower back problems should use the abdominal crunch exercise in its place.

Leg Curl

Action: Lie on the floor face down. Cross the right ankle over the left heel. Apply resistance with your right foot, while you bring the left foot up to 90° at the knee joint. (Apply enough resistance so that the left foot can only be brought up slowly.) Repeat the exercise, crossing the left ankle over the right heel.

Muscles Developed: Hamstrings (and quadriceps).

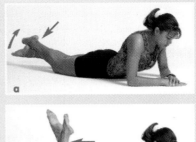

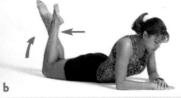

Modified Dip

Action: Place your hands and feet on opposite chairs with knees slightly bent (make sure that the chairs are well stabilized). Dip down at least to a 90° angle at the elbow joint, then return to the initial position. To increase the resistance, have someone else hold you down by the shoulders on the way up (see illustration c). You may also perform this exercise using a gymnasium bleacher or box and with the help of a partner, as illustrated in photo d.

Muscles Developed: Triceps, deltoid, and pectoralis major.

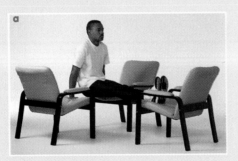

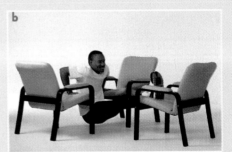

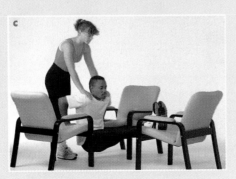

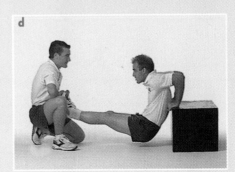

Pull-Up

Action: Suspend yourself from a bar with a pronated grip (thumbs in). Pull your body up until your chin is above the bar, then lower the body slowly to the starting position. If you are unable to perform the pull-up as described, either have a partner hold your feet to push off and facilitate the movement upward (illustrations c and d) or use a lower bar and support your feet on the floor (illustration e).

Muscles Developed: Biceps, brachioradialis, brachialis, trapezius, and latissimus dorsi.

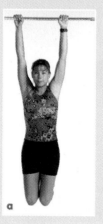
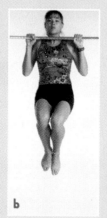
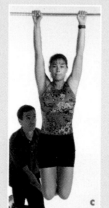
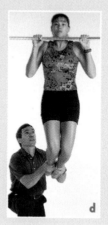
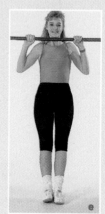

Arm Curl

Action: Using a palms-up grip, start with the arm completely extended, and with the aid of a sandbag or bucket filled (as needed) with sand or rocks, curl up as far as possible, then return to the initial position. Repeat the exercise with the other arm.

Muscles Developed: Biceps, brachioradialis, and brachialis.

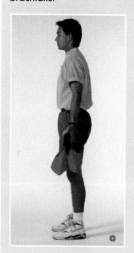
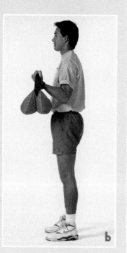

Heel Raise

Action: From a standing position with feet flat on the floor, raise and lower your body weight by moving at the ankle joint only (for added resistance, have someone else hold your shoulders down as you perform the exercise).

Muscles Developed: Gastrocnemius and soleus.

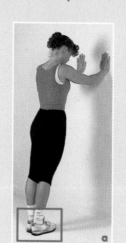
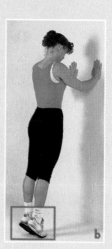

Leg Abduction and Adduction

Action: Both participants sit on the floor. The subject on the left places the feet on the inside of the other partici-pant's feet. Simultaneously, the subject on the left presses the legs laterally (to the outside — abduction), while the subject on the right presses the legs medially (adduction). Hold the contraction for five to ten seconds. Repeat the exercise at all three angles, and then reverse the pressing sequence. The subject on the left places the feet on the outside and presses inward, while the subject on the right presses outward.

Muscles Developed: Hip abductors (rectus femoris, sar-tori, gluteus medius and minimus), and adductors (pectineus, gracilis, adductor magnus, adductor longus, and adductor brevis).

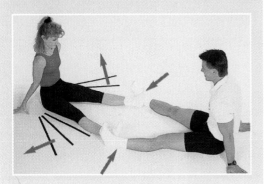

Reverse Crunch

Action: Lie on your back with arms crossed on your chest and knees and hips flexed at 90° (a). Now attempt to raise the pelvis off the floor by lifting vertically from the knees and lower legs (b). This is a challenging exercise that may be difficult for beginners to perform.

Muscles Developed: Abdominals.

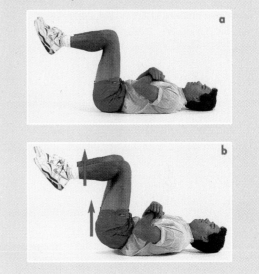

Pelvic Tilt

Action: Lie flat on the floor with the knees bent at about a 90° angle (a). Tilt the pelvis by tighten-ing the abdominal muscles, flattening your back against the floor, and raising the lower gluteal area ever so slightly off the floor (b). Hold the final position for several seconds. The exercise can also be performed against a wall (c).

Areas Stretched: Low-back muscles and ligaments.

Areas Strengthened: Abdominal and glu-teal muscles.

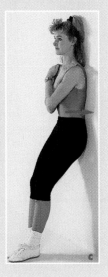

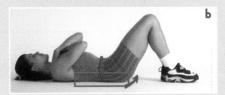

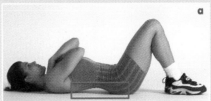

Strength-Training Exercises With Weights

13

Arm Curl

Action: Use a supinated or palms-up grip, and start with the arms almost completely extended. Now curl up as far as possible, then return to the starting position.

Muscles Developed: Biceps, brachioradialis, and brachialis.

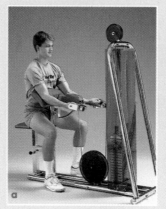 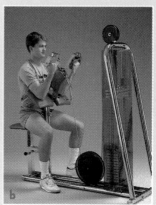

14

Bench Press

Action: Lie down on the bench with the head by the weight stack, the bench press bar above the chest, and place the feet on the bench. Grasp the bar handles and press upward until the arms are completely extended, then return to the original position. Do not arch the back during this exercise.

Muscles Developed: Pectoralis major, triceps, and deltoid.

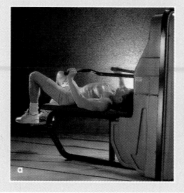 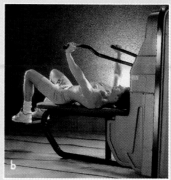

15

Abdominal Crunch

Action: Sit in an upright position and grasp the handles over your shoulders and crunch forward. Slowly return to the original position.

Muscles Developed: Abdominals.

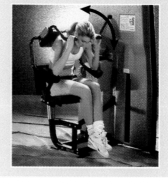

Leg Extension

Action: Sit in an upright position with the feet under the padded bar and grasp the handles at the sides. Extend the legs until they are completely straight, then return to the starting position.

Muscles Developed: Quadriceps.

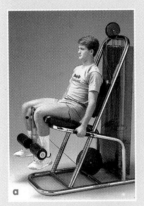
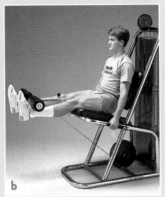

Leg Curl

Action: Lie with the face down on the bench, legs straight, and place the back of the feet under the padded bar. Curl up to at least 90°, and return to the original position.

Muscles Developed: Hamstrings.

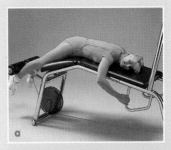
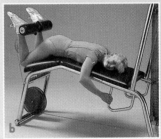

Lat Pull-Down

Action: Start from a sitting position, and hold the exercise bar with a wide grip. Pull the bar down until it touches the base of the neck, then return to the starting position.

Muscles Developed: Latissimus dorsi, pectoralis major, and biceps.

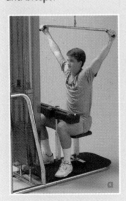

Heel Raise

Action: Start with your feet either flat on the floor or the front of the feet on an elevated block, then raise and lower yourself by moving at the ankle joint only. If additional resistance is needed, you can use a squat strength-training machine.

Muscles Developed: Gastrocnemius and soleus.

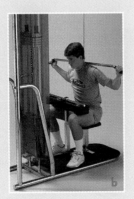
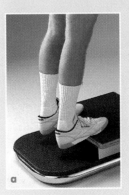
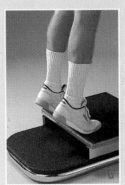

20 Triceps Extension

Action: Using a palms-down grip, grasp the bar slightly closer than shoulder width, and start with the elbows almost completely bent (a). Extend the arms fully (b), then return to starting position.

Muscles Developed: Triceps.

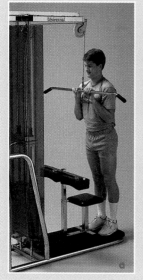
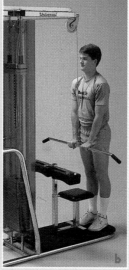

21 Rotary Torso

Action: Sit upright into the machine and place the elbows behind the padded bars (a). Rotate the torso as far as possible to one side (b) and then return slowly to the starting position. Repeat the exercise to the opposite side.

Muscles Developed: Internal and external obliques (abdominal muscles).

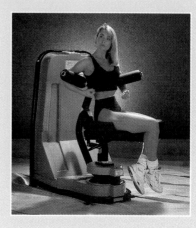

22 Seated Back

Action: Sit in the machine with your trunk flexed and the upper back against the shoulder pad. Place the feet under the padded bar and hold on with your hands to the bars on the sides (a). Start the exercise by pressing backward, simultaneously extending the trunk and hip joints (b). Slowly return to the original position.

Muscles Developed: Erector spinae and gluteus maximus.

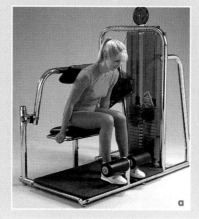
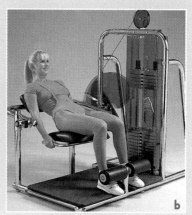

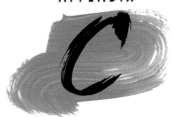

Flexibility Exercises

23 Lateral Head Tilt

Action: Slowly and gently tilt the head laterally. Repeat several times to each side.

Areas Stretched: Neck flexors and extensors and ligaments of the cervical spine.

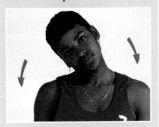

24 Arm Circles

Action: Gently circle your arms all the way around. Conduct the exercise in both directions.

Areas Stretched: Shoulder muscles and ligaments.

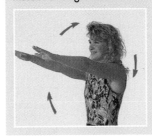

25 Side Stretch

Action: Stand straight up, feet separated to shoulder width, and place your hands on your waist. Now move the upper body to one side and hold the final stretch for a few seconds. Repeat on the other side.

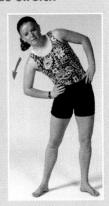

Areas Stretched: Muscles and ligaments in the pelvic region.

26 Body Rotation

Action: Place your arms slightly away from your body and rotate the trunk as far as possible, holding the final position for several seconds. Conduct the exercise for both the right and left sides of the body. You can also perform this exercise by standing about two feet away from the wall (back toward the wall), and then rotate the trunk, placing the hands against the wall.

Areas Stretched: Hip, abdominal, chest, back, neck, and shoulder muscles; hip and spinal ligaments.

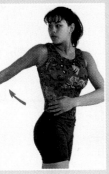

27 Chest Stretch

Action: Kneel down behind a chair and place both hands on the back of the chair. Gradually push your chest downward and hold for a few seconds.

Areas Stretched: Chest (pectoral) muscles and shoulder ligaments.

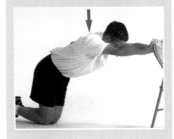

28 Shoulder Hyperextension Stretch

Action: Have a partner grasp your arms from behind by the wrists and slowly push them upward. Hold the final position for a few seconds.

Areas Stretched: Deltoid and pectoral muscles, and ligaments of the shoulder joint.

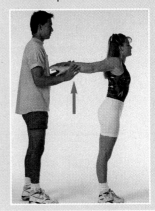

29 Shoulder Rotation Stretch

Action: With the aid of surgical tubing or an aluminum or wood stick, place the tubing or stick behind your back and grasp the two ends using a reverse (thumbs-out) grip. Slowly bring the tubing or stick over your head, keeping the elbows straight. Repeat several times (bring the hands closer together for additional stretch).

Areas Stretched: Deltoid, latissimus dorsi, and pectoral muscles; shoulder ligaments.

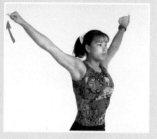

30 Quad Stretch

Action: Lie on your side and move one foot back by flexing the knee. Grasp the front of the ankle and pull the ankle toward the gluteal region. Hold for several seconds. Repeat with the other leg.

Areas Stretched: Quadriceps muscle, and knee and ankle ligaments.

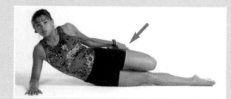

31 Heel Cord Stretch

Action: Assume a push-up position, then bend one knee and stretch the opposite heel cord. Hold the stretched position for a few seconds. Alternate legs. You may also perform this exercise leaning against a wall or standing at the edge of a step, then stretch the heel downward.

Areas Stretched: Heel cord (Achilles tendon), gastrocnemius, and soleus muscles.

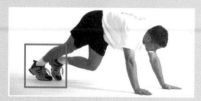

32 Adductor Stretch

Action: Stand with your feet about twice shoulder width and place your hands slightly above the knee. Flex one knee and slowly go down as far as possible, holding the final position for a few seconds. Repeat with the other leg.

Areas Stretched: Hip adductor muscles.

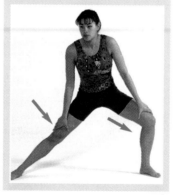

33 Sitting Adductor Stretch

Action: Sit on the floor and bring your feet in close to you, allowing the soles of the feet to touch each other. Now place your forearms (or elbows) on the inner part of the thigh and push the legs downward, holding the final stretch for several seconds.

Areas Stretched: Hip adductor muscles.

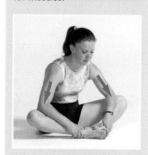

34 Sit-and-Reach Stretch

Action: Sit on the floor with legs together and gradually reach forward as far as possible. Hold the final position for a few seconds. This exercise may also be performed with the legs separated, reaching to each side as well as to the middle.

Areas Stretched: Hamstrings and lower back muscles, and lumbar spine ligaments.

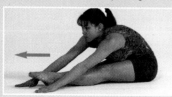

35 Triceps Stretch

Action: Place the right hand behind your neck. Grasp the right arm above the elbow with the left hand. Gently pull the elbow backward. Repeat the exercise with the opposite arm.

Areas Stretched: Back of upper arm (triceps muscle) and shoulder joint.

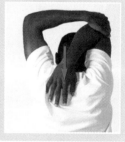

Exercises for the Prevention and Rehabilitation of Low-Back Pain

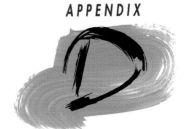

36 — Single-Knee to Chest Stretch

Action: Lie down flat on the floor. Bend one leg at approximately 100° and gradually pull the opposite leg toward your chest. Hold the final stretch for a few seconds. Switch legs and repeat the exercise.

Areas Stretched: Lower back and hamstring muscles, and lumbar spine ligaments.

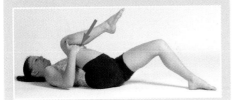

37 — Double-Knee to Chest Stretch

Action: Lie flat on the floor and then slowly curl up into a fetal position. Hold for a few seconds.

Areas Stretched: Upper and lower back and hamstring muscles; spinal ligaments.

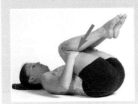

38 — Upper and Lower Back Stretch

Action: Sit on the floor and bring your feet in close to you, allowing the soles of the feet to touch each other. Hold on to your feet and gently bring your head and upper chest toward your feet.

Areas Stretched: Upper and lower back muscles and ligaments.

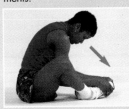

39 — Sit-and-Reach Stretch

See Exercise 34 in Appendix C.

40 — Gluteal Stretch

Action: Sit on the floor, bend the left leg and place your left ankle slightly above the right knee. Grasp the right thigh with both hands and gently pull the leg toward your chest. Repeat the exercise with the opposite leg.

Areas Stretched: Buttock area (gluteal muscles).

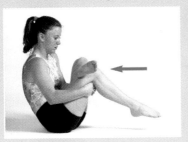

41 — Back Extension

Action: Lie face down on the floor with the elbows by the chest, forearms on the floor, and the hands beneath the chin. Gently raise the trunk by extending the elbows until you reach an approximate 90° angle at the elbow joint. Be sure that the forearms remain in contact with the floor at all times. Hold the stretched position for a few seconds. DO NOT extend the back beyond this point. Hyperextension of the lower back may lead to or aggravate an already existing back problem.

Area Stretched: Abdominal region.

Additional Benefit: Restore lower back curvature.

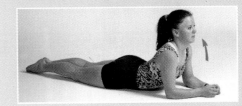

42

Trunk Rotation and Lower Back Stretch

Action: Sit on the floor and bend the right leg, placing the right foot on the outside of the left knee. Place the left elbow on the right knee and push against it. At the same time, try to rotate the trunk to the right (clockwise). Hold the final position for a few seconds. Repeat the exercise with the other side.

Areas Stretched: Lateral side of the hip and thigh; trunk, and lower back.

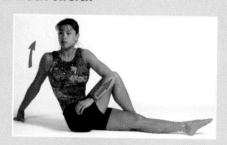

43

Pelvic Tilt

Action: Lie flat on the floor with the knees bent at about a 90° angle. Tilt the pelvis by tightening the abdominal muscles, flattening your back against the floor, and raising the lower gluteal area ever so slightly off the floor (see illustration b). Hold the final position for several seconds. The exercise can also be performed against a wall (as shown in illustration c).

Areas Stretched: Low back muscles and ligaments.

Areas Strengthened: Abdominal and gluteal muscles.

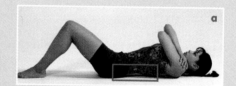

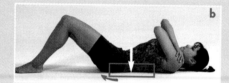

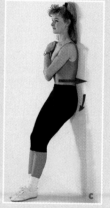

44

Cat Stretch

Action: Kneel on the floor and place your hands in front of you (on the floor) about shoulder width apart. Relax your trunk and lower back (a). Now arch the spine and pull in your abdomen as far as you can and hold this position for a few seconds (b). Repeat the exercise 4–5 times.

Areas Stretched: Low back muscles and ligaments.

Areas Strengthened: Abdominal and gluteal muscles.

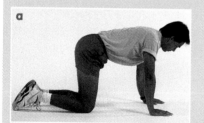

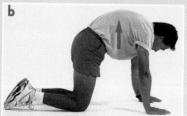

45

Abdominal Crunch or Bent-Leg Curl-Up

(see Exercise 4 in Appendix B)

It is important that you do not stabilize your feet when performing either of these exercises, because doing so decreases the work of the abdominal muscles. Also, remember not to "swing up" but rather to curl up as you perform these exercises.

Caloric, Protein, Fat, Saturated Fat, Cholesterol, and Carbohydrate Content of Selected Foods*

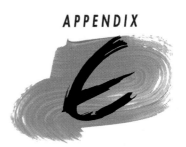

Code	Food	Amount	Weight gm	Calories	Protein gm	Fat gm	Sat. Fat gm	Cholesterol mg	Carbohydrate gm
1.	Almond Joy, candy bar	1.5 oz.	42	227	2.5	12	10.2	0	28
2.	Almonds, shelled	1/4 c	36	213	6.6	19	1.4	0	9
3.	Apple, raw, unpared	1 med	150	80	0.3	1	0.0	0	20
4.	Apple juice, canned or bottled	1/2 c	124	59	0.1	0	0.0	0	15
5.	Apple Pie, McDonald's	1	307	260	2	15	10.0	6	30
6.	Applesauce, canned, sweetened	1/2 c	128	116	0.3	0	0.0	0	31
7.	Apricots, canned, heavy syrup	3 halves; 1¾ tbsp. liq.	85	73	0.5	0	0.0	0	19
8.	Apricots, dried, sulfured, uncooked	10 med halves	35	91	1.8	0	0.0	0	23
9.	Apricots, raw	3 (12 per lb)	114	55	1.1	0	0.0	0	14
10.	Arby Q, Arby's	1	190	389	18	15	5.5	29	48
11.	Arby Sauce, Arby's	.5 oz.	14	15	0	0	0.0	0	3
12.	Asparagus, cooked green spears	4 med	60	12	1.3	0	0.0	0	2
13.	Avocado, raw	1/2 med	120	185	2.4	19	3.2	0	7
14.	Bacon, cooked, drained	2 slices	15	86	3.8	8	2.7	30	1
15.	Bacon, lettuce, tomato sandwich	1	130	327	11.6	19	4.7	21	31
16.	Bagel	1 3½ in.	68	180	7.0	1	0.2	0	35
17.	Banana, raw	1 sm (7¼")	140	81	1.0	0	0.0	0	21
18.	Banana, nut bread	1 slice	50	169	3.0	8	1.5	33	22
19.	BBQ Sauce, McDonald's	1.12 oz.	32	50	0	0.6	0.2	0	12
20.	Beans, green snap, cooked	1/2 c	65	16	1.0	0	0.0	0	3
21.	Beans, lentils	1/4 c	50	53	3.9	0	0.0	0	10
22.	Beans, lima (Fordhook), froz., cooked	1/2 c	85	84	6.0	0	0.0	0	17
23.	Beans, red kidney, cooked	1 c	185	218	14.4	1	0.0	0	40
24.	Beans, refried	1/2 c	145	148	9.0	1	0.2	0	25
25.	Bean sprouts, mung, raw	1/2 c	52	18	2.0	0	0.0	0	4
26.	Beef, chuck, cooked,	3 oz.	85	212	25.0	12	7.8	80	0
27.	Beef, corned, canned	3 oz.	85	163	21.0	10	8.0	70	0
28.	Beef, ground, lean	3 oz.	85	186	23.3	10	5.0	81	0
29.	Beef, lite roast deluxe, Arby's	1	182	294	18	10	3.5	42	33
30.	Beef, meatloaf	1 piece	111	246	20.0	15	6.1	125	6
491.	Beef, meatloaf, traditional Healthy Choice	1	340	320	16.0	8	4.0	35	46
31.	Beef N' Cheddar, Arby's	1	194	508	25	27	7.7	52	43
32.	Beef, round steak, cooked, trimmed	3 oz.	85	222	24.3	13	6.0	77	0
33.	Beef, rump roast	3 oz.	85	177	24.7	9	4.0	80	0
34.	Beef, sirloin, cooked	3 oz.	85	329	19.6	27	13.0	77	0
493.	Beef, sirloin tips, Healthy Choice	1	334	280	23.0	8	0.0	65	30
500.	Beef stroganoff, Weight Watchers	1	238	290	22.0	9	4.0	25	26
35.	Beef, T-bone steak	3 oz.	85	403	16.7	37	15.6	66	0
36.	Beef, thin, sliced	3 oz.	85	105	18.5	3	1.4	36	0
37.	Beer	12 fl. oz.	360	151	1.1	0	1.1	0	14
38.	Beer, light	12 fl. oz.	354	96	0.7	0	0.0	0	4
39.	Beets, red, canned, drained	1/2 c	80	32	0.8	0	0.0	0	8
40.	Beet greens, cooked	1/2 c	73	13	1.3	0	0.0	0	2
41.	Biscuits, baking powder	1 med	35	114	2.5	6	1.1	0	18
42.	Blueberries, fresh cultivated	1/2 c	73	45	0.5	0	0.0	0	11

From *Lifetime Physical Fitness & Wellness: A Personalized Program*, by W. W. K. Hoeger, Morton Publishing Company, 1998.

Code	Food	Amount	Weight gm	Calo- ries	Pro- tein gm	Fat gm	Sat. Fat gm	Cho- les- terol mg	Car- bohy- drate gm
43.	Bologna	1 slice (1 oz.)	28	86	3.4	8	3.0	15	0
44.	Bologna, turkey	2 slices	57	113	7.8	9	3.0	56	1
45.	Bouillon, broth	1 cube	4	5	0.8	0	0.0	0	0
46.	Brandy	1 oz.	28	69	0.0	0	0.0	0	11
47.	Bread, corn	1 slice	78	161	5.8	6	0.1	0	23
48.	Bread, cracked wheat	1 slice	25	65	2.3	1	0.2	0	12
49.	Bread, French enriched	1 slice	35	102	3.2	1	0.2	0	19
50.	Bread, oatmeal	1 slice	25	65	2.1	1	0.2	0	12
51.	Bread, pita pocket	1 piece	60	165	6.2	1	0.1	0	33
52.	Bread, pumpernickel	1 slice	32	80	2.9	1	0.2	0	15
53.	Bread, rye (American)	1 slice	25	61	2.3	0	0.0	0	13
54.	Bread, white enriched	1 slice	25	68	2.2	1	0.2	0	13
55.	Bread, whole wheat	1 slice	25	61	2.6	1	0.6	0	12
56.	Broccoli, cooked drained	1 sm stalk	140	36	4.3	0	0.0	0	6
57.	Broccoli, raw	1 sm stalk	114	38	4.1	0	0.0	0	7
58.	Brownies, with nuts	1	20	95	1.3	6	2.3	18	11
59.	Brussels sprouts, frozen, cooked, drained	1/2 c	78	28	3.2	0	0.0	0	5
60.	Bulgur, wheat	1 c	135	227	8.4	1	0.0	0	47
61.	Burrito, bean	1	166	307	12.5	9.5	3.6	14	45
62.	Burrito, combination, Taco Bell	1	175	404	21.0	16	0.0	0	43
482.	Burrito, 7 layer, Taco Bell	1	234	458	14.0	20	5.9	17	55
483.	Burrito, 7 layer light, Taco Bell	1	276	440	19.0	9	3.5	8	67
63.	Butter	1 tsp	5	36	0.0	4	0.4	12	0
64.	Buttermilk, cultured	1 c	245	88	8.8	0	1.3	5	12
65.	Cabbage, boiled, drained wedge	1/2 c	85	16	0.9	0	0.0	0	3
66.	Cabbage, raw chopped	1/2 c	45	11	0.6	0	0.0	0	3
67.	Cake, angel food, plain	1 piece	60	161	4.3	0	0.0	0	36
68.	Cake, carrot	1 piece	96	385	4.2	21	4.1	74	48
69.	Cake, cheesecake	1 piece (3½")	85	257	4.6	16	9.0	150	24
70.	Cake, chocolate, w/icing	1 piece	69	235	3.0	8	3.6	37	40
71.	Cake, coffee	1 piece	72	230	4.5	7	2.5	47	38
72.	Cake, devil's food, iced	1 piece	99	365	4.5	16	5.0	68	55
73.	Cake, pound	1 piece	30	120	2.0	5	1.0	32	15
74.	Cake, white, choc. icing	1 piece	71	268	3.5	11	3.7	2	48
75.	Candy, hard	1 oz.	28	109	0.0	0	0.0	0	28
76.	Cantaloupe	1/4 melon 5" diam.	239	35	2.0	0	0.0	0	10
77.	Caramel (candy, plain or choc.)	1 oz.	28	113	1.1	3	1.6	0	22
78.	Carrots, cooked, drained	1/2 c	73	23	0.7	0	0.0	0	5
79.	Carrots, raw	1 carrot 7½" long	81	30	0.8	0	0.0	0	7
80.	Cashew, roasted, unsalted	2 oz.	57	326	9.2	27	5.4	0	16
81.	Cauliflower, cooked, drained	1/2 c	63	14	1.5	0	0.0	0	3
82.	Celery, green, raw, long	1 outer stalk 8"	40	7	0.4	0	0.0	0	2
83.	Cereal, All-Bran	1/4 c	21	53	3.0	0	0.1	0	16
84.	Cereal, Alpha Bits	1 c	28	111	2.2	1	0.0	0	25
85.	Cereal, Bran	1/2 c	30	72	3.8	1	0.0	0	22
86.	Cereal, Cheerios	1 c	23	89	3.4	1	1.2	0	16
87.	Cereal, Corn Chex	1 c	28	111	2.0	0	0.1	0	25
88.	Cereal, Corn Flakes	1 c	25	97	2.0	0	0.0	0	21
89.	Cereal, Cream of Wheat	1 c	244	140	3.6	1	0.1	0	29
90.	Cereal, Frosted Mini-Wheats	4 biscuits	31	111	3.2	0	0.0	0	26
91.	Cereal, Fruit & Fibre w/dates	1 c	56	180	6.0	2	0.3	0	42
92.	Cereal, Granola, Nature Valley	1/2 c	57	252	5.8	10	7.0	0	38
93.	Cereal, Grape Nuts	1/2 c	57	202	6.6	0	0.0	0	47
94.	Cereal, Life	1 c	44	162	8.1	1	0.1	0	32
95.	Cereal, Nutri-Grain Wheat	1 c	44	158	3.8	1	0.1	0	37
96.	Cereal, Oatmeal, quick, cooked	1/2 c	120	66	2.4	1	0.2	0	12
97.	Cereal, Raisin Bran	1 c	49	160	4.0	1	0.2	0	40
98.	Cereal, Rice Krispies	3/4 c	22	85	1.4	0	0.0	0	19
99.	Cereal, Shredded Wheat	1 c	19	65	2.1	0	0.0	0	11
100.	Cereal, Special K	1 c	21	83	4.2	0	0.0	0	16

Code	Food	Amount	Weight gm	Calories	Protein gm	Fat gm	Sat. Fat gm	Cholesterol mg	Carbohydrate gm
101.	Cereal, Sugar Corn Pops	1 c	28	108	1.4	0	0.0	0	26
102.	Cereal, Sugar Frosted Flakes	1 c	35	133	1.8	0	0.0	0	32
103.	Cereal, Sugar Smacks	1 c	37	141	2.7	1	0.1	0	32
104.	Cereal, Total	1 c	33	116	3.3	1	0.1	0	26
105.	Cereal, Wheat Chex	1 c	46	169	4.5	1	0.2	0	38
106.	Cereal, whole wheat, cooked	1/2 c	123	55	2.2	0	0.0	0	12
107.	Cereal, whole wheat flakes, ready-to-eat	1 c	30	106	3.1	1	0.0	0	24
108.	Cereal, 40% Bran Flakes	1 c	39	125	4.9	1	0.1	0	31
109.	Cereal, 100% Bran	1/2 c	33	89	4.2	2	0.3	0	24
110.	Champagne	4 oz.	113	87	0.2	0	0.1	0	2
111.	Cheese, American	1 oz. slice	28	100	6.0	8	5.6	27	0
112.	Cheese, bleu	1 oz.	28	100	6.0	8	5.3	25	1
113.	Cheese, cheddar	1 oz.	28	114	7.0	9	6.0	30	0
114.	Cheese, cottage, 2%	1/2 c	113	103	15.5	2	1.4	10	4
115.	Cheese, cottage, creamed	1/2 c	105	112	14.0	5	6.4	15	3
116.	Cheese, creamed	1 oz.	28	99	6.0	8	3.0	31	1
117.	Cheese, feta	1 oz.	28	75	4.5	6	4.2	25	1
118.	Cheese, monterey jack	1 oz.	28	106	6.9	9	5.4	26	0
119.	Cheese, mozzarella, skim	1 oz.	28	80	7.6	5	3.1	15	1
120.	Cheese, parmesan	1 tbsp	5	23	2.1	2	1.0	4	0
121.	Cheese, ricotta, part skim	1 oz.	28	39	3.2	2	1.4	9	1
122.	Cheese, souffle	1 portion	110	240	10.9	19	9.5	189	7
123.	Cheese, swiss	1 oz.	28	107	8.0	8	5.0	26	1
124.	Cheese puffs, Cheetos	1 oz.	28	158	2.2	10	4.8	5	14
125.	Cheeseburger, McDonald's	1	115	321	15.2	16	6.7	40	29
126.	Cherries	10	75	47	0.9	0	0.0	0	12
127.	Chicken, BK Broiler sandwich, Burger King	1 sandwich	168	379	24.0	18	3.0	53	31
128.	Chicken Breast Filet, Arby's	1	204	445	22	23.0	3.0	45	52
129.	Chicken breast, roast w/skin	1	98	193	29.2	8	2.1	83	0
501.	Chicken burrito w/vegetables Weight Watchers	1	216	330	15.0	14	4.0	65	36
484.	Chicken cacciatore, Budget Gourmet	1	312	300	20.0	13	0.0	60	27
496.	Chicken cacciatore, Lean Cuisine	1	308	280	22.0	7	2.0	45	31
130.	Chicken chow mein	1 c	250	255	31.0	11	3.6	75	10
488.	Chicken chow mein, Healthy Choice	1	241	220	18.0	3	0.8	45	31
497.	Chicken chow mein, Lean Cuisine	1	255	240	14.0	5	1.0	30	34
502.	Chicken chow mein Weight Watchers	1	255	200	12.0	2	0.5	25	34
131.	Chicken club sandwich, Wendy's	1	220	520	30	25	6.0	75	44
132.	Chicken Cordon Bleu, Arby's	1	225	518	30	27	5.3	92	52
133.	Chicken, drumstick, Kentucky Fried	1	54	136	14.0	8	2.2	73	2
134.	Chicken, drumstick, roasted	1	52	112	14.1	6	1.6	48	0
135.	Chicken McNuggets	6	111	329	19.5	21	5.2	64	15
136.	Chicken Nuggets, Wendy's	6 pc.	94	280	14	20	5.0	50	12
137.	Chicken, patty sandwich	1	157	436	24.8	23	6.1	68	34
138.	Chicken, wing, Kentucky Fried	1	45	151	11.0	10	2.9	70	4
139.	Chicken, roast, light meat without skin	3 oz.	85	141	27.0	3	0.4	45	0
140.	Chicken, roast, dark meat without skin	3 oz.	85	149	24.0	5	0.8	50	0
141.	Chicken, Roast Deluxe, Arby's	1	195	276	24	7	1.7	33	33
510.	Chicken, Rotisserie, dark w/skin Kentucky Fried	1/4 chicken	146	333	30.0	24	6.6	163	1
511.	Chicken, Rotisserie, light w/skin Kentucky Fried	1/4 chicken	176	335	40.0	19	5.4	157	1

Code	Food	Amount	Weight gm	Calo-ries	Pro-tein gm	Fat gm	Sat. Fat gm	Cho-les-terol mg	Car-bohy-drate gm
142.	Chicken Sandwich, breaded Wendy's	1	208	450	26	20	4.0	60	44
143.	Chicken Sandwich, Grilled, Wendy's	1	177	290	24	7	1.0	60	35
144.	Chicken Sandwich, McChicken	1	187	415	19	19	9.0	50	39
485.	Chicken, Teriyaki, Budget Gourmet	1	340	360	20.0	12	0.0	55	44
145.	Chili con carne	1 c	255	339	19.1	16	5.8	28	31
146.	Chocolate fudge	1 oz.	28	115	0.6	3	2.1	1	21
147.	Chocolate, milk	1 oz.	28	147	2.0	9	3.6	5	16
148.	Chocolate, milk w/almonds	1 oz.	28	150	2.9	10	4.4	5	15
149.	Clam, canned, drained	3 oz.	85	83	13.0	2	0.2	50	2
150.	Cocoa, hot, with whole milk	1 c	250	218	9.1	9	6.1	33	26
151.	Cocoa, plain, dry	1 tbsp	5	14	0.9	1	0.0	0	3
152.	Coconut, shredded, packed	1/2 c	65	225	2.3	23	20.0	0	6
153.	Cod, batter fried	3.5 oz.	100	199	19.6	10	3.9	55	8
154.	Cod, cooked	3 oz.	85	144	24.3	4	1.5	60	0
155.	Cod, poached	3.5 oz.	100	94	20.9	1	0.3	60	0
156.	Coffee	3/4 cup	180	1	0.0	0	0.0	0	0
157.	Coleslaw	1 c	120	173	1.6	17	1.0	5	6
158.	Collards, leaves without stems, cooked, drained	1/2 c	95	32	3.4	1	2.0	0	5
159.	Cookies, chocolate chip, homemade	2 2¼" diam.	20	103	1.0	6	1.7	14	12
160.	Cookies, fig bars	4 bars	56	210	2.0	4	1.0	27	42
161.	Cookies, oatmeal raisin	2 2" diam.	26	122	1.5	5	1.3	1	18
162.	Cookies, peanut butter, homemade	2 cookies	24	123	2.0	7	2.0	11	14
163.	Cookies, sandwich, all	4 cookies	40	195	2.0	8	2.0	0	29
164.	Cookies, shortbread	4 cookies	32	155	2.0	8	2.9	27	20
165.	Cookies, vanilla	5 1¾" diam.	20	93	1.0	3	0.8	10	15
166.	Cookies, vanilla wafers	10 wafers	40	185	2.0	7	1.8	25	29
167.	Corn, boiled on cob	1 ear 5" long	140	70	2.5	1	0.0	0	16
168.	Corn, canned, drained	1/2 c	83	70	2.2	1	0.0	0	16
169.	Corn chips	1 oz.	28	155	2.0	9	1.8	0	16
170.	Cornmeal, degermed, yellow, enriched, cooked	1/2 c	120	60	1.3	0	0.0	0	13
171.	Crab, canned	1 c	135	135	23.0	3	0.5	135	1
172.	Crackers, cheese	10 crackers	10	50	1.0	3	0.9	6	5
173.	Crackers, graham	2 squares	14	55	1.1	1	0.3	0	10
174.	Crackers, Ritz	1 cracker	3	15	0.2	1	0.2	0	2
175.	Crackers, Ryewafers, whole grain	2 crackers	14	55	1.0	1	0.3	0	10
176.	Crackers, saltines	4 squares	11	48	1.0	1	0.3	0	8
177.	Crackers, soda	1	3	13	0.3	0	0.1	0	2
178.	Crackers, Triscuits	1	5	23	0.4	1	0.3	0	3
179.	Crackers, Wheat Thins	1	2	9	0.2	0	0.1	0	1
180.	Cranberry juice	1 c	253	145	0.1	0	0.0	0	36
181.	Cream, light coffee or table	1 tbsp	15	20	0.5	2	0.5	5	1
182.	Cream, heavy whipping	1 tbsp	15	53	0.3	6	1.3	12	1
183.	Croissant	1	57	235	4.7	12	4.0	13	27
184.	Croissants (Sara Lee)	1 roll	18	59	1.6	2	0.3	0	8
185.	Croissan'wich, egg, cheese Burger King	1 sandwich	110	315	13.0	20	7.0	222	19
186.	Cucumbers, raw pared	9 sm slices	28	4	0.3	0	0.0	0	1
187.	Danish, Apple, McDonald's	1	115	390	6	17	11.0	25	51
188.	Danish, Cinnamon Raisin	1	110	440	6	21	13.0	34	58
189.	Dates hydrated	5	46	110	0.9	0	0.0	0	29
190.	Doughnut, plain	1	42	164	1.9	8	2.0	19	22
191.	Doughnut, yeast raised	1	27	235	4.0	13	5.2	21	26
192.	Dressing, Bleu cheese	1 tbsp	15	77	0.7	8	1.9	4	1
193.	Dressing, French	1 tbsp	16	83	0.1	9	1.4	0	1

Code	Food	Amount	Weight gm	Calo- ries	Pro- tein gm	Fat gm	Sat. Fat gm	Cho- les- terol mg	Car- bohy- drate gm
194.	Dressing, French, low cal	1 tbsp.	15	24	0.0	2	0.2	0	2
195.	Dressing, Italian	1 tbsp.	15	69	0.1	9	1.3	0	2
196.	Dressing, Italian, low cal	1 tbsp.	15	10	0.0	1	0.0	0	1
197.	Dressing, Ranch style	1 tbsp.	15	54	0.4	6	0.9	6	1
198.	Dressing, Thousand island	1 tbsp.	15	60	0.2	6	1.0	4	2
199.	Dressing, Thousand island, low cal	1 tbsp.	15	25	0.1	2	0.2	2	3
200.	Egg, hard cooked	1 large	50	72	6.0	5	1.6	212	1
201.	Egg, fried with butter	1	46	95	5.4	7	2.4	240	1
202.	Egg McMuffin	1	138	327	18.5	15	5.9	259	31
203.	Egg salad sandwich	1	111	325	10.0	19	3.9	215	28
204.	Egg, scrambled, with milk, butter	1 egg	64	95	6.0	7	3.0	244	1
205.	Egg, white	1 large	33	17	3.6	0	0.0	0	0
206.	Egg, yolk, raw	1 yolk	17	63	2.8	5	1.6	212	0
207.	Enchilada, beef	1	200	487	21.8	23	8.8	63	26
208.	Enchilada, cheese	1	230	632	25.3	34	17.6	82	31
209.	Figs, dried	1 large	21	60	1.0	0	0.0	0	15
210.	Filet of Fish, McDonald's	1	131	402	15.0	23	7.9	43	34
489.	Fish, fillet, florentine, Healthy Choice	1	273	220	26.0	7	3.0	65	13
211.	Fish sandwich, Wendy's	1	182	460	16	25	5.0	55	42
494.	Fish, Sole Au Gratin, Healthy Choice	1	312	270	16.0	5	0.0	55	40
212.	Fish, sticks	2	56	140	12.0	6	1.6	52	8
213.	Flounder	3 oz.	85	171	25.5	7	1.0	60	0
214.	Flour, all purpose enriched	1 c	125	455	13.0	1	0.0	0	95
215.	Flour, whole wheat	1 c	120	400	16.0	2	0.0	0	85
216.	Frankfurter, cooked	1	57	176	7.0	16	5.6	45	1
217.	Frankfurter, turkey, cooked	1	45	102	6.4	8	2.7	39	1
218.	French Dip, Arby's	1	154	368	22	15	5.6	43	35
219.	French toast	1 piece	65	123	4.9	4	1.1	73	15
220.	Fries, Curly, Arby's	1 small	99	337	4	18	7.4	0	43
221.	Fruit cocktail	1 c	245	91	1.0	0	0.0	0	24
222.	Fruit cocktail, juice pack	1 c	248	115	1.1	0	0.0	0	29
223.	Grapefruit, raw white	1/2 med	301	56	1.0	0	0.0	0	15
224.	Grapefruit juice, unsweet. canned	1/2 c	124	50	0.6	0	0.0	0	12
225.	Grapes, seedless, European	10 grapes	50	34	0.3	0	0.0	0	9
226.	Grape juice, unsweetened bottled	1/2 c	127	84	0.3	0	0.0	0	21
227.	Gravy, beef, homemade	1 tbsp	17	19	0.3	2	1.0	1	1
228.	Haddock, fried (dipped in egg, milk, bread crumbs)	3 oz.	85	141	17.0	5	1.0	54	5
229.	Halibut, broiled with butter or margarine	3 oz.	85	144	21.0	6	2.1	55	0
230.	Ham (cured pork)	3 oz.	85	318	20.0	26	9.4	77	0
231.	Ham, lunch meat	1 slice	28	37	5.5	1	0.5	13	.3
508.	Hamburger, Arch Deluxe, McDonalds	1	242	560	27.0	32	11.0	90	42
509.	Hamburger, Arch Deluxe w/bacon, McDonalds	1	253	610	31.0	36	13.0	105	42
232.	Hamburger, Big Classic, Wendy's	1	251	480	27	23	7.0	75	44
233.	Hamburger, Big Mac	1	204	581	25.1	36	12.0	85	40
234.	Hamburger bun	1 bun	40	129	3.7	2	1.0	0	23
235.	Hamburger, Jr. Bacon Cheeseburger, Wendy's	1	170	440	22	25	8.0	65	33
236.	Hamburger, McDonald's	1	99	257	13.0	9	3.7	26	30
237.	Hamburger, McLean Deluxe	1	206	320	22	10	5.0	60	35
238.	Hamburger, McLean Deluxe, w/cheese	1	219	370	24	14	8.0	75	35
239.	Hamburger, Quarter pounder	1 burger	160	427	24.6	24	9.1	80	29
240.	Hamburger, Quarter pounder, with cheese	1 burger	186	525	29.6	32	12.8	107	31

Code	Food	Amount	Weight gm	Calories	Protein gm	Fat gm	Sat. Fat gm	Cholesterol mg	Carbohydrate gm
241.	Hamburger, Wendy's	1	219	440	26	23	7.0	75	36
242.	Ham N' Cheese, Arby's	1	169	355	25	14	5.1	55	35
243.	Honey	1 tbsp	21	64	0.0	0	0.0	0	17
244.	Honeydew melon	1 slice (1/10 melon)	129	45	0.6	0	0.0	0	12
245.	Horsey Sauce, Arby's	.5 oz.	14	55	0	5	2.0	0	3
246.	Hotcakes w/Margarine & Syrup, McDonald's	1 serving	174	440	8	12	5.0	8	74
247.	Hotdog bun	1 bun	40	115	3.3	2	1.0	0	20
248.	Ice cream, vanilla	1/2 c	67	135	3.0	7	4.4	27	14
249.	Ice cream cone	1 small	115	185	4.3	5	2.2	24	30
250.	Ice cream cone, Dairy Queen	medium	142	230	6.0	7	4.6	15	35
251.	Ice cream, hot fudge sundae	1	164	357	7.0	11	5.4	27	58
252.	Ice milk, vanilla	1/2 c	61	100	3.0	3	1.8	13	15
253.	Instant breakfast, whole milk	1 c	281	280	15.0	8	5.1	33	34
254.	Instant breakfast, skim milk	1 c	282	216	15.4	0	0.0	4	35
255.	Jams or preserves	1 tbsp	7	18	0.0	0	0.0	0	5
256.	Jelly	1 tbsp	18	49	0.0	0	0.0	0	13
257.	Kale, fresh cooked, drained	1/2 c	55	22	2.5	0	0.0	0	3
258.	Kiwi fruit, raw	1 med	76	46	1.0	0	0.0	0	11
259.	Kool Aid, with sugar	1 c	240	100	0.0	0	0.0	0	25
260.	Lamb leg, roast, trimmed	3 oz.	85	237	22.0	16	7.3	60	0
261.	Lamb loin chop, broiled, lean	3 oz.	84	183	25.0	8	3.4	78	0
490.	Lasagna, Healthy Choice	1	284	260	18.0	5	0.0	20	37
262.	Lasagna, homemade	1 piece	220	357	23.6	18	8.3	50	27
498.	Lasagna, Lean Cuisine	1	291	260	19.0	5	2.0	25	34
263.	Lemon juice, fresh	1 tbsp	15	4	0.1	0	0.0	0	1
264.	Lemonade (concentrate)	12 oz.	340	137	0.2	0	0.1	0	36
265.	Lentils, cooked	1/2 c	100	106	8.0	0	0.0	0	19
266.	Lettuce, crisp head	1 c sm chunks	75	10	0.7	0	0.0	0	2
267.	Lettuce, cos or romaine	1 c chopped	55	10	0.7	0	0.0	0	2
268.	Liver, beef, fried	1 slice 3 oz.	85	195	22.0	9	2.5	345	5
269.	Liverwurst, fresh	1 slice 1 oz.	28	87	5.0	7	3.5	50	1
270.	Lobster	1 c	145	138	27.0	2	1.0	293	0
271.	M&M's, chocolate, plain	1 oz.	28	140	1.9	6	3.3	0	19
272.	M&M's, chocolate, w/peanuts	1 oz.	28	145	3.2	7	3.2	0	17
273.	Macaroni, enriched, cooked	1/2 c	70	78	2.4	0	0.0	0	16
274.	Macaroni and cheese	1/2 c	100	215	8.2	11	4.0	21	20
275.	Margarine	1 tsp	5	34	0.0	4	0.7	2	0
276.	Mars bar	1 bar	50	240	4.0	11	4.8	0	30
277.	Matzo	1 piece	30	117	3.0	0	0.0	0	2
278.	Mayonnaise	1 tsp	5	36	0.0	4	0.7	3	0
513.	Mayonnaise, light	1 tsp.	5	17	0.0	2	0.3	2	1
507.	Milk, 1% fat	1 c	244	102	8.0	3	1.6	10	12
279.	Milk, chocolate, 2%	1 c	250	180	8.0	5	3.1	17	26
280.	Milk, evaporated whole	1/2 c	126	172	9.0	10	5.8	40	13
281.	Milk, lowfat 2% fat	1 c	244	121	8.0	5	2.9	18	12
282.	Milk shake, chocolate	1 (10 fluid oz.)	340	433	11.5	13	7.8	45	70
283.	Milk shake, Frosty, Wendy's	16 oz.	324	460	13	13	7.0	55	76
284.	Milk shake, strawberry	1 (10 fluid oz.)	340	383	11.4	10	6.0	37	64
285.	Milk shake, vanilla, McDonald's	1	289	323	10	8	5.1	29	52
286.	Milk, skim	1 c	245	85	8.0	1	0.3	4	12
287.	Milk, whole 3.5% fat	1 c	244	149	8.0	8	5.1	33	11
288.	Milky Way bar	1 bar	60	260	3.2	9	5.4	14	43
289.	Molasses, medium	1 tbsp	20	50	0.0	0	0.0	0	13
290.	Muffin, apple bran, fat free, McDonald's	1	75	180	5	0	0.0	0	40
291.	Muffin, blueberry	1	45	135	3.0	5	1.5	19	20
292.	Muffin, bran	1	45	125	3.0	6	1.4	24	19
293.	Muffin, cornmeal	1	45	145	3.0	5	1.5	23	21
294.	Muffin, English, plain	1	57	140	4.5	1	0.3	0	26
295.	Muffin, English w/butter	1	63	186	5.0	5	2.3	15	30

Code	Food	Amount	Weight gm	Calo- ries	Pro- tein gm	Fat gm	Sat. Fat gm	Cho- les- terol mg	Car- bohy- drate gm
296.	Mushrooms, fresh cultivated	1/2 c sliced	35	12	1.0	0	0.0	0	2
297.	Mustard greens, cooked drained	1/2 c	70	16	1.7	0	0.0	0	3
298.	Noodles, egg, enriched cooked	1/2 c	80	100	3.3	1	0.0	0	19
299.	Nuts, brazil	1 oz. (6-8 nuts)	28	185	4.1	19	4.8	0	3
300.	Nuts, pecans	1 oz.	28	195	2.6	20	1.4	0	4
301.	Nuts, walnuts	1 oz. (14 halves)	28	185	4.2	18	1.0	0	5
302.	Oil, corn	1 tbsp.	15	125	0.0	14	1.8	0	0
303.	Oil, olive	1 tbsp.	15	125	0.0	14	1.9	0	0
304.	Oil, safflower	1 tbsp.	15	125	0.0	14	1.3	0	0
305.	Oil, soybean	1 tsp.	5	44	0.0	5	2.0	0	0
306.	Okra, cooked, drained	1/2 c	80	23	1.6	0	0.0	0	5
307.	Olives, black, ripe	10 extra large	55	61	0.5	7	1.0	0	1
308.	Onions, mature,	1/2 c sliced	105	31	1.3	0	0.0	0	7
309.	cooked, drained								
310.	Onion rings, fried	3	30	122	1.6	8	2.3	0	11
311.	Onion rings (Brazier) Dairy Queen	1 serving	85	360	6.0	17	6.0	15	33
312.	Orange juice, froz., reconstituted	1/2 c	125	61	0.9	0	0.0	0	15
313.	Orange, raw (medium skin),	1 med	180	64	1.3	0	0.0	0	16
314.	Oysters, Eastern, breaded, fried	1 oyster	45	90	5.0	5	1.4	35	5
315.	Oysters, raw, Eastern	1/2 c (6-9 med)	120	79	10.0	2	1.3	60	4
316.	Pancakes	1 6" diam x 1/2" thick	73	169	5.2	5	1.0	36	25
317.	Pancakes, buckwheat	1 4 in. diam.	27	55	2.0	2	0.9	20	6
318.	Pancakes w/butter, syrup	1 large	100	250	4.0	5	1.9	24	47
319.	Papaya, raw	1/2 med	227	60	0.9	0	0.0	0	15
320.	Parsnips, cooked	1 large 9" long	160	106	2.4	1	0.0	0	24
503.	Pasta primavera, Weight Watchers	1	238	260	15.0	11	0.8	5	22
321.	Peaches, canned, heavy syrup	1 half 2⅛ tbsp liq.	96	75	0.4	0	0.0	0	19
322.	Peaches, canned, juice pack	1 half	77	34	0.5	0	0.0	0	9
323.	Peaches, raw, peeled	1 2¾" diam.	175	58	0.9	0	0.0	0	15
324.	Peanut butter	2 tbsp	32	188	8.0	16	1.0	0	6
325.	Peanut butter, jam sandwich	1	100	340	11.4	14	2.6	0	45
326.	Peanuts, roasted	1 oz.	28	166	7.0	14	1.0	0	5
327.	Pears, canned, heavy syrup	1 half 2¼ tbsp liq.	103	78	0.2	0	0.0	0	20
328.	Pears, canned, juice pack	1 half	77	38	0.3	0	0.0	0	10
329.	Pears, raw	1 pear	180	100	1.1	1	0.0	0	25
330.	Peas, canned, drained	1/2 c	85	75	4.0	0	0.0	0	14
331.	Peas, frozen, cooked drained	1/2 c	80	55	4.1	0	0.0	0	10
332.	Peppers, sweet, raw	1 pepper 3¼" x 3" diam.	200	36	2.0	0	0.0	0	8
333.	Pickles, dill	1 large 4" long	135	15	0.9	0	0.0	0	3
334.	Pickles, sweet	1 large 3" long	35	51	0.2	0	0.0	0	13
335.	Pie, Apple	1 piece (3½")	118	302	2.6	13	3.5	120	45
336.	Pie, Apple, fried	1 pie	85	255	2.2	14	5.8	14	32
337.	Pie, Blueberry	1 piece (3½")	158	380	4.0	17	4.0	0	55
338.	Pie, Cherry	1 piece (3½")	118	308	3.1	13	5.0	137	45
339.	Pie, Cherry, fried	1 pie	85	250	2.0	14	5.8	13	32
340.	Pie, Chocolate cream	1 piece (1/6 pie)	175	311	7.4	13	4.5	15	42
341.	Pie, Lemon meringue	1 piece (1/6 pie)	140	355	4.7	14	3.5	137	53
342.	Pie, Pecan	1 piece (1/6 pie)	138	583	6.3	24	3.9	13	92
343.	Pie, Pumpkin	1 (3½")	114	241	4.6	13	3.0	70	28
344.	Pineapple, canned, heavy syrup	1/2 c	128	95	0.4	0	0.0	0	25
345.	Pineapple, canned, juice pack	1/2 c	125	75	0.5	0	0.0	0	20
346.	Pineapple, raw	1/2 c diced	78	41	0.3	0	0.0	0	11
347.	Pizza, cheese, thin 'n crispy, Pizza Hut	1/2 10" pie	*	450	25.0	15	7.0	125	54
348.	Pizza, Cheese, Thick 'n Chewy, Pizza Hut	1/2 10" pie	*	560	34.0	14	6.0	110	71
504.	Pizza, Cheese, Weight Watchers	1	164	300	22.0	7	3.0	35	37

Code	Food	Amount	Weight gm	Calo- ries	Pro- tein gm	Fat gm	Sat. Fat gm	Cho- les- terol mg	Car- bohy- drate gm
505.	Pizza, deluxe comb. Weight Watchers	1	200	330	26.0	10	3.0	25	35
506.	Pizza, Pepperoni, Weight Watchers	1	171	320	26.0	10	3.0	35	31
480.	Pizza, pepperoni, pan, Pizza Hut	2 pieces	211	540	29.0	22	9.2	42	62
481.	Pizza, supreme, pan, Pizza Hut	2 pieces	255	589	32.0	30	13.8	48	53
349.	Plums, Japanese and hybrid, raw	1 plum 2⅛" diam.	70	32	0.3	0	0.0	0	8
350.	Popcorn, cooked, oil	1 c	11	55	0.9	3	0.5	0	6
351.	Popcorn, popped, plain, large kernel	1 c	6	12	0.8	0	0.0	0	5
352.	Pork, roast, trimmed	2 slices 3 oz.	85	179	24.0	8	2.2	65	0
353.	Pork, sausage, cooked	1 sm link	17	72	2.8	6	2.1	13	1
354.	Potato, au gratin	1 c	245	228	5.6	10	6.3	12	32
355.	Potato, baked in skin	1 potato 2⅓ x 4¼"	202	145	4.0	0	0.0	0	33
356.	Potato chips	10 chips	20	114	1.1	8	2.1	0	10
357.	Potato, French fried long	10 strips 3½-4"	78	214	3.4	10	1.7	0	28
358.	Potato, hashbrowns, McDonald's	1 patty	55	144	1.4	9	3.0	4	15
359.	Potato, mashed, milk added	1/2 c	105	69	2.2	1	0.4	8	14
360.	Potato salad w/eggs, mayo	1/2 c	125	179	3.4	10	7.8	85	14
361.	Potato, hash brown	1/2 c	78	170	2.5	9	3.5	0	22
362.	Pretzel, thin, twists	1 oz.	28	113	2.8	1	0.3	0	23
363.	Prunes, dried "softenized" without pits	5 prunes	61	137	1.1	0	0.0	0	36
364.	Prune juice, canned or bottled	1/2 c	128	99	0.5	0	0.0	0	24
365.	Pudding, chocolate, canned	5 oz.	142	205	3	11	9.5	1	30
366.	Pudding, tapioca, canned	5 oz.	142	160	3	5	4.8	1	28
367.	Pudding, vanilla, canned	5 oz.	142	220	2	10	9.5	1	33
368.	Quiche, Lorraine	1 piece	242	825	18	66	31.9	392	40
369.	Raisins, unbleached, seedless	1 oz.	28	82	0.7	0	0.0	0	22
370.	Raspberries, fresh	1 c	123	60	1.1	1	0.0	0	14
371.	Raspberries, frozen	1 c	250	255	1.7	1	0.0	0	62
495.	Ravioli, baked cheese, Lean Cuisine	1	241	240	13.0	8	3.0	55	30
372.	Rice, brown, cooked	1/2 c	96	116	2.5	1	0.0	0	25
373.	Rice, white enriched, cooked	1/2 c	103	113	2.1	0	0.0	0	25
374.	Rice, wild, cooked	1/2 c	100	92	3.6	0	0.0	0	19
375.	Roast beef sand., regular, Arby's	1	155	383	22	18	7.0	43	35
376.	Roast beef sub, Arby's	1	305	623	38	32	11.5	73	47
377.	Roll, hard, white	1 roll	50	155	5	2	0.0	0	30
378.	Reuben sandwich	1	237	488	28.7	28	10.4	85	30
379.	Salad, caesar side, Wendy's	1	130	160	10	6	1.0	10	18
380.	Salad, chef, Burger King	1 serving	273	178	17	9	4.0	103	7
381.	Salad, chef, McDonald's	1	265	170	17	9	4.0	111	8
382.	Salad, chicken, Burger King	1 serving	258	142	20	4	1.0	49	8
383.	Salad, chicken w/celery	1/2 c	78	266	10.5	25	4.1	48	1
384.	Salad, deluxe Garden, Wendy's	1	271	110	7	5	1.0	0	9
385.	Salad, garden, Arby's	1	330	117	7	5	2.7	12	11
386.	Salad, grilled Chicken, Wendy's	1	338	200	25	8	1.0	55	9
387.	Salad, tuna	1 c	205	375	33	19	3.3	80	19
388.	Salami, dry	1 oz.	28	128	7.0	11	1.6	24	0
389.	Salmon, broiled with butter or margarine	3 oz.	85	156	23.0	6	2.2	53	0
390.	Salmon, canned Chinook	3 oz.	85	179	16.6	12	0.8	30	0
514.	Salsa	1 tbsp.	15	5	0.0	0	0.0	0	1
391.	Sardines, canned drained	1 oz.	28	58	7.0	3	1.0	20	0
392.	Sauerkraut, canned	1/2 c	118	21	1.2	0	0.0	0	5
393.	Sausage biscuit w/egg, McDonald's	1	175	505	19	33	20.0	260	33
394.	Sausage McMuffin, McDonald's	1	135	345	15	20	11.0	57	27
395.	Sausage McMuffin, w/Egg	1	159	430	21	25	14.0	270	27
396.	Sausage, smoked link, pork	1	68	265	15	22	7.7	46	1

Code	Food	Amount	Weight gm	Calo- ries	Pro- tein gm	Fat gm	Sat. Fat gm	Cho- les- terol mg	Car- bohy- drate gm
397.	Scallops, breaded, cooked	6 pieces	90	195	15	10	2.5	70	10
398.	Sherbet	1/2 c	97	135	1.1	2	1.3	7	29
399.	Shrimp, boiled	3 oz.	85	99	18.0	1	0.1	128	1
400.	Shrimp, fried	7 medium	85	200	16.0	10	2.5	168	11
487.	Shrimp, linguini, Budget Gourmet	1	284	330	15.0	15	0.0	75	33
401.	Snickers bar	1 bar	61	290	6.6	4	5.4	0	37
402.	Soda pop, cola	12 oz.	369	144	0.0	0	0.0	0	37
403.	Soda pop, diet	12 oz.	340	2	0.1	0	0.0	0	0
404.	Soda pop, Ginger ale	12 oz.	366	113	0.0	0	0.0	0	29
405.	Soda pop, Lemon-lime	12 oz.	340	138	0.0	0	0.0	0	35
406.	Soda pop, Root beer	12 oz.	340	140	0.0	0	0.0	0	36
407.	Soup, chicken, cream	1 c	248	191	7.5	12	4.6	27	15
408.	Soup, chicken noodle	1 c	241	75	4.0	2	0.7	7	9
409.	Soup, clam chowder, Manhattan	1 c	244	78	4.2	2	0.4	2	12
410.	Soup, clam chowder, north east	1 c	248	163	9.5	7	3.0	22	16
411.	Soup, cream of mushroom condensed, prepared with equal volume of milk	1 c	245	216	7.0	14	5.4	15	16
412.	Soup, minestrone	1 c	241	80	4.3	3	0.5	2	11
413.	Soup, split pea, condensed, prepared with equal volume of water	1 c	245	145	9.0	3	1.1	0	21
414.	Soup, tomato, condensed, prepared with equal volume of water	1 c	245	88	2.0	3	0.5	0	16
415.	Soup, tomato with milk	1 c	248	160	6.0	6	2.9	17	22
416.	Soup, vegetable beef, condensed, prepared with equal volume of water	1 c	245	78	5.0	2	0.0	0	10
417.	Soup, Vegetarian vegetable	1 c	250	70	2.1	2	0.3	0	12
418.	Sour cream	1 tbsp	14	30	0.4	3	1.8	6	1
419.	Soup cream, imitation	1 tbsp.	14	29	0.3	3	2.5	0	1
492.	Spaghetti, Healthy Choice	1	284	280	14.0	6	0.0	20	42
420.	Spaghetti, in tomato sauce with cheese	1 c	250	260	8.8	9	2.0	10	37
421.	Spaghetti, plain, cooked	1 c	140	155	5.0	1	0.1	0	32
422.	Spaghetti, whole wheat, cooked	1 c	125	151	6.6	1	0.1	0	32
423.	Spaghetti, with meatballs and tomato sauce	1 c	248	332	18.6	11.7	3.0	75	39
499.	Spaghetti w/meatballs, Lean Cuisine	1	290	280	19.0	7	2.0	35	35
424.	Spareribs, cooked	3 oz.	85	377	17.8	33	12.0	73	0
425.	Spinach, canned, drained	1/2 c	103	25	2.3	1	0.0	0	4
426.	Spinach, frozen, cooked, drained	1/2 c	103	24	3.1	0	0.0	0	4
427.	Spinach, raw, chopped	1 c	55	14	1.8	0	0.0	0	2
428.	Squash, summer, cooked	1/2 c	90	13	0.8	0	0.0	0	3
429.	Squash, winter, baked mashed	1/2 c	103	70	1.9	0	0.0	0	18
430.	Strawberries, frozen, sweetened	1 c	250	245	1.4	0	0.0	0	66
431.	Strawberries, raw	1 c	149	55	1.0	1	0.0	0	13
432.	Stuffing, bread, prepared	1/2 c	70	250	4.6	15	3.1	0	25
433.	Sundae, chocolate, Dairy Queen	medium	184	300	6.0	7	4.9	79	53
434.	Sugar, brown granulated	1 tsp	5	17	0.0	0	0.0	0	5
435.	Sugar, white granulated	1 tsp	4	15	0.0	0	0.0	0	4
436.	Super roast beef, Arby's	1	254	552	24	28	7.6	43	54
437.	Sweet n' sour sauce, McDonald's	1.12 oz.	32	60	0	0.2	0.1	0	14
438.	Sweet potato, baked	1 potato 5" long	146	161	2.4	1	0.0	0	37
439.	Syrup (maple)	1 tbsp	20	50	0.0	0	0.0	0	13
440.	Taco salad, Wendy's	1	510	640	34	30	12.0	80	70
441.	Taco shell	1 shell	10	60	1.1	3	0.3	0	9

Code	Food	Amount	Weight gm	Calories	Protein gm	Fat gm	Sat. Fat gm	Cholesterol mg	Carbohydrate gm
512.	Taco, soft, Taco Bell	1	92	225	12.0	12	5.4	32	18
442.	Taco, Taco Bell	1	83	186	15.0	8	0.0	0	14
443.	Tangerine	1 med 2⅛" diam.	116	39	0.7	0	0.0	0	10
444.	Tartar sauce	1 tbsp.	14	74	0.2	8	1.2	4	1
445.	Tea, brewed	1/4 c	180	0	0.0	0	0.0	0	0
446.	Tomato juice, canned	1 c	244	42	1.9	0	0.1	0	10
447.	Tomato sauce (catsup)	1 tbsp	15	16	0.3	0	0.0	0	4
448.	Tomato, canned	1/2 c	121	26	1.2	0	0.0	0	5
449.	Tomato, raw	1 tomato 3½ oz.	100	20	1.0	0	0.0	0	4
450.	Tortilla chips	1 oz.	28	139	2.2	8	1.1	0	17
451.	Tortilla, corn, lime	1 6" diam.	30	63	1.5	1	0.0	0	14
452.	Tortilla, flour	1	35	105	2.6	3	0.4	0	19
453.	Tostada	1	148	206	9.2	18	3.0	14	25
454.	Trout, broiled w/butter, lemon	3 oz.	85	175	21.0	9	4.1	71	0
455.	Tuna, canned, oil pack, drained	3 oz.	85	167	25.0	7	1.7	60	0
456.	Tuna, canned, water pack, solids and liquid	3½ oz.	99	126	27.7	1	0.0	55	0
457.	Turkey, lite roast deluxe, Arby'	1	195	260	20	6	1.6	33	33
458.	Turkey, roast (light and dark mixed)	3 oz.	85	162	27.0	5	1.5	73	0
459.	Turnip, cooked, drained	1/2 c cubed	78	18	0.6	0	0.0	0	4
460.	Turnip greens, cooked drained	1/2 c	73	19	2.1	0	0.0	0	3
461.	Veal, cooked loin	3 oz.	85	199	22.0	11	4.0	90	0
462.	Veal cutlet, braised, broiled	3 oz.	85	185	23.0	9	4.0	109	0
486.	Veal parmigiana, Budget Gourmet	1	340	440	26.0	20	0.0	165	39
463.	Vegetables, mixed, cooked	1 c	182	116	5.8	0	0.0	0	24
464.	Waffles	1 waffle	75	205	6.9	8	2.7	59	27
465.	Watermelon	1 c diced	160	42	0.8	0	0.0	0	10
466.	Wheat germ, plain toasted	1 tbsp	6	23	1.8	1	0.0	0	3
467.	Whiskey, gin, rum, vodka 90 proof	1/2 11 oz (jigger)	42	110	0	0	0.0	0	0
468.	Whopper, Burger King	1 sandwich	270	614	27.0	36	12.0	90	45
469.	Whopper with cheese, Burger King	1 sandwich	294	706	32.0	44	16.0	115	47
470.	Whopper, double, Burger King	1 sandwich	351	844	46.0	53	19.0	169	45
471.	Wine, dry table 12% alc.	3½ fl. oz.	102	87	0.1	0	0.0	0	4
472.	Wine, red dry 18.8% alc.	2 oz.	59	81	0.1	0	0.0	0	5
473.	Yeast, brewers	1 tbsp	8	23	3.1	0	0.0	0	3
474.	Yogurt, fruit	1 c	227	231	9.9	2	1.6	10	43
475.	Yogurt, nonfat, TCBY	4 oz.	113	110	4	0	0	0	23
476.	Yogurt, plain low fat	1 8-oz. container	226	113	7.7	4	2.3	15	12
477.	Yogurt, regular, TCBY	4 oz.	113	120	4	3	2.0	13	23
478.	Yogurt, sugar free, TCBY	4 oz.	113	80	4	0	0	0	18
479.	Yogurt, vanilla lowfat, McDonald's	3 oz.	85	105	4	1	0.3	3	22

"0" represents both less than 1 and 0

Sources:

Nutritive Value of American Foods in Common Units. *Agriculture Handbook No. 456.* U.S. Dept. of Agriculture. Washington, D.C. 1988.

Young, E. A., E. H. Brennan, and C. L. Irving, Guest Eds. Perspectives on Fast Foods. *Public Health Currents,* 19(1), 1979, Published by Ross Laboratories, Columbus, OH.

Dennison, D. *The Dine System: the Nutrition Plan For Better Health.* C. V. Mosby Company St. Louis, Missouri, 1982.

Pennington, S. A. T. and H. N. Church. *Food Values of Portions Commonly Used.* Harper and Row Publishers, New York, 1985.

Kullman, D. A. *ABC Milligram Cholesterol Diet Guide.* Merit Publications, Inc. North Miami Beach, Florida 1978.

Food Processor nutrient analysis software by Esha Corporation, P.O. Box 13028, Salem, Oregon, 97309. With permission.

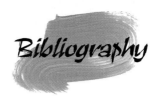

Bibliography

Allsen, P. E. *Strength Training: Beginners, Bodybuilders, and Athletes.* Dubuque, IA: Kendall/Hunt Publishing, 1996.

Allsen, P. E., J. M. Harrison, and B. Vance. *Fitness for Life: An Individualized Approach.* Madison, WI: Brown & Benchmark, 1997.

American College of Sports Medicine. *Guidelines for Exercise Testing and Prescription.* Baltimore: William & Wilkins, 1995.

American Diabetes Association and American Dietetic Association. *Exchange Lists for Meal Planning.* Chicago: American Dietetic Association and American Diabetes Association, 1995.

Bouchard, C., et al. *Physical Activity, Fitness, and Health.* Champaign, IL: Human Kinetics, 1994.

Brownell, K., and F. Kramer. "Behavioral Management of Obesity." *Medical Clinics of North America,* 73)1989), 185–202.

Byrne, K. *Understanding and Managing Cholesterol: A Guide for Wellness Professionals.* Champaign, IL: Human Kinetics Books, 1991.

Carroll, C. R. *Drugs in Modern Society.* Madison, WI: Brown & Benchmark, 1996.

Coleman, E. *Eating for Endurance.* Palo Alto, CA: Bull Publishing, 1997.

Fleck, S. J., and W. J. Kraemer. *Designing Resistance Training Programs.* Champaign, IL: Human Kinetics Publishers, 1997.

Goldberg, R. *Drugs Across the Spectrum.* Englewood, CO: Morton Publishing, 1997.

Greenberg, J. S. *Comprehensive Stress Management.* Madison, WI: Brown & Benchmark, 1996.

Hafen, B. Q., and W. W. K. Hoeger. *Wellness: Guidelines for a Healthy Lifestyle.* Englewood, CO: Morton Publishing, 1998.

Hesson, J. L. *Weight Training for Life.* Englewood, CO: Morton Publishing, 1998.

Hoeger, W. W. K., and S. A. Hoeger. *Principles & Labs for Fitness & Wellness.* Englewood, CO: Morton Publishing, 1997.

Hoeger, W. W. K., and S. A. Hoeger. *Lifetime Fitness & Wellness: A Personalized Program.* Englewood, CO: Morton Publishing, 1998.

Mazzeo, K. *Fitness Through Aerobics & Step Training.* Englewood, CO: Morton Publishing, 1996.

National Institute of Health. *NIH Consensus Statement: Physical Activity and Cardiovascular Health.* Washington, DC: NIH Consensus Statement Vol. 13(3), 1995.

Pfeiffer, R. P., and B. C. Mangus. *Concepts of Athletic Training.* Boston: Jones and Bartlett, 1998.

Plowman, S. A., and D. L. Smith. *Exercise Physiology for Health, Fitness, and Performance.* Needham Heights, MA: Allyn and Bacon, 1997.

President's Council on Physical Fitness and Sport. Government Printing Office, June 1995. *Physical Activity and Cancer: Physical Activity and Fitness Research Digest.*

Rosato, F. *Jogging and Walking for Health and Fitness.* Englewood, CO: Morton Publishing, 1995.

Schafer, W. *Stress Management for Wellness.* Fort Worth, TX: HBJ College Publishers, 1995.

Selye, H. *The Stress of Life.* New York: McGraw-Hill Book, 1978.

Silvester, L. J. *Weight Training for Strength and Fitness.* Boston: Jones and Bartlett Publishers, 1992.

U. S. Department of Health and Human Services. *Physical Activity and Health: A Report of the Surgeon General."* Atlanta: U.S. Department of Health and Human Services, Centers for Disease Control and Prevention, National Cancer for Chronic Disease Prevention and Health Promotion, 1996.

U. S. Department of Health and Human Services, Public Health Service. *Healthy People 2000: National Health Promotion and Disease Prevention Objectives.* Boston: Jones and Bartlett Publishers, 1992.

"Wellness Facts." *University of California at Berkeley Wellness Letter.* Palm Coast, FL: The Editors, April 1995.

Wescott, W. *Strength Fitness: Physiological Principles and Training Techniques.* Madison, WI: Brown & Benchmark, 1995.

Whitney, E. N., and S. R. Rolfes. *Understanding Nutrition.* St. Paul: West Publishing, 1996.

Wilmore, J. H., and D. L. Costill. *Physiology of Sport and Exercise.* Champaign, IL: Human Kinetics,

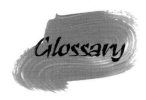

Glossary

Acquired immunodeficiency syndrome End stage of infection by the human immunodeficiency virus (HIV).

Addiction Compulsive and uncontrollable behavior(s) or use of substance(s), most frequently drugs.

Adipose tissue Fat cells.

Aero-belt® (Aerobic Endurance Resistance Overloader) Belt with an elastic band that slides freely through the belt and attaches to the wrists.

Aerobic dance Series of exercise routines performed to music.

Aerobic exercise Activity that requires oxygen to produce the necessary energy to carry out the activity.

Agility Ability to quickly and efficiently change body position and direction.

AIDS *See* Acquired immunodeficiency syndrome.

Altruism True concern for and action on behalf of others (opposite of egoism) or a sincere desire to serve others above one's personal needs.

Amenorrhea Cessation of regular menstrual flow.

Amino acids Chemical compounds that contain nitrogen, carbon, hydrogen, and oxygen; the basic building blocks the body uses to form different types of protein.

Anabolic steroids Synthetic version of the male sex hormone testosterone, which promotes muscle development and hypertrophy.

Anaerobic exercise Exercise that does not require oxygen to produce the necessary energy to carry out the activity.

Angiogenesis Formation of blood vessels.

Anorexia nervosa Condition of self-imposed starvation to lose and then maintain very low body weight.

Antioxidants Compounds such as the vitamins C, E, beta-carotene, and the mineral selenium, which prevent oxygen

from combining with other substances so that it may cause damage; thought to play a key role in preventing heart disease and cancer.

Atherosclerosis Harmful accumulation of plaque in the arteries.

Balance Ability to maintain the body in proper equilibrium.

Ballistic (or dynamic) stretching Exercises performed using jerky, rapid, and bouncy movements.

Basal metabolic rate (BMR) Lowest level of caloric intake necessary to sustain life.

Behavior modification A process to change destructive or negative behaviors permanently to positive behaviors that will lead to better health and well-being.

Benign Noncancerous.

Beta-carotene A precursor to vitamin A; an antioxidant that plays a role in disease prevention.

Blood lipids Fat-soluble substances in the body.

Blood pressure The force of the blood exerted against artery walls.

Body composition Fat and nonfat components of the human body.

Body Mass Index (BMI) Index that incorporates height and weight to estimate critical fat values at which risk for disease increases.

Breathing techniques Stress management method in which the individual concentrates on "breathing away" the tension and inhaling fresh air to the entire body.

Bulimia nervosa Eating disorder characterized by a pattern of binge eating and purging.

Calorie Unit to measure energy value of food and physical activity; the amount of heat necessary to raise the

temperature of 1 gram of water 1 degree Centigrade; short term for kilocalorie.

Cancer Group of diseases characterized by uncontrolled growth and spread of abnormal cells into malignant tumors.

Carbohydrates Compounds composed of carbon, hydrogen, and oxygen used by the body as its major source of energy.

Carcinogens Substances that contribute to formation of cancers.

Carcinoma in situ An encapsulated malignant tumor.

Cardiorespiratory endurance Ability of the lungs, heart, and blood vessels to deliver adequate amounts of oxygen to the cells to meet the demands of prolonged physical (aerobic) activity.

Cardiorespiratory training zone The range of intensity at which a person should exercise to develop the cardiorespiratory system.

Cardiovascular diseases Array of conditions that affect the heart and blood vessels.

Cellulite Term frequently used in reference to lumpy fat deposits; actually enlarged fat cells resulting from excessive accumulation of body fat.

CHD *See* Coronary heart disease.

Cholesterol A waxy substance, technically a steroid alcohol, found only in animal fats and oil; used in making cell membranes, as a building block for some hormones, in the fatty sheath around nerve fibers, and in other necessary substances.

Chronic diseases Illnesses that develop over a long time, usually associated with unhealthy lifestyle factors (e.g., hypertension, atherosclerosis, coronary disease, strokes, diabetes, and cancer).

Chronic obstructive pulmonary disease (COPD) Any of the several diseases that limit air flow, such as chronic bronchitis and emphysema (also called chronic obstructive lung disease (COLD)).

Chronological age Actual, numerical age of the individual.

Concentric muscle contraction A dynamic contraction in which the muscle shortens as it develops tension.

Cool-down A period at the end of an exercise session when exercise is tapered off.

Coordination Integration of nervous and muscular systems to produce correct, graceful, and harmonious body movements.

Coronary heart disease (CHD) Condition caused by obstruction of coronary arteries by plaque formation.

Criterion referenced standard See Health-fitness standard.

Cross-training Combination of aerobic activities that contribute to overall fitness.

Cruciferous vegetables Plants that produce cross-shaped leaves (cauliflower, broccoli, cabbage, Brussels sprouts, and kohlrabi); seem to have a protective effect against cancer.

Daily Values (DVs) Percentages of recommended daily amounts of vitamins, minerals, total fat, saturated fat, cholesterol, sodium, carbohydrates, fiber, and sugar.

Dehydration Loss of body water below normal volume.

Deoxyribonucleic acid (DNA) Genetic material in the nucleus of each body cell.

Diabetes mellitus Disease in which the body doesn't produce or properly utilize insulin.

Dietary fiber Material in plant foods that the human body cannot digest; a necessary carbohydrate.

DNA See Deoxyribonucleic acid.

Distress Negative or harmful stress under which health and performance begin to deteriorate.

Duration of exercise Time exercising per session.

Dynamic exercise Strength training that involves a muscle contraction with movement.

Dynamic stretching See Ballistic stretching.

Dysmenorrhea Painful menstruation.

Eccentric muscle contraction A dynamic contraction in which the muscle fibers lengthen while developing tension.

ECG See Electrocardiogram.

EKG See Electrocardiogram.

Electrocardiogram (ECG or EKG) A recording of the electrical impulses that stimulate the heart to contract.

Endurance See Cardiorespiratory endurance; Muscular endurance.

Energy-balancing equation Body weight formula stating that when caloric intake equals caloric output, weight remains unchanged.

Epidemiology Science that studies the relationship between diverse factors (lifestyle and environmental) and occurrence of disease.

Essential fat Minimal amount of body fat needed for normal physiological functions; about 3% of total weight in men and 12% in women.

Eustress Positive stress.

Exercise Type of physical activity that requires planned, structured, and repetitive bodily movement done to improve or maintain one or more components of physical fitness.

Exercise ECG A recording of heart activity during high-intensity activity.

Exercise intolerance Physical aversion to exercise conducted at intensity levels beyond a person's functional capacity.

Exercise tolerance test See Exercise electrocardiogram.

Fats (lipids) A class of nutrients used by the body as a source of energy.

Fiber A general term used to denote plant material that cannot be digested by human digestive enzymes.

Fight or flight A series of physical responses activated automatically in response to environmental stressors.

Flexibility The ability of a joint to move freely through its full range of motion.

Free fatty acids (FFA) See Triglycerides.

Free radicals See Oxygen free radicals.

Frequency of exercise How often a person engages in an exercise session.

Functional age Physiological age of the individual; usually lower than chronological (actual) age in fit people and vice versa in unfit people.

HDL See High density lipoprotein.

Health fitness standards Lowest fitness requirements for maintaining good health, decreasing risk for chronic diseases, and lowering incidence of muscular-skeletal injuries.

Health-related fitness Physical state encompassing cardiorespiratory endurance, muscular strength and endurance, muscular flexibility, and body composition.

Heart rate reserve Difference between maximal heart rate (MHR) and resting heart rate (RHR).

Heat cramps Muscle spasms caused by heat-induced changes in electrolyte balance in muscle cells.

Heat exhaustion Heat-related condition; symptoms include fainting, dizziness, profuse sweating, cold clammy skin, headaches, and a rapid, weak pulse.

Heat stroke Heat-related emergency; symptoms include serious disorientation, warm dry skin, no sweating, rapid pulse, vomiting, diarrhea, unconsciousness, and high body temperature.

Hemoglobin Substance in blood that carries oxygen from lungs to all body tissues.

High-density lipoproteins (HDL) Cholesterol-transporting molecules in the blood (the "good" cholesterol); offers protection against some forms of cardiovascular disease.

High-impact aerobics (HIA) Exercises incorporating movements in which both feet are off the ground at the same time momentarily.

High physical-fitness standards Required criteria to achieve a high level of physical fitness.

HIV See Human Immunodeficiency Virus.

Homocysteine An amino acid used to build proteins and carry out cell metabolism.

Human immunodeficiency virus (HIV) A chronic infectious disease, the end result of which is AIDS, spread by exchange of bodily fluids through sexual contact and shared needles in drug use.

Hypertension Chronically elevated blood pressure; blood pressures above 140/90, according to the American Heart Association.

Hypertrophy *See* Muscle hypertrophy.

Hypokinetic diseases Illnesses associated with lack of physical activity (e.g., hypertension, coronary heart disease, obesity, diabetes).

Hypothermia A breakdown in the body's ability to generate heat and a drop in body temperature below 95°F.

Intensity (in flexibility exercise) Degree of stretch.

Intensity of exercise (cardiorespiratory) How hard a person has to exercise to improve cardiorespiratory endurance.

Interval training A repeated series of exercise work bouts (intervals) interspersed with low-intensity or rest intervals.

Isokinetic exercise Strength training in which the equipment accommodates resistance to match the user's force through the full range of motion.

Isometric exercise Strength training that entails muscle contraction producing little or no movement.

Kilocalorie The amount of heat necessary to raise the temperature of 1 kilogram of water 1 degree Centigrade; usually shortened to "calorie."

LDL *See* Low density lipoprotein.

Lean body mass Nonfat component of the body.

Locus of control Extent to which a person believes he or she can influence the external environment.

Low-density lipoproteins (LDL) Cholesterol-transporting molecules in the blood (the "bad" cholesterol) that increases the risk of some forms of cardiovascular disease.

Low-impact aerobics Exercises in which at least one foot is in contact with the ground or floor at all times.

Macronutrients Nutrients that the body requires in proportionately large amounts daily.

Malignant Cancerous.

Malignant melanoma Deadliest of all types of skin cancer. Tumors grow at a rapid rate and readily spread to other parts of the body if not treated at an early stage.

Maximal oxygen uptake (VO$_{2max}$) Maximum amount of oxygen the human body is able to utilize per minute of physical activity.

Melanoma Malignant skin cancer.

Meditation Mental exercise in which the objective is to gain control over one's attention, clearing the mind and blocking out stressor(s).

Metabolic fitness Denotes improvements in the metabolic profile through a moderate-intensity exercise program.

Metabolic profile Used in the assessment of diabetes and cardiovascular disease risk by measuring plasma insulin, glucose, lipid, and lipoprotein levels.

Metabolism All energy and material transformations that take place within living cells.

Metastasis Movement of bacteria or body cells from one part of the body to another; usually refers to spread of cancer.

METs (metabolic equivalent) An alternative method of prescribing exercise intensity; 1 MET represents body's energy requirement at rest, or equivalent of VO$_2$ of 3.5 ml/kg/min.

Micronutrients Vitamins and minerals that the body requires in small amounts.

Minerals Inorganic elements found in the body and in food, essential for normal body functions.

Mode of exercise Form of exercise (e.g., aerobic).

Motivation Desire and will to do something.

Muscle hypertrophy An increase in muscle mass or size.

Muscular endurance (localized muscular endurance) Ability of a muscle to exert submaximal force repeatedly over a period of time (for example, 30 repetitions on a bench-press exercise); usually implies a specific muscle group (e.g., chest, thighs, abdominals).

Muscular flexibility Ability of a joint to move freely through its full range of motion.

Muscular strength Ability to exert maximum force against resistance.

Nonmelanoma skin cancer Cancer that grows directly from original site but does not metastasize to other regions of body.

Nutrient Substance found in food that provides energy, regulates metabolism, and helps with growth and repair of body tissues.

Nutrition Science that studies the relationship of foods to optimal health and performance.

Obesity Chronic disease characterized by an excessively high amount of body fat (about 20% or more above recommended weight).

Oligomenorrhea Irregular menstrual cycles.

One repetition maximum (1 RM) Maximal amount of resistance a person is able to lift in a single effort.

Osteoporosis Softening, deterioration, or loss of total body bone.

Overload principle Training concept holding that the demands placed on a body system must be increased systematically and progressively over time to cause physiologic adaptation.

Overweight Excess weight when compared to a given standard such as height or recommended percent body fat.

Oxygen free radicals Substances formed during metabolism that attack and damage proteins and lipids, in particular the cell membrane and DNA, leading to development of diseases such as heart disease, cancer, and emphysema.

Percent body fat (fat mass) Total amount of fat in the body based on person's weight; includes both essential and storage fat.

Physical activity Bodily movement produced by skeletal muscles that requires energy expenditure and produces progressive health benefits.

Physical fitness General capacity to adapt and respond favorably to physical effort, capable of meeting the ordinary as well as the unusual demands of daily life safely and effectively without being overly fatigued and still have energy left for leisure and recreational activities.

Phytochemicals Compounds found in vegetables and fruits with cancer-fighting properties.

Plyometric training Form of aerobic exercise that requires forceful jumps or springing off the ground immediately after landing from a previous jump.

PNF *See* Proprioceptive neuromuscular facilitation.

Progressive muscle relaxation Relaxation technique that involves contracting, then relaxing muscle groups in the body in succession.

Proprioceptive neuromuscular facilitation (PNF) Stretching technique in which muscles are stretched out progressively with intermittent isometric contractions.

Proteins Complex organic compounds containing nitrogen and formed by combinations of amino acids; the main substances used in the body to build and repair tissues such as muscles, blood, internal organs, skin, hair, nails, and bones; also part of hormones, antibodies, and enzymes.

Quackery/fraud Conscious promotion of unproven claims for profit.

RDA *See* Recommended dietary allowances.

Reaction time Time required to initiate a response to a given stimulus.

Recommended body weight Weight at which there appears to be no harm to human health.

Recommended Dietary Allowances (RDAs) Daily nutrient intakes suggested for healthy people.

Repetitions Number of times a movement is performed.

Resistance (in strength training) Amount of weight lifted.

Resting metabolic rate Amount of energy (expressed in milliliters of oxygen per minute or total calories per day) required during nonactive conditions to sustain proper body function.

Risk factors Characteristics that predict the development of a certain disease.

Set (in strength training) The number of repetitions performed for a given exercise.

Setpoint Weight control theory that indicates that each body has an established weight and strongly attempts to maintain that weight.

Sexually transmitted diseases (STDs) Communicable diseases spread through sexual contact.

Shin splint Injury to the lower leg characterized by pain and irritation at the front of the leg.

Side stitch Sharp pain in the side during exercise.

Skill-related fitness Refers to fitness components beyond health-related fitness that enhance athletic performance (agility, balance, coordination, reaction time, power, and speed).

Skinfold thickness Technique to assess body composition, including percent body fat, by measuring the thickness of a fold of skin at different body sites.

Slow-sustained (static) stretching (flexibility) Technique in which the muscles are lengthened gradually through a joint's complete range of motion and the final position is held for a few seconds.

Specificity of training Principle holding that, for a muscle to increase in strength or endurance, the training program must be specific to obtain the desired effects.

Speed Ability to rapidly propel the body or a part of the body from one point to another.

Spirituality An affirmation of life in a relationship with God, self, community, and environment that nurtures and celebrates wholeness (National Interfaith Coalition on Aging).

Spot reducing Fallacious theory that claims that exercising a specific body part will result in significant fat reduction in that area.

Static stretching *See* Slow-sustained stretching.

STDs *See* Sexually transmitted diseases.

Step aerobics Form of exercise that combines stepping up and down from a bench with arm movements.

Storage fat Body fat stored in adipose tissue.

Stress Mental, emotional, and physiological response of the body to any situation that is new, threatening, frightening, or exciting.

Stress ECG *See* Exercise ECG.

Stressor Stress-causing event or agent.

Tolerable weight Realistic body weight that is close to the health-fitness percent-body fat standard.

Transtheoretical Model Stages-of-change model that provides a framework for studying intentional behavior change.

Triglycerides Fats formed by glycerol and three fatty acids.

Type A Behavior pattern characteristic of a hard-driving, overambitious, aggressive, at times hostile, and overly competitive person.

Type B Behavior pattern characteristic of a calm, casual, relaxed, and easy going individual.

Variable-resistance training Exercise that utilizes special equipment with mechanical devices that provide differing amounts of resistance through the range of motion.

Very low density lipoprotein (VLDL) Proteins that transport cholesterol and triglycerides in the bloodstream.

Vitamins Organic substances essential for normal bodily metabolism, growth, and development.

VLDL *See* Very low density lipoprotein.

VO$_{2max}$ *See* Maximal oxygen uptake.

Waist-to-hip ratio Test designed to assess potential risk for diseases associated with obesity.

Warm-up A period preceding exercise when exercise begins slowly.

Water The most important nutrient, involved in almost every vital bodily process.

Wellness The constant and deliberate effort to stay healthy and achieve the highest potential for well-being.

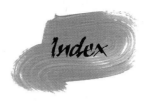

Index